STUDY GUIDE AND WORKBOOK

TO ACCOMPANY

McCance & Huether's

PATHOPHYSIOLOGY

The Biologic Basis for Disease
in Adults and Children

STUDY GUIDE AND WORKBOOK
TO ACCOMPANY
McCance & Huether's

PATHOPHYSIOLOGY
The Biologic Basis for Disease in Adults and Children

SECOND EDITION

Clayton Parkinson

Professor, College of Health Professions
Weber State University, Ogden, Utah

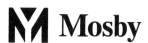 Mosby

St. Louis Baltimore Boston Chicago London Madrid Philadelphia Sydney Toronto

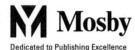

Editor: Sally Schrefer
Developmental Editor: Penny Rudolph
Editorial Assistant: Brian Dennison
Project Manager: Karen Edwards
Production Editor: Gail Brower

Design and Layout: Ken Wendling

Printed in the United States of America
Composition by Wordbench
Printing/binding by Plus Communications

Mosby–Year Book, Inc.
11830 Westline Industrial Drive
St. Louis, MO 63146

International Standard Book Number 0-8151-6710-5

93 94 95 96 97   9 8 7 6 5 4 3 2 1

Contributors

**Pediatric content
contributed by**

Dorian G. Blevins, RN, MS
Clinical Instructor
College of Nursing
University of Utah
Salt Lake City, Utah

Reviewers

Kathryn L. McCance, RN, PhD
Professor
College of Nursing
University of Utah
Salt Lake City, Utah

Sue E. Huether, RN, PhD
Associate Professor
College of Nursing
University of Utah
Salt Lake City, Utah

Preface

The study of pathophysiology is complex, ever expanding, and challenging. It provides linkage between basic science and clinical application by health-care providers and, as such, gives substance to educational efforts.

This study guide is designed for students as an adjunct to *Pathophysiology: The Biologic Basis for Disease in Adults and Children*, Second Edition, by Kathryn L. McCance and Sue E. Huether. The textual material was planned to reinforce learning and synthesize connections that students otherwise may not make. It hopes to dissuade tedious memorization of factual material and encourage an understanding of the consequences of pathologic processes on the structure and function of the human body. The design of the guide provides directed study for understanding of the complex processes presented in the main text.

The guide has 42 chapters and follows the organization of the text. The chapters have two different formats, one for normal anatomy and physiology and another for anatomic and physiologic alterations. The normal anatomy and physiology chapters assume prior study and foundational knowledge. Thus they are short and direct or guide review of principles and concepts that are both informative and essential for understanding the specific diseases that follow. Each of these chapters is followed by a practice examination to give students an opportunity to assess their understanding of normality. The format of the longer chapters on physiologic alterations directs the learner's study by the use of (1) prerequisite and study objectives with narrative and charts that are consistent with the text, (2) practice examinations that require factual knowledge and synthesis of essential concepts related to disease mechanisms, and (3) case studies that link concept and reality. The selected, directed objectives for chapters on both normal and altered states are referenced to corresponding pages in McCance and Huether's text. The learner also is referred to figures and tables in the text.

I acknowledge and give special thanks to some special individuals. My first acknowledgement goes to Kathryn L. McCance and Sue E. Huether. Their philosophy that students who grasp basic laws and principles can understand how alterations occur led them to develop a conceptually integrated text. McCance and Huether's text piques appreciation of this philosophy, since an instructor can select portions from their text appropriate to student needs that will promote conceptual learning rather than rote factual memorization. Thank you, authors!

Next, no textual endeavor is without helpful contributors. I am grateful to Dorian Blevins for her preparation of the eight chapters on alterations in children. Her clinical expertise in writing about her own specialty provided an integration of theoretic and empirical bases. Thank you, Dorian!

Lastly, I had the pleasure of working with Mosby, particularly Sally Schrefer, Penny Rudolph, and Brian Dennison. They ensured that my efforts were developed into a creative, professional, and pleasing style for student learners, my hope for the future. Without Klaus Gurgel, a sales representative for Mosby who saw my earlier pathophysiology study guide and encouraged me, the joint effort between me and Mosby would not have happened. Thank you, Mosby!

I wish to dedicate my efforts during the preparation of this study guide to Kimberly Jo, who makes teaching pleasurable and inspires teachers to search for ultimate truth and a better way to convey it to students.

Clayton F. Parkinson

Contents

CHAPTER 1

Cellular Biology

Objectives

After successful study of this chapter, the learner will be able to:

1. **Identify the location of the three principle parts of a typical eucaryotic cell.**
   Refer to Figure 1-1.

2. **State the function of the nucleus, the cytoplasm, the cytoplasmic organelles, and the plasma membrane.**
   Review text pages 6-14.

3. **Describe the structure and composition of the plasma membrane.**
   Review text pages 15-16; refer to Figure 1-11.

4. **Categorize plasma membrane functions; state examples of each category of functions.**
   Refer to Table 1-1.

5. **Classify cellular receptors on the basis of location and function.**
   Review text pages 18-19; refer to Figure 1-12.

6. **Describe cellular catabolism and the transfer of energy to drive other cellular processes.**
   Refer to Figure 1-16.

7. **Classify cellular micromolecular transport as active or passive; give examples of each.**
   Refer to Table 1-3.

8. **Describe macromolecular transport and endocytosis and exocytosis.**
   Refer to Figure 1-23.

9. **Describe the changes in the plasma membrane which result in an action potential.**
   Review text page 32; refer to Figure 1-25.

10. **Identify the phases of mitosis and cytokinesis; state the purposes of mitosis. Give examples of growth factors.**
    Refer to Figure 1-26 and Table 1-4.

11. **Compare two theories of tissue formation.**
    Refer to Figure 1-27.

12. **Identify the functions of cell junctions.**
    Review text pages 36-37; refer to Figure 1-28.

13. **Identify the location and a major function for each type of tissue: epithelial, connective, muscle, and nervous.**
    Review tissue summary, text pages 50-51.

Practice Examination

1. Which are principle parts of a eucaryotic cell?
   a. fat, carbohydrate, protein
   b. minerals and water
   c. organelles
   d. phospholipids and protein
   e. protoplasm and nucleus

2. The current description of the cell membrane is the fluid mosaic model. Proteins have a degree of mobility within the lipid bilayer.
   1. The first sentence is true.
   2. The first sentence is false.
   3. The second sentence is true.
   4. The second sentence is false.
   5. The second sentence is relevant to the first.
   6. The second sentence is irrelevant to the first.

   a. 1, 4, 6
   b. 1, 3, 6
   c. 2, 3, 6
   d. 2, 4, 5
   e. 1, 3, 5

3. Which particle can penetrate cell membranes most easily?
   a. lipid soluble, carrier present
   b. neutral charge, water soluble
   c. smaller, water soluble
   d. uncharged, larger
   e. All of the above are correct.

4. In order for a cell to engage in active transport processes, it requires
   a. mitochondria.
   b. appropriate fuel.
   c. ATP.
   d. enzymes.
   e. All of the above are correct.

5. Which is inconsistent with the other choices?
   a. diffusion
   b. osmosis
   c. filtration
   d. phagocytosis
   e. facilitated diffusion

6. Which of these can transport substances "uphill" against the concentration gradient?
   a. active transport
   b. osmosis
   c. dialysis
   d. facilitated diffusion
   e. None of the above is correct.

7. Imagine that you have aqueous (water) solution A and aqueous solution B separated by a membrane that is permeable to the solvent but is not permeable to the solute. If solution A is isotonic to human blood and solution B is hypotonic to human blood, then
   a. net diffusion of the solute will occur from side B to side A.
   b. net diffusion of the solute will occur from side A to side B.
   c. net osmosis will occur from side B to side A.
   d. net osmosis will occur from side A to side B.
   e. None of the above is correct.

8. Which is true for cytoplasm?
   a. It is located outside the nucleus.
   b. It provides support for organelles.
   c. It is mostly water.
   d. All of the above are true.
   e. Both a and b are true.

Match the term with its descriptor.

9. anaphase
10. chromatin
11. metaphase
12. mitochondria
13. prophase
14. ribosome
15. telophase

   a. 75-90% H_2O, lipids and protein
   b. within the nucleus, stored RNA
   c. compartmentalizes cellular activity
   d. single strand of DNA, non-dividing cell
   e. "generation plant" for ATP
   f. centriole migration
   g. chromatid pair alignment
   h. chromatid migration
   i. daughter nuclei
   j. protein synthesis site

16. A major function of connective tissue is
    a. to form glands.
    b. support and binding.
    c. covering and lining.
    d. movement.
    e. to conduct nerve impulses.

17. Which are typical of epithelial tissue?
    1. non-innervated
    2. avascular
    3. abundant matrix
    4. closely-packed cells

    a. 1, 3
    b. 2, 4
    c. 2, 3, 4
    d. 1, 2, 3

Match the location with the tissue type found.

18. lining kidney tubules
19. lining urinary bladder
20. lining upper respiratory tract

    a. simple squamous
    b. simple cuboidal
    c. simple columnar, ciliated
    d. stratified squamous
    e. transitional

21. Ligands that bind with membrane receptors include
    1. hormones.
    2. antigens.
    3. neurotransmitters.
    4. drugs.
    5. infectious agents.

    a. 1, 3
    b. 5
    c. 2, 5
    d. 4
    e. 1, 2, 3, 4, 5

22. The products from the metabolism of glucose include
    1. kilocalories.
    2. CO_2.
    3. H_2O.
    4. ATP.

    a. 1, 4
    b. 2, 3
    c. 3
    d. 4
    e. 1, 2, 3, 4

23. Identify the correct sequence of events for initiation and conduction of a nerve impulse.
    1. Sodium rushes inside.
    2. Potassium rushes outside.
    3. Sodium permeability changes.
    4. Resting potential is reestablished.
    5. Potassium permeability changes.

    a. 1, 3, 2, 5, 4
    b. 3, 1, 5, 2, 4
    c. 5, 2, 3, 1, 4
    d. 4, 5, 2, 3, 1

24. Chemotaxis
    a. causes one cell to adhere to another.
    b. involves founder cells.
    c. is attraction of migrant cells along a chemical gradient.
    d. All of the above are correct.
    e. None of the above is correct.

25. Cell junctions
    a. coordinate activities of cells within tissues.
    b. are an impermeable part of the plasma membrane.
    c. prevent the leakage of small molecules between the plasma membranes of adjacent cells.
    d. Both a and c are correct.
    e. Both b and c are correct.

Altered Cellular and Tissue Biology

Prerequisite Objectives

a. Describe processes of cellular intake and output.
   Review text pages 23-32.

> ### Remember!
>
> - The intact, normally functioning plasma membrane is selectively or differentially permeable to substances; it allows some substances to pass while excluding others. Water and small, uncharged substances move through pores of the lipid bilayer by passive transport which requires no expenditure of energy. This process is driven by the forces of osmosis, hydrostatic pressure, and diffusion. Larger molecules and molecular complexes are moved into the cell by active transport which requires the expenditure of energy or ATP by the cell. In active transport, materials move from low concentrations to high concentrations. The largest molecules and fluids are ingested by endocytosis and expulsed by exocytosis after cellular synthesis of smaller building blocks. When the plasma membrane is injured, it becomes permeable to virtually everything and substances move into and out of the cells in an unrestricted manner. Notably, such substances may affect (a) the nucleus and its genetic information or (b) the cytoplasmic organelles and their varied functions; then, there is altered cellular physiology and pathology.

b. Identify the relationship between homeostasis, stress, and disease.
   Review text page 301.

> ### Remember!
>
> - Homeostasis is the concept of a dynamic steady state, turnover of bodily substances, that maintains physiologic parameters within narrow limits. Stressors cause reactions that alter this dynamic steady state or homeostasis. Deviations from normal values, or homeostasis, cause disease.

Objectives

After successful study of this chapter, the learner will be able to:

1. Describe the cellular adaptations occurring in atrophy, hypertrophy, hyperplasia, dysplasia, and metaplasia. Identify the condition under which each can occur.

Study text pages 54-57; refer to Figure 2-1.

When confronted with stresses that disrupt normal structure and function, the cell undergoes adaptive changes that permit survival and maintain function. An adapted cell is neither normal nor injured — it is somewhere between these two states. These changes may lead to atrophy, hypertrophy, hyperplasia, metaplasia, or dysplasia. These adaptive responses occur in response to need and an appropriate stimulus. Once the need is no longer present, the adaptive response ceases.

Cellular atrophy decreases the cell substance and results in cell shrinkage. The size of all the structural components of the cell usually decreases as the cell atrophies. Causes of atrophy include disuse, denervation, lack of endocrine stimulation, decreased nutrition, or ischemia. Disuse atrophy is seen in muscles that are not used. Denervation atrophy occurs in the muscles of paralyzed limbs. Lack of endocrine stimulation causes changes that may occur in reproductive structures during menopause. During prolonged periods of malnutrition, the body may undergo a generalized wasting of tissue mass. Ischemia reduces blood flow and delivery of oxygen and nutrients to tissues.

Hypertrophy increases the amount of functioning mass by increasing cell size. This allows the cell to achieve an equilibrium between demand and function. Hypertrophy is commonly seen in cardiac and skeletal muscle tissue. These tissues cannot adapt to increased workload by mitotic division to form more cells. The increase in cell components is related to a increased rate of protein synthesis. However, the extent of hypertrophy may be related to limitations in blood flow. Hypertrophy may be either physiologic or pathologic. In myocardial hypertrophy, initial enlargement is caused by dilation of the cardiac chambers in response to valvular disease or hypertension. This adaptation is short-lived and is followed by increased synthesis of cardiac muscle proteins which allows cardiac muscle fibers to do more work. Ultimately, advanced hypertrophy becomes pathologic and can lead to heart failure.

Hyperplasia is an increase in the number of cells of a tissue or organ. It occurs in tissues where cells are capable of mitotic division. Hyperplasia is a controlled response to an appropriate stimulus and ceases once the stimulus has been removed. Breast and uterine enlargement during pregnancy are examples of a physiologic hyperplasia that is hormonally regulated. A pathologic hyperplasia occurs when the endometrium enlarges with excessive estrogen production. Then, abnormally thickened uterine layer may bleed excessively and frequently. Compensatory hyperplasia enables certain organs, like the liver, to regenerate after loss of substance.

Dysplasia is deranged cell growth that results in cells that vary in size, shape, and appearance and is related to hyperplasia. Minor degrees of dysplasia occur in association with chronic irritation or inflammation in the uterine cervix, oral cavity, gallbladder, and respiratory passages. Dysplasia is potentially reversible once the irritating cause has been removed. Dysplastic changes may progress to neoplastic disease. This makes dysplasia a phenomenon of importance.

Metaplasia is a reversible conversion from one adult cell type to another adult cell type. It allows for replacement with cells that are better able to tolerate environmental stresses. In metaplasia, one type of cell may be converted to another type of cell within its tissue class; an epithelial cell cannot change to a connective tissue cell. An example of metaplasia is the substitution of stratified squamous epithelial cells for ciliated columnar epithelial cells in the airways of the person who is a habitual cigarette smoker.

2. Identify the mechanism of cellular injury for the following causes:

Hypoxia (Study text pages 57-59; refer to Figure 2-5), **chemicals** (Study text pages 59-61), **infectious agents** (Study text pages 63-66; refer to Figure 2-10 and Table 2-1), **immunological and inflammatory responses** (Study text pages 66-67), **genetic factors** (Study text page 67), **nutritional imbalances** (Study text pages 67-68), and **physical trauma** (Study text pages 68-72; refer to Figure 2-11).

Hypoxia deprives the cell of oxygen and interrupts oxidative metabolism and the generation of ATP. As oxygen tension within the cell falls, oxidative metabolism ceases and the cell reverts to anaerobic metabolism. One of the earliest effects of reduced ATP is acute cellular swelling caused by failure of the sodium-potassium membrane pump. With impaired function of this pump, intracellular potassium levels decrease and sodium and water accumulate within the cell. As fluid and ions move into the cell, there is dilatation of the endoplasmic reticulum, increased membrane permeability, and decreased mitochondrial function as extracellular calcium accumulates in the mitochondria. If the oxygen supply is not restored, there is continued loss of essential enzymes, proteins, and ribonucleic acid through the very permeable membrane of the cell. Hypoxia can result from inadequate oxygen in the air, respiratory disease, decreased blood flow due to circulatory disease, anemia, or inability of the cells to utilize oxygen. In edema, the distance for diffusion of oxygen may become too great.

Toxic chemical agents can injure the cell membrane, and cell structures, block enzymatic pathways, coagulate cell proteins, and disrupt the osmotic and ionic balance of any cell. Chemicals may injure cells during the process of metabolism or elimination. Carbon tetrachloride, for example, causes little damage until it is metabolized by liver enzymes to a highly reactive free radical and then it is extremely toxic to liver cells. Carbon monoxide has a special affinity for the hemoglobin molecule and reduces its ability to carry oxygen.

Alcohol (ethanol) is the favorite mood-altering drug in the United States. Liver and nutritional disorders are serious consequences of alcohol abuse. The hepatic changes, initiated by ethanol conversion to acetaldehyde, include deposition of fat, enlargement of the liver, interruption of transport of proteins and their secretion, increase in intracellular water, depression of fatty acid oxidation, increased membrane rigidity, and acute liver cell necrosis. In the CNS, alcohol is a depressant, initially affecting subcortical structures. Consequently, motor and intellectual activity become disoriented. At high blood alcohol levels, respiratory medullary centers become depressed.

Infectious agents that survive and proliferate in the body may produce substances that injure cells and tissues. Some clostridial bacteria produce destructive enzymes such as collagenases and lecithinases. These powerful enzymes destroy connective tissues and cellular membranes. Other gram-positive bacteria release **exotoxins** which are proteins having highly specific effects. These toxins may inactivate enzymes critical to protein synthesis, produce neurotoxins, block motor inhibition which can cause spasm or depression of the respiratory muscles, or cause severe food poisoning.

Endotoxins are contained in the cell walls of gram-negative bacteria and are released from cell walls during lysis or destruction of the bacteria. These toxins are phospholipids or polysaccharides. Endotoxin can be released during treatment with antibiotics; the antibiotic is unable to prevent the toxic effects of endotoxin. Once in the blood, endotoxins cause the release of vasoactive peptides that affect blood vessels. One vascular effect is vasodilation that reduces blood pressure which in turn causes decreased oxygen delivery and subsequent cardiovascular shock.

Viruses are intracellular parasites that take over the metabolic machinery of host cells and use it for their own survival and replication. This results in decreased synthesis of macromolecules vital to the host. Viruses cause the most common afflictions of humans. Their disease mechanisms range from the "cold sore" of herpes simplex to cancer. Viruses do not produce exotoxins or endotoxins but injure cellular structure in other cytopathic ways. Once inside the host cell, virions may do any of the following:

- Cause cessation of protein synthesis.
- Disrupt lysosomal membranes which result in release of lysosomal enzymes that can kill the host cell.
- Form inclusion bodies where synthesis of viral nucleic acids or proteins is involved.
- Fuse host cells which produce multinucleated giant cells.
- Alter the antigenic properties or the "identity" of the host cell; then, the host's immune system attacks the cell as if it were a foreign protein.
- Transform host cells into cancerous cells.

Immunologic and inflammatory injury is an important cause of cellular injury. Cellular membranes are injured by direct contact with cellular and chemical components of the immune and inflammatory responses. Such mediators are lymphocytes and macrophages and chemicals such as histamine, antibodies, lymphokines, complement, and proteases. Complement, a serum protein, is responsible for many of the membrane alterations that occur during immunologic injury. Membrane alterations are associated with rapid leakage of potassium out of the cell and rapid influx of water. Antibodies can interfere with membrane function by binding to and occupying receptor molecules on the plasma membrane. (Later chapters will deal with these injurious consequences as well as with hypersensitivity and autoimmune disease.)

Genetic disorders may alter the cell's nucleus and the plasma membrane's structure, shape, receptors, or transport mechanisms. (Mechanisms causing genetic abnormalities will be discussed in later chapters.)

Nutritional imbalances are important because cells require adequate amounts of proteins, carbohydrates, lipids, vitamins, and minerals to function normally. If inadequate or excessive amounts of nutrients are consumed and transported, pathophysiologic cellular effects can develop.

Proteins are the major structural units of the cell and participate in many enzymatic and hormonal functions. With lowered plasma proteins, particularly albumin, fluids move into the interstitium and produce edema. Children suffering from protein malnutrition are very susceptible and often die from infectious diseases.

Glucose is the major carbohydrate obtained from the breakdown of starch. Hyperglycemia, excessive glucose in the blood, if caused by excessive carbohydrate intake may lead to obesity. Deficiencies of glucose result from starvation or from inadequate use, as in diabetes. In both of these conditions, the body compensates by metabolizing lipids to obtain cellular energy. In lipid deficiency, the body compensates by mobilizing fatty acids from adipose tissue. This causes an increase in the production and circulation of acidic ketone bodies. Severe increases in ketone bodies can cause coma or death. Hyperlipidemia, or an increase in lipoproteins in the blood, results in deposits of fat in the heart, liver, and muscle.

Vitamins are involved in many reactions including metabolism of visual pigments (vitamin A), calcium and phosphate metabolism (vitamin D), prothrombin synthesis (vitamin K), and antioxidation reactions (vitamin E). Vitamin B affects amino acid transfer reactions; FAD, FMN, and NAD help transfer electrons. Deficiencies in vitamin C cause poor wound healing and scurvy. Vitamin D deficiency causes rickets and problems with healing of fractures. Folate deficiency is associated with plasma and membrane changes of the red blood cell and is particularly a problem in individuals with severe liver dysfunction. Vitamin deficiencies are associated with several other disease states including cancer.

Injurious physical agents include temperature extremes, changes in atmospheric pressure, radiation, illumination, mechanical factors, noise, and prolonged vibration. Physical injury is often environmental.

The **temperature extremes** of chilling or freezing of cells cause hypothermic injury directly by creating high intracellular sodium concentrations. This results from the formation and dissolution of ice crystals. Indirect forms of injury like vasoconstriction paralyze vasomotor control and vasodilation follows with increased membrane permeability. This causes cellular and tissue swelling. Hyperthermic injury, excessive heat, varies depending on the nature, intensity, and duration of the heat. Burns cause extensive loss of fluids and plasma proteins. Also, intense heat damages temperature-sensitive enzymes and the vascular endothelium and causes coagulation of the blood vessels.

Sudden increases or decreases in **atmospheric pressure** cause blast injury. In air blast or explosive injuries, tissue injury is due to compressive waves of air against the body. The pressure changes may collapse the thorax, rupture solid internal organs, or cause widespread hemorrhage. In increased pressure caused by immersion blast, water pressure is applied suddenly to the body, and the body is forced up out of the water. The positive pressure compresses the abdomen and ruptures hollow internal organs such as the spleen, kidneys, and liver. With sudden decreases in pressure, carbon dioxide and nitrogen normally dissolved in the blood leave solution and form tiny bubbles, gas emboli, which obstruct blood vessels. This is seen in rapidly ascending deep sea divers and underwater workers. At low atmospheric pressure, such as occurs at altitudes above 15,000 feet, there is a decrease in available oxygen; this causes hypoxic injury. The compensatory vasoconstriction shunts the blood from the peripheral circulation to the visceral organs including the lungs. The combination of increases in pulmonary blood flow and systemic hypoxia causes pulmonary edema, interstitial water excess.

Ionizing radiation is any form of radiation capable of removing orbital electrons from atoms. Ionizing radiation is emitted by x-rays, gamma rays, and the process of radioactive decay. Radiant energy from sunlight can also injure cells. DNA is the most vulnerable target of radiation, particularly the bonds within the DNA molecule. Irradiation during mitosis produces chromosome aberrations. Membrane molecules and enzymes are also damaged by radiation. Radiosensitivity depends on rate of mitosis and cellular maturity. The more numerous the mitotic figures, the greater the sensitivity; more maturity, less sensitivity. Particularly vulnerable cells are embryonic germ cells which are precursors of ova and sperm. Throughout life, cells of the bone marrow, intestinal mucosa, testicular seminiferous epithelium, and ovarian follicles are susceptible to injury because they are always undergoing mitosis.

The harmful effects of **illumination** in fluorescent lighting include eye-strain, obscured vision, and possible cataract formation. Emission of ultraviolet radiation from halogen lamps is thought to be in the range of wavelength responsible for inducing melanoma, a malignant skin growth.

Mechanical injury is caused by physical impact or irritation; e.g., a head injury when a worker is struck in the head by a falling object. Most mechanical stresses, however, are subtle and can cause accumulative injuries and disorders over time.

Noise is sound that has the potential for inflicting bodily harm. Noise trauma can be caused by acute loud noise or by the cumulative effects of various intensities, frequencies, and durations of noise.

3. Identify the various cellular accumulations occurring in response to injury and the subsequent manifestation of cellular damage.

Study text pages 72-76.

Acoustic trauma is instantaneous damage and can rupture the eardrum, displace the ossicles of the middle ear, or damage the organ of Corti in the inner ear. Structural changes associated with prolonged, loud exposure include intracellular changes in the sensor cells, swelling of the auditory nerve endings, and cochlear blood flow impairment. Noise-induced hearing loss is gradual and painless. Symptoms of noise-induced hearing loss include soft sounds not being heard and tinnitus.

Cellular Accumulations

Accumulation	Cause	Injury
H_2O	Extracellular H_2O shifts into cell, reduced ATP and ATPase, sodium accumulates in cell	Cellular swelling, vacuolation, hydropic degeneration
Lipids, Carbohydrates	Imbalance in production, utilization or mobilization of lipid or carbohydrates	Vacuolation, displaced nucleus and organelles, leads to fibrosis and scarring
Glycogen	Genetic disorders, diabetes mellitus	Cytoplasmic vacuolation
Proteins	Enzymes digest cellular organelles, renal disorders, plasma cell tumor	Disrupted function and intracellular communication, displaced cellular organelles
Pigments	Exogenous particle ingestion, UV light stimulates melanin production, cellular metabolism, malignancy loss of hormonal feedback, genetic defects, burning and hemorrhage increases hemosiderin, liver dysfunction	Membrane injury, disrupted
Calcium	Altered membrane permeability, influx of extracellular calcium, excretion of H^+ leading to more OH^- which precipitates Ca^{++}, endocrine disturbances	Hardening of cellular structure, interferes with function
Urate	Absence of enzymes	Crystal deposition, inflammation

4. Identify the major types of cellular necrosis and cite examples of the tissues involved in each type. Compare necrosis with apoptosis.
Study text pages 76-79.

Necrosis is local cell death and involves the process of cellular self-digestion known as autodigestion or autolysis. As necrosis progresses, most organelles are disrupted and karyolysis, nuclear dissolution from the action of hydrolytic enzymes, becomes evident. There are four major types of necrosis: coagulative, liquefactive, caseous, and fatty. Gangrenous necrosis is not a distinctive type of cell death but refers to large areas of tissue death.

Coagulative necrosis occurs primarily in the kidneys, heart, and adrenal glands and usually results from hypoxia caused by severe ischemia. Protein denaturation causes coagulation. An increased intracellular level of calcium may be a critical event in coagulation necrosis.

Liquefactive necrosis is common following ischemic injury to neurons and glial cells in the brain. Because brain cells are rich in digestive hydrolytic enzymes and lipids, the brain cells are digested by their own hydrolases. The brain tissue becomes soft, liquefies, and is walled off from healthy tissue to form cysts. Liquefactive necrosis can also result from bacterial infections. Here, the hydrolases are released from the lysosomes of phagocytic neutrophils which are attracted to the infected area to kill the bacteria; these hydrolases also destroy brain tissue. The accumulation of pus is present in liquefaction necrosis.

Caseous necrosis is commonly seen in tuberculous pulmonary infection and is a combination of coagulative and liquefactive necrosis. The necrotic debris is not digested completely by hydrolases, so tissues appear soft, granular, and resemble clumped cheese. A granulomatous inflammatory wall may enclose the central areas of caseous necrosis.

The **fatty necrosis** found in the breast, pancreas, and other abdominal structures is a specific cellular dissolution caused by lipases. Lipases break down triglycerides and release free fatty acids which then combine with calcium, magnesium, and sodium ions to create soaps, or saponification. The necrotic tissue appears opaque and chalk white.

Gangrenous necrosis refers to death of tissue, usually in considerable mass and putrefaction. It results from severe hypoxic injury subsequent to arteriosclerosis or blockage of major arteries followed by bacterial invasion. Dry gangrene is usually due to a coagulative necrosis while wet gangrene develops when neutrophils invade the site and cause liquefaction necrosis. Gas gangrene, a special type of gangrene, is due to bacterial infection of injured tissue by species of Clostridium. These anaerobic bacteria produce hydrolytic enzymes and toxins that destroy connective tissue and cellular membrane; bubbles of gas likely form in muscle cells.

Apoptosis is an important, distinct type of cell death that differs from necrosis. It is an active process of cellular self-destruction in both normal and pathologic tissue changes. Apoptosis likely plays a major role in endocrine-dependent tissues that are undergoing atrophic change. It may occur spontaneously in malignant tumors and in normal, rapidly proliferating cells treated with cancer chemotherapeutic agents and ionizing radiation. Unlike necrosis, apoptosis affects scattered, single cells and results in shrinkage of a cell; whereas in necrosis, cells swell and lyse.

5. Compare some of the different theories of aging.
Study text pages 82-84; refer to Table 2-6.

Much of the confusion about aging arises from the difficulty of distinguishing between normal aging and changes that are secondary to disease. Health and longevity are affected by a number of factors such as heredity, culture, race, and nutrition. No one theory answers all the questions of aging. Each of the following theories, while not inclusive of all possibilities, provides clues to the aging process and certain interrelationships.

Waste Product Theory

The waste product theory is associated with the observation of increased pigment in aging cells. This pigment, known as lipofuscin, appears to occur as a result of autophagocytosis, oxidation of lipids, and copolymerization of organic molecules. It is considered likely that lipofuscin forms as an end product of free radical-induced peroxidations. This theory provides a connection between oxygen consumption, free radicals, lipofuscin, and aging.

Free Radical Theory

The free radical theory proposes that free radicals serve as central agents in the changes observed with aging. Free radicals are parts of molecules or molecules that have had an electron stripped from their structure. Diffusible free radicals damage or alter the original structure or function of other molecules by attaching to these other molecules. This theory has been linked to the idea of oxygen toxicity since oxidation of carbohydrate, fat, protein, and other elements in the body results in the formation of free radicals.

Since the cell membrane is the key to cellular survival, the greatest damage likely could be perpetrated by free radicals at this level by altering ingress and egress of nutrients or wastes. When DNA is irradiated, it responds with free radical formation and establishes aberrant cellular development. Free radical activity is promoted in the body by such environmental factors as smog, by-products of industry, gasoline, and atmospheric ozone. Vitamin E and coenzyme Q are thought to protect the mitochondria from the hazards of free radical activity. Vitamin E may also serve as an antioxidant and binding agent in the antioxidation process.

Cross-Link Theory

The cross-link theory, also known as the collagen theory, states that strong chemical reactions create strong bonds between molecular structures that are normally separate. Collagen, a tissue protein, maintains strength, support, and structural form. As a result of chemical crosslinkage, aging collagen becomes more insoluble and rigid. This process decreases cell permeability and passage of nutrients, metabolites, antibodies, and gases through epithelium.

Elastin, another fibrillar protein of connective tissue, is also prone to cross-linkage. Aging elastin becomes frayed, fragmented, and brittle which leads to many changes in connective tissue.

Cross-linkage also affects cell division because it can prevent divisions of the strands of DNA. If the linking molecule attaches itself to both sides of the DNA, cellular division is prevented; whereas if only one strand of DNA is affected, no damage results.

Genetic Aging Theory

The genetic aging theory proposes that the life span and number of time cells can replicate themselves is programmed in the genes of the DNA molecule; there exists a limited possible number of cellular doubling. This means that a person having short-lived parents or grandparents has a life expectancy shorter than a person having long-lived parents or grandparents.

Innate gender genetic material favors the longevity of the female over the male. Race is also a factor of longevity; whites of both sexes live longer than blacks.

Immunologic Theory

The immunologic theory asserts that aging is an autoimmune process. In this process, the body's immune system fails to recognize its own cells as the cells change with age. Immune responses then damage or destroy the cells of one's own body.

Aging affects all of the immune system but especially the T cell lymphocytes. A decline in T cells begins at sexual maturity with involution of the thymus gland. The involution of the thymus gland appears to be the key to the aging of the immune system. As the immune system ages, there is increased frequency of diseases such as cancer and autoimmune diseases. The B cell lymphocytic numbers remain normal but responsiveness to stimulation by antigens, foreign invaders or nonself, decreases markedly because of B cell dependence on T cell stimulation. Fortunately, macrophages that play a major role in protecting the body against infection do not seem to decrease in number as the body ages.

6. Characterize somatic death and its manifestations.

Study text page 85.

Somatic death is death of the entire organism. Unlike the changes that follow cellular death in a viable body, somatic death is diffuse and does not involve components of the inflammatory response, a vascular response to injury. The most notable manifestations of somatic death are complete cessation of respiration and circulation, the surface of the skin usually becomes pale and yellowish, and body temperature falls gradually until, after 24 hours, body temperature equals that of the environment. Notably, within 6 hours after death, depletion of ATP interferes with ATP-dependent detachment of the contractile proteins, and muscle stiffening or rigor mortis develops. Within 12 to 14 hours, rigor mortis usually affects the entire body. Rigor mortis gradually diminishes as the body becomes flaccid because of the release of enzymes and lytic dissolution.

Practice Examination

1. A cellular adaptation observable in uterine cervical epithelium is
   a. atrophy.
   b. hyperplasia.
   c. hypertrophy.
   d. dysplasia.
   e. metaplasia.

2. What are the consequences when a cell is forced into anaerobic glycolysis?
   1. insufficient glucose production   a. 1, 2
   2. excessive pyuric acid retention   b. 3, 4
   3. increased lactic acid   c. 4, 5
   4. inadequate ATP production   d. 3, 5
   5. excessive CO_2 production

Match the following.

3. low oxygen tension   a. anoxia
4. may deposit in areas of unresolved healing b. melanin
                                               c. lipids
                                               d. hypoxia
                                               e. calcium

5. Viruses cause cellular injury by
   a. decreasing protein synthesis.
   b. altering host cell antigenic properties; then, activating immune response.
   c. transforming host cells into malignant cells.
   d. Both a and c are correct.
   e. a, b, and c are correct.

Match the characteristic with the toxin.

6. gram-negative bacteria   a. endotoxin
7. heat stable   b. exotoxin
8. protein
9. generalized, systemic effects

10. What is the probable cause of cellular swelling in the early stages of cell injury?
    a. fat inclusion
    b. loss of genetic integrity
    c. hydrolytic enzyme activation
    d. Na-K pump fails to remove intracellular Na^+
    e. None of the above is correct.

11. Dystropic calcification
    a. occurs in dying or dead tissues.
    b. is the result of too much calcium in the blood.
    c. is observed in chronic lesions.
    d. Both a and c are correct.
    e. a, b, and c are correct.

12

12. Cellular swelling is
    a. irreversible.
    b. evident early in all types of cellular injury.
    c. manifested by decreased intracellular sodium.
    d. None of the above is correct.
    e. Both b and c are correct.

13. Which is not reversible?
    a. karyolysis
    b. fatty infiltration
    c. hydropic degeneration
    d. All of the above are reversible.

14. Aging
    a. is easy to distinguish from pathology.
    b. does not have a genetic relationship.
    c. is more advanced in primitive societies
    d. None of the above is correct.
    e. a, b, and c are correct.

15. Of the following theories of aging, the cross-linking theory implies that
    a. the life span and number of times a cell can replicate is programmed.
    b. the number of cell doubling is limited.
    c. there is oxygen toxicity.
    d. cell permeability decreases.
    e. Both a and b are correct.

Match the manifestation with the appropriate condition.

16. necrosis produced by clostridia	a. liquefactive
17. rigidity of muscles after somatic death	b. rigor mortis
18. increased tissue mass because of increased cell numbers	c. gas gangrene
	d. hyperplasia
19. necrosis resulting from lysosomal release	e. metaplasia
20. replacement of one cell type for another, more suitable type	f. cloudy swelling
	g. coagulation

Match the manifestation with the appropriate condition.

21. decreased cell size	a. fatty necrosis
22. related to pancreatic necrosis	b. gangrene
23. combination of coagulative and liquefactive necrosis	c. atrophy
	d. caseous necrosis
24. large areas of tissue death	e. apoptosis
25. a normal and pathologic cellular self-destruction	f. algor mortis
	g. hypertrophy

The Cellular Environment: Fluids and Electrolytes, Acids and Bases

Prerequisite Objectives

a. Describe the different compartments for body fluids and identify the fluid distribution changes occurring with age.
    Review text pages 92-93; refer to Tables 3-1, 3-2, and 3-3.

b. Describe the factors which affect water movement.
    Review text pages 93-94; refer to Figure 3-2.

c. Identify the distribution of electrolytes in body compartments.
    Refer to Table 3-4.

Remember!

- m Eq/L = $\dfrac{\text{milligrams of ion per liter of solution} \times \text{number of charges of one ion}}{\text{atomic weight of ion}}$

- m Eq/L expresses the concentration of chemicals dissolved in body fluids; they relate to chemical activity.

---

d. Identify the role of ADH, aldosterone, and natriuretic hormone on water and electrolyte balance.
    Review text pages 96-97.

e. Identify body mechanisms to buffer excessive hydrogen ion/acid and explain the mechanics of the most important buffer. Distinguish between short-term and long-term adjustments.
    Review text pages 110-113; refer to Table 3-9.

Remember !

- Pulmonary acid/base regulation of blood involves CO_2 and is rapid.

$$CO_2 + H_2O \leftrightarrow H_2CO_3 \leftrightarrow H^+ + HCO_3^-$$

An increase in CO_2 tension liberates hydrogen ions; thus, the pH decreases. A decrease in CO_2 tension results in fewer hydrogen ions; thus, the pH increases.

- Renal acid/base regulation of blood involves HCO_3^- conservation and H^+ and NH_3 excretion and is slow. This process essentially secretes H^+ into the urine and returns HCO_3^- to the blood plasma.

Objectives

After successful study of this chapter, the learner will be able to:

1. Identify the mechanisms causing edema.
Refer to Figure 3-3.

Osmotic/oncotic pressure is responsible for keeping fluids (water) inside the blood vessels. The osmotic pressure is normally greater within the blood vessels than it is in the interstitial fluid compartment. If this pressure differential is lost, fluid will leave the blood vessels by osmosis. Conversely, if the osmotic/oncotic pressure is increased in the blood, interstitial fluids will be drawn into the blood vessels resulting in tissue dehydration. The two major substances in the blood that most greatly regulate the blood's osmotic or oncotic pressure are sodium and proteins respectively. Since alterations of blood protein levels affect oncotic pressure, the blood level of sodium should be inversely proportional to the blood protein concentration. Individuals with very elevated blood protein levels, such as in multiple myeloma, would be expected to have decreased blood sodium levels. Individuals suffering conditions which cause decreased blood protein levels would be expected to have slightly increased blood sodium levels or hypernatremia. Decreases in blood osmotic pressure will cause tissue edema. Increases will cause tissue dehydration.

Common Causes of Edema (an excess of interstitial fluid due to fluids leaving the capillaries in response to low osmotic/oncotic pressure in the blood):

- High capillary pressure, high hydrostatic pressure, venous obstruction or arteriolar dilation
- Low blood protein or plasma-filtered oncotic pressure, albumin loss from kidney disease or burns, protein malnutrition
- Lymphatic blockage, filtered proteins from the blood failing to re-enter the capillaries thus drawing water from capillaries, cancer therapy with removal of lymph nodes and vessels (mastectomy) and increased edema
- Increased capillary permeability to histamine, inflammation

Common Causes of Dehydration (water depletion leading to hypernatremia or hypertonic imbalance):

- Vomiting, diarrhea, or gastric suction
- Inadequate fluid intake
- Hyperventilation (loss of H_2O vapor)
- Evaporation of perspiration during heavy exercise, diaphoresis
- Evaporation from burned surfaces

- Diuresis drugs
- Diabetes insipidus
- Third space losses as in ascites

Fluid movement can be explained by the following formula:

$$Q = (BHP + IFOP) - (IFHP + BOP)$$
$$\text{[from vessel]} \qquad \text{[to vessel]}$$

Q = fluid movement, BHP = blood hydrostatic pressure, IFOP = interstitial fluid osmotic pressure, IFHP = interstitial fluid hydrostatic pressure, and BOP = blood osmotic pressure.

Remember!

- Water moves from high concentration to low concentration and to dilute the solute.

---

2. Define isotonic, hypertonic, and hypotonic water and solute alterations.
Refer to Table 3-5.

Isotonic Imbalances
Extracellular fluid loss or gain is accompanied by proportional changes of electrolytes in these alterations. Losses are seen in hemorrhage or excessive sweating. Gains occur in administration of intravenous normal saline or renal retention of sodium and water. Cells do not shrink or swell in isotonic fluids.

Hypertonic Imbalances
Water loss or solute gain occurs in these changes. These alterations are seen in administration of hypertonic saline solutions, hyperaldosteronism, Cushing syndrome, diabetes, diarrhea, or insufficient water intake. Cells shrink in hypertonic fluid.

Hypotonic Imbalances
Water gain or solute loss occurs in these changes. These alterations may be caused by vomiting, diarrhea, burns, diuretic users, excessive sweating, or renal failure to excrete water. Cells swell in hypotonic fluid.

3. Identify the major consequences of abnormal levels of sodium, potassium, calcium, phosphate, and magnesium. Define the terms associated with excess or deficit of each electrolyte.
Study text pages 98-100; refer to Tables 3-6 and 3-7.

Clinical Manifestations of Excess and Deficit States of Major Electrolytes

Excess	*Deficit*
Sodium	
Hypernatremia > 147 mEq/L	**Hyponatremia** < 135 mEq/L
Cellular shrinking due to hypertonic extra-cellular fluid, may cause central nervous system irritability, tachycardia, dry, flushed skin, hypotension, thirst, elevated temperature, rapid pulse, weight loss, oliguria, anuria	Cellular swelling, may cause cerebral edema, headache, stupor, coma, peripheral edema, polyuria, absence of thirst, decreased body temperature, rapid pulse, hypotension, nausea, vomiting
Potassium	
Hyperkalemia > 5.5 mEq/L	**Hypokalemia** < 3.5 mEq/L
Depressed conductivity in heart, muscle cramping, paresthesias, nausea, diarrhea, associated with metabolic acidosis	Cardiac irritability, dysrhythmias, vomiting, paralytic ileus, thirst, associated with metabolic alkalosis, inability to concentrate urine
Calcium	
Hypercalcemia > 12 mg/dl	**Hypocalcemia** < 8.5 mg/dl
Decreased neuromuscular excitability, muscle weakness, central nervous system depression, stupor to coma, increased risk of bone fracture, vomiting, constipation, kidney stones	Increased neuromuscular excitability, skeletal muscle cramps, tetany, laryngospasm, asphyxiation, death
Phosphate	
Hyperphosphatemia > 4.5 mg/dl	**Hypophosphatemia** < 2.0 mg/dl
See Hypocalcemia	Anorexia, weakness, osteomalacia, muscle weakness, tremors, seizures, coma, anemia, bleeding disorders, leukocytic alterations
Magnesium	
Hypermagnesemia > 2.5 mEq/L	**Hypomagnesemia** < 1.5 mEq/L
Skeletal muscle depression, muscle weakness, hypotension, bradycardia, respiratory depression	Hypocalcemia and hypokalemia, neuro-muscular irritability, tetany, convulsions, tachycardia, hypertension

4. Differentiate between metabolic/respiratory acidosis and metabolic/respiratory alkalosis.

Refer to Figures 3-12, 3-13, 3-14, 3-15, and 3-16.

Comparison of Common Acid-Base Disturbances

Disturbance	Primary Disturbance	Correction/ Compensation	Usual Causes
Metabolic Acidosis ($HCO_3^- < 24$ mEq/L)	Excess endogenous acid depletes bicarbonate or bicarbonate is lost by kidneys	Hyperventilation lowers pCO_2, kidneys excrete more hydrogen ions and retain more bicarbonate	Renal failure, ketosis, aspirin poisoning, over-production of lactic acid
Respiratory Acidosis ($pCO_2 > 45$ mmHg)	Inefficient excretion of carbon dioxide by lungs	Additional bicarbonate retention and H^+ excretion by kidneys	Chronic pulmonary disease, drug depression of respiratory center
Metabolic Alkalosis ($HCO_3^- > 26$ mEq/L)	Excess plasma bicarbonate	Hypoventilation raises pCO_2 to acidify blood, kidneys increase H^+ retention and excrete HCO_3^-	Loss of gastric juice, chloride depletion, excess corticosteroid hormones, ingestion of excessive bicarbonate or other antacids
Respiratory Alkalosis ($pCO_2 < 35$ mmHg)	Hyperventilation lowers pCO_2	Increased excretion of bicarbonate and retention of H^+ by kidneys	Severe anxiety with hyperventilation, central nervous system disease, hypoxia, pulmonary imbalances

Important Values to Remember:

pH = 7.35 - 7.45

K^+ = 5 mEq/L

Na^+ = 142 mEq/L

Cl^- = 104 mEq/L

HCO_3^- = 24 mEq/L

pCO_2 = 35-45 mm/Hg

CO_2 = 28 mEq/L

5. Describe what is meant by the "anion gap" and explain the significance of an abnormal anion gap in metabolic acidosis.

Study text pages 114-115.

The blood and cellular electrolytes must maintain osmotic neutrality; i.e., the number of cations must equal the number of anions present. Routine measurement of serum electrolytes usually involves only Na^+ and K^+ cations and the anions of Cl^- and HCO_3^- as total CO_2. There are about 12 mEq/L of other anions present in the blood that are not routinely measured; i.e., phosphates, sulfates, and protein anions. Therefore, assuming that no abnormal anions are present, an individual's serum sodium and potassium should equal the chloride + bicarbonate + 12 mEq/L of unmeasured, normal anions. If this is true, then the individual would have a normal **anion gap**. The "gap" therefore represents the unmeasured anions. Another way of saying this is that the sum of the chloride and bicarbonate should be about 12 mEq/L less than the sum of the sodium and potassium cations. The anion gap is therefore 12 mEq/L when no abnormal anions are present. This may be expressed by the following formula:

$$Na^+ + K^+ = Cl^- + HCO_3^- + 12 \text{ mEq/L}$$
of unmeasured anions

Since the amount of potassium present in the blood is very small relative to the large amount of sodium, the equation may be simplified to:

Na +/- 5 mEq/L =
Chloride + Bicarbonate + 12 mEq/L

If this latter equation is followed during electrolyte studies, the individual is said to have a normal anion gap. Another way of thinking about this is that the individual's chloride shift is normally operating and that there are no abnormal, unmeasured anions present. If no abnormal anions are present, even though an individual may have a low bicarbonate level, the chloride shift will cause the chloride level to proportionately increase to maintain a normal anion gap.

The significance of an abnormally large anion gap is that an abnormal anion is present in the blood from lactic acid, ketone bodies, salicylates, etc. When this is the case, the individual will have a low bicarbonate but there is not a corresponding increase in chloride. The anion gap will be greater then 12 mEq/L. If the anion gap is normal but the Cl^- has increased and the HCO_3^- is low, the metabolic acidosis may be due to diarrhea, ammonium chloride ingestion, or renal dysfunction.

Interestingly enough, there is also a shift between cellular and plasma cations. The most noteworthy shift is with potassium as a function of pH. This is known as the potassium shift. As the pH of the blood becomes more acid, the pH decreases, the hydrogen ions shift into cells while potassium ions shift out of the cell to maintain electrolyte neutrality. We, therefore, expect to see higher serum K^+ levels when an individual is in acidosis and lower serum K^+ levels in alkalosis.

Practice Examination

1. The total water loss per day in the adult is approximately
   a. 0.8 liter.
   b. 1.2 liter.
   c. 1.8 liter.
   d. 2.2 liter.
   e. 2.8 liter.

2. Of the 60% of the body weight made up of water, about 3L is
   a. extracellular water.
   b. intracellular water.
   c. intravascular water.
   d. interstitial water.
   e. None of the above is correct.

3. Because fat is hydrophobic, very little water is contained in adipose cells.
   1. The first part of the sentence is true.   a. 1, 4, 6
   2. The first part of the sentence is false.   b. 1, 3, 6
   3. The second part of the sentence is true.   c. 2, 3, 6
   4. The second part of the sentence is false.   d. 2, 4, 5
   5. The second part of the sentence is relevant to the first.   e. 1, 3, 5
   6. The second part of the sentence is irrelevant to the first.

4. A milliequivalent is a unit of
   a. mass.
   b. physical activity.
   c. chemical activity.
   d. osmotic concentration.

5. The principle of body electroneutrality implies that
   a. the number of cations and anions in the body must be equal.
   b. intravascular molecules of protein are without charge.
   c. the number of sodium ions must be united with chloride ions.
   d. the positive and negative charges in any particular body compartment must be equal to each other.

6. Aldosterone controls ECF volume by
    a. carbohydrate, fat, and protein catabolism.
    b. sodium reabsorption.
    c. potassium reabsorption.
    d. water reabsorption.
    e. Both b and d are correct.

7. The release of ADH is stimulated by all except
    a. stress.
    b. hyponatremia.
    c. hypernatremia.
    d. an increase in plasma osmolality.
    e. a decrease in plasma volume.

Match the term with its definition.

8. hydrostatic pressure
9. oncotic/osmotic pressure

    a. water-pulling effect of plasma proteins
    b. pressure of blood within the capillaries
    c. mechanism to move fluid to lymph glands
    d. movement of fluid through semipermeable membrane

10. In laboratory findings of an adult:
    Plasma sodium - 110 mEq/L
    Plasma chloride - 85 mEq/L
    Plasma potassium - 4.8 mEq/L
    Plasma calcium - 5.2 mEq/L
    Plasma bicarbonate - 26 mEq/L

The most likely alteration is
    a. base bicarbonate deficit (metabolic acidosis).
    b. hypokalemia.
    c. hyponatremia.
    d. base bicarbonate excess (metabolic alkalosis).
    e. calcium deficit.

11. An individual suffers from weakness, dizziness, irritability, and intestinal cramps. Laboratory studies reveal:
    Plasma sodium - 138 mEq/L
    Plasma potassium - 6.8 mEq/L
    Blood pH - 7.38
    Plasma bicarbonate - 25 mEq/L
    An EKG with tall, peaked T wave but otherwise normal

    The individual is suffering from
    a. hypernatremia.
    b. hyponatremia.
    c. hypercalcemia.
    d. hyperkalemia.
    e. hypokalemia.

12. An acid is
    a. an anion.
    b. a cation.
    c. a substance/chemical that combines with a hydrogen ion to lower pH.
    d. a substance/chemical that donates a hydrogen ion or proton.

13. Strong acids
    1. ionize easily.
    2. contribute many H^+ to the solution.
    3. have a pH of 7.
    4. have a pH of 14.
    5. are highly dissociated.
    6. are good buffers.

    a. 1, 2 ,3
    b. 1, 2, 4
    c. 1, 2, 5
    d. 2, 3, 5
    e. 2, 3, 6

14. The blood pH is maintained near 7.4 by systems. The sequence from the fastest acting to the slowest acting system is, respectively,
    a. lungs, kidney, blood buffers.
    b. blood buffers, lungs, kidneys.
    c. blood buffers, kidneys, lungs.
    d. lungs, blood buffers, kidneys.

15. The pH of saliva is about 7 and the pH of gastric juice is about 2. How many times more concentrated is the hydrogen ion in gastric juice than in saliva?
    a. 5
    b. 50
    c. 100
    d. 10,000
    e. 100,000

16. Which of the following would not shift the blood pH toward alkalosis?
    a. hydrogen ion secretion into urine
    b. exhalation of carbon dioxide
    c. bicarbonate ion secretion into urine
    d. All of the above would shift the blood pH toward alkalosis.
    e. None of the above would do so.

17. A young female individual became quite agitated and apprehensive and eventually lost consciousness. At the hospital emergency room, the following laboratory values were obtained:

    Plasma sodium - 137 mEq/L   Her immediate diagnosis was
    Plasma potassium - 5.0 mEq/L   a. hypokalemia.
    Blood pH - 7.53   b. metabolic acidosis.
    Serum CO_2 - 22 mmHg   c. metabolic alkalosis.
    Plasma bicarbonate - 24 mEq/L   d. respiratory acidosis.
                                             e. respiratory alkalosis.

18. As HCO_3^- shifts from the red blood cell to the blood plasma, it is expected that the plasma
    a. Na^+ increases.
    b. Cl^- shifts into the red blood cell.
    c. K^+ increases.
    d. pH decreases.

Match the acid-base imbalance with the probable cause.

19. respiratory acidosis   a. severe anxiety
20. respiratory alkalosis   b. diabetes
21. metabolic alkalosis   c. chronic diarrhea
                                         d. emphysema
                                         e. excessive baking soda ingestion

Match the acid-base imbalance with the compensatory mechanism.

22. respiratory acidosis   a. kidneys retain H^+ and excrete HCO_3^-
23. respiratory alkalosis   b. kidneys excrete H^+ and retain HCO_3^-
24. metabolic acidosis   c. respirations increase, more CO_2 is eliminated
                              d. respirations decrease, more CO_2 is retained

25. An elevated anion gap is associated with an accumulation of
    a. chloride anions.
    b. lactate anion.
    c. Both a and b are correct.
    d. Neither a nor b is correct.

Genes and Genetic Diseases

Prerequisite Objectives

a. Describe the interrelationships of DNA, RNA, and proteins.
    Review text pages 127-134; refer to Figure 4-1.

Remember!

• The gene consists of a particular sequence of nucleotides in the deoxyribonucleic acid (DNA) of the chromosome. The sequence of nucleotides in a gene determines either the structure or function of a cell. Thus, the genes dictate which proteins are found in a cell and these proteins determine the form and function of the cell.

• Genetic information flows from DNA to RNA proteins. Three major processes are involved in the preservation and transmission of genetic information. The first is replication, or the copying of DNA to form identical daughter molecules. The second is transcription, in which the genetic message encoded within DNA is transcribed into the form of RNA and is carried to the ribosomes, the sites of protein synthesis. The third is translation, in which the genetic message is decoded and converted into the 20-letter alphabet of protein structure. Because the sequence of nucleotides in the DNA bears a linear correspondence to the sequence of amino acids in the formed proteins, genetic information is preserved and transmitted to progeny.

---

b. Define general genetic terms.
    Review text pages 134-135, 143-144, and 147.

Remember!

Genetic Term	Definition
Progeny	Offspring
Chromosomes	Structures in the nucleus that contain DNA, which transmits genetic information; each chromosome composed of thousands of genes arranged in linear order

(Continued)

Remember! *(cont'd)*

Genetic Term	Definition
Gene	DNA, the basic unit of heredity, located at a particular place on the chromosome
Allele	One of two or more different genes that contain specific inheritable characteristics (such as eye color) and occupy corresponding positions on paired chromosomes — one gene from each parent; a different version of the same paired gene
Gamete	A mature male or female reproductive cell
Gametogenesis	Development of gametes
Homozygous	A trait of an organism produced by identical or nearly identical alleles
Heterozygous	Possessing different alleles at a given chromosomal location
Karyotype	A display of human chromosomes based on their length and the location of the centromere
Genotype	The basic combination of genes of an organism
Phenotype	The expression of the gene or trait in an individual (e.g., physical appearance such as eye color)
Dominant traits	Traits for which one of a pair of alleles is necessary for expression (e.g., brown eyes)
Recessive traits	Traits for which two alleles of a pair are necessary for expression (blue eyes, a recessive gene on the male's X chromosome, will be expressed because it is not matched by a corresponding gene on the Y chromosome).
Pedigree chart	A schematic method for classifying genetic data
Expressivity	The extent of variation in phenotype for a particular genotype
Penetrance	The percentage of individuals with a specific genotype who exhibit the expected phenotype

Single-gene disorders are known to be caused by mutation in a single gene. The mutated gene may be present on one or both chromosomes of a pair.

Multifactorial disorders result from a combination of small variations in genes that, when combined with environmental factors, produce serious defects. Multifactorial disorders tend to cluster in families.

Objectives

After successful study of this chapter, the learner will be able to:

1. Characterize chromosome disorders.

Study text pages 136-143; refer to Figures 4-10, 4-15, and 4-18.

In **chromosome disorders**, the defect is due to an abnormality in chromosome number or structure. The structure of the genes in chromosome disorders may be normal but the genes may be present in multiple copies or be situated on a different chromosome. For example, Down syndrome results from the presence of an extra chromosome 21, trisomy 21.

Normal somatic cells having two sets of 23 chromosomes are said to be diploid (double) or 2N. Gametes with a single set of 23 chromosomes are haploid (single) or N. A cell with an exact multiple of the haploid number is euploid. Euploid numbers may be 2N, 3N (triploid), or 4N (tetraploid). Chromosome numbers that are exact multiples of N but greater than 2N are called polyploid. Aneuploid refers to a chromosome complement that is abnormal in number but is not an exact multiple of N. An aneuploid cell may be trisomic (2N + 1 chromosome) or monosomic (2N - 1 chromosome). Any cell with a chromosome number that deviates from the characteristic N and 2N is heteroploid.

Disjunction is the normal separation and migration of chromosomes during cell division. Failure of the process, or nondisjunction, in a meiotic division results in one daughter cell receiving both homologous chromosomes and the other receiving neither. It is the primary cause of aneuploidy. If this deviation in normal processes occurs during the first meiotic division, half of the gametes will contain 22 chromosomes and half will contain 24. If joined with a normal gamete, a gamete produced in this manner will produce either a monosomic (2N - 1) or trisomic (2N + 1) zygote.

Deviations in the **normal structure** of chromosomes result from the chromosome material breaking and reassembling in an abnormal arrangement. These changes in structure may be stable and persist through future cell divisions. Stable types of structural abnormalities include deletion, duplication, inversion, or translocation.

In **deletion,** or loss of a portion of a chromosome, the missing segment may be a terminal portion of the chromosome resulting from a single break or an internal section resulting from two breaks. Cri-du-chat syndrome is such a deletion and is manifested by the "cry of the cat" in an affected child.

Duplication is the presence of a repeated gene or gene sequence. A deleted segment of one chromosome may become incorporated into its homologous chromosome.

Inversion is the reversal of gene order. The linear arrangement of genes on a chromosome is broken and the order of a portion of the gene complement is reversed in the process of reattachment.

Translocation is the transfer of part of one chromosome to a nonhomologous chromosome. This occurs when two chromosomes break and the segments are rejoined in an abnormal arrangement.

2. Cite examples of chromosome disorders.

Refer to Figures 4-11, 4-13, 4-14, and 4-16.

A common example of a disorder that results from an abnormality of chromosome number is trisomy 21 or **Down syndrome**. This disorder can result when nondisjunction of chromosome 21 occurs at meiosis, producing one gamete with an extra chromosome 21 (N + 1 = 24) and one gamete with no chromosome 21 (N - 1 = 22). Union of the 24-chromosome gamete with a normal sperm produces a 47-chromosome zygote or trisomy 21.

The overall incidence of Down syndrome is 1 per 800 live births. The incidence increases with increasing maternal age. Clinical diagnosis of trisomy 21 is often based on facial appearance. The palpebral fissures are upslanting with speckling of the edge of the iris, the nose is small, and the facial profile is flat. The simian crease, a single midpalmar fold, is found in approximately 50 percent of persons with Down syndrome and in approximately 5 to 10 percent of nonafflicted persons. Mental retardation is consistent in children with Down syndrome but its degree may vary. The average IQ is approximately 50. Infrequently, IQ values may range towards 70 or 80.

Two other chromosomal disorders are **Turner syndrome** and **Klinefelter syndrome**. The most common genotype showing female phenotype is 45 X; the male phenotype is 47 XXY.

The overall incidence of Turner syndrome is 1 per 5000 female births. The frequency at conception is higher but 99 percent spontaneously abort. The diagnosis is suggested in the newborn by the presence of redundant neck skin and peripheral lymphedema. Later, the presence of short stature or primary amenorrhea is suggestive.

The incidence of Klinefelter syndrome is 1 per 1000 males. This syndrome is the most common cause of hypogonadism and infertility in men. Other manifestations include long lower extremities, sparse body hair with female distribution, and female breast development in about 50 percent of the cases.

3. Characterize single-gene disorders.
Study text pages 144-154; refer to Figures 4-20 through 4-27.

Single-gene disorders are caused by the genetic code, the sequence of nucleotides, in a single gene. Each gene has a specific site or locus on a specific chromosome. The inherited gene may be present on one or both chromosomes of a pair. The pedigree patterns of inherited traits are dependent on whether the gene is located on an autosomal chromosome, any chromosome other than a sex chromosome, or on the X chromosome and whether the gene is dominant or recessive. There are no known Y-linked genetic disorders. These factors allow four basic patterns of inheritance for single-gene traits, whether normal or abnormal: autosomal dominant, autosomal recessive, X-linked dominant, and X-linked recessive.

In **autosomal dominant** inheritance of genetic defect, the abnormal allele is dominant and the normal allele is recessive. The phenotype is the same whether the allele is present in either a homozygous of heterozygous state.

Characteristics of autosomal dominant inheritance are (1) affected persons have an affected parent, (2) affected persons mating with normal persons have affected and unaffected offspring in equal proportion, (3) unaffected children born to affected parents will have unaffected children, and (4) males and females are equally affected.

In **autosomal recessive** disorders, the abnormal allele is recessive. For the trait to be expressed, a person must be homozygous for the abnormal allele. Because the dominant or normal allele masks the trait, most persons who are heterozygous for an autosomal recessive allele go undetected. When two heterozygous individuals mate and an offspring receives the recessive allele from each parent, the trait is expressed. Procreation by persons who are blood relatives may increase the probability of expression.

Characteristics of autosomal recessive inheritance are (1) the trait usually appears in siblings only, not in the parents; (2) males and females are equally likely to be affected; (3) for parents of one affected child, the recurrence risk is one in four for every subsequent birth; (4) both parents of an affected child carry the recessive allele; and (5) the parents of the affected child may be consanguineous or blood relatives.

Of the 23 pairs of chromosomes that determine the karyotype of the human, 22 are autosomes and 1 is the sex chromosome. Unlike the 44 autosomes that can be arranged in 22 homologous pairs, the two sex chromosomes in the female are XX and in the male are XY. Because the ovum must contain an X chromosome, if it is fertilized by a sperm containing an X chromosome, the progeny will be a female (XX). If the sperm contributes a Y chromosome, the progeny will be male (XY).

Traits determined by either dominant or recessive X-linked genes are expressed in the male. The genes on the X chromosome cannot be transmitted from father to son (fathers contribute a Y chromosome to sons) but are transmitted from father to all daughters through one X chromosome. Recessive abnormal genes on the X chromosome of a female may not be expressed because they are matched by normal genes inherited with the other X chromosome.

X-linked dominant disorders are rare. The main characteristic of this inheritance pattern is that an affected male transmits the gene to all his daughters and to none of his sons. The affected female may transmit the gene to offspring of either sex. Characteristics of X-linked dominant inheritance are (1) affected males have normal sons and affected daughters, (2) affected females (heterozygous) have a 50 percent risk of transmitting the abnormal gene to each daughter or son, and (3) the disorder tends to be more severe in males than in females.

In **X-linked recessive disorders**, the recessive gene located on the one X chromosome of the male is not balanced by the dominant allele on the Y chromosome and is thus expressed. Only matings between an affected male and a carrier or affected female should result in an affected female.

Males affected with an X-linked recessive disorder cannot transmit the gene to sons but transmit it to all daughters. An unaffected female who is heterozygous for the recessive gene transmits it to 50 percent of her sons and daughters.

Characteristics of the X-linked recessive inheritance are (1) males are predominantly affected, (2) affected males cannot transmit the gene to sons but transmit the gene to all daughters, (3) sons of female carriers have a 50 percent risk of being affected, and (4) daughters of female carriers have a 50 percent risk of being carriers.

4. Cite examples of single-gene disorders.
Study text pages 137-140 and figures in Objective 3.

One of the most well-known autosomal dominant diseases is **Huntington disease**, a neurologic disorder which exhibits progressive dementia and increasingly uncontrollable movements of the limbs. One of the key features of this disease is that its symptoms are not usually seen until after age 40. Thus, those who develop the disease often have had children before they are aware that they have the gene.

The severity of an autosomal dominant disease can vary greatly. An example of variable expressivity in an autosomal dominant disease is **neurofibro-**

matosis, or von Recklinghausen disease, which has been mapped to the long arm of chromosome 17. The expression of this gene can vary from a few harmless "cáfe au lait" spots on the skin to numerous malignant neurofibromas, scoliosis, seizures, gliomas, neuromas, hypertension, and mental retardation.

The **cystic fibrosis** gene, the cause of a lethal autosomal recessive gene, has been mapped to the long arm of chromosome 7. In this disease, defective transport of chloride ions leads to a salt imbalance that results in secretions of abnormally thick, dehydrated mucus. Some of the digestive organs, particularly the pancreas, become obstructed with mucus, resulting in malnutrition. The lung airways tend to become clogged with mucus, making them highly susceptible to bacterial infections.

The most common and severe of all X-linked recessive disorders is **Duchenne muscular dystrophy**, which affects males. This disorder is characterized by progressive muscle degeneration; individuals are usually unable to walk by age 10 or 12. The disease also affects the heart and respiratory muscles, and death due to respiratory or cardiac failure may occur before age 20. These cases are generally due to frameshift deletions, in which all of the amino acids are altered following the deletion.

Hemophilia is genetically transmitted through an X-linked recessive gene and it affects males almost exclusively. Hemophilia is characterized by spontaneous or traumatic subcutaneous or intramuscular hemorrhage.

5. Characterize multifactorial inheritance and cite examples.

Study text pages 160-161; refer to Figure 4-30.

Not all traits are produced by single genes; some traits are the result of several genes acting together.

When several genes act together, the trait is referred to as polygenic. When environmental factors also influence the expression of the trait, the term multifactorial inheritance is used. Both genes and environment contribute to variation in traits. Multifactorial disorders tend to cluster in families. Although both height and IQ are determined by genes, they are also influenced by environment. For example, height has increased by 5 to 10 cm since the turn of the century because of improvements in nutrition and health care. Also, IQ scores can be improved by exposing children to enriched learning environments.

A number of diseases do not follow the bell-shaped distribution of polygenic and multifactorial traits. Instead, a certain threshold of liability must be crossed before the disease is expressed. A well-known example of a threshold trait is pyloric stenosis, a disorder characterized by a narrowing or obstruction of the pylorus. Chronic vomiting, constipation, weight loss, and electrolyte imbalance can result from this condition. Pyloric stenosis is much more common in males than females. The reason for this difference is that the threshold of liability is much lower in males than females. Thus, fewer defective alleles are required to generate the disorder in males. This also means that the offspring of affected females are more likely to have pyloric stenosis because affected females carry more disease-causing alleles than do most affected males.

Other multifactorial diseases include cleft lip and/or cleft palate, neural tube defects, clubfeet, and some forms of congenital heart disease. Hypertensive heart disease and diabetes mellitus likely can be grouped in the category of multifactorial disorders.

Practice Examination

1. Which genetic disease is caused by an abnormal karyotype?
   a. Down syndrome
   b. Huntington disease
   c. PKU
   d. neurofibromatosis
   e. cystic fibrosis

2. Which is not characteristic of Down syndrome?
   a. It is an autosomal aneuploidy.
   b. It is a genetic error of metabolism.
   c. The presence of mental retardation is consistently expressed.
   d. Clinical diagnosis is often based on facial appearance.
   e. The genotype is 47 XY, + 21.

3. Cri-du-chat syndrome is an abnormality of chromosomal structure involving
   a. translocation.
   b. an inversion.
   c. duplication.
   d. deletion.

4. An individual's karyotype lacks a homologous X chromosome and has only a single X chromosome present. Which is not true?
   a. There is a meiotic failure in the father.
   b. The genotype is 45 XO.
   c. Features include ribbed neck and short stature.
   d. The genotype is 46 XY.
   e. The disorder is a sex chromosome aneuploidy.

5. If homologous chromosomes fail to separate during meiosis, the disorder is
   a. polyploidy.
   b. aneuploidy.
   c. disjunction.
   d. nondisjunction.
   e. translocation.

6. A clinically useful, early technique for prenatal diagnosis of chromosomal abnormalities is
   a. pedigree analysis.
   b. gene mapping.
   c. amniocentesis.
   d. chorionic villi biopsy.

7. In autosomal dominant inherited disorders,
   a. affected individuals do not have an affected parent.
   b. affected persons mating with normal persons have a 50 percent risk of having an affected offspring.
   c. male offspring are most often affected.
   d. unaffected children born to affected parents will have affected children.

8. In X-linked recessive inherited disorders,
   a. affected males have normal sons.
   b. affected males have affected daughters.
   c. sons of female carriers have a 50 percent risk of being affected.
   d. the affected female may transmit the gene to both sons and daughters.

9. Which disease is not an autosomal dominant disease?
   a. Huntington disease
   b. neurofibromatosis
   c. Duchenne muscular dystrophy
   d. von Recklinghausen disease
   e. pyloric stenosis

10. Once environmental influences cause variation in the phenotype for different genotypes, a blended spectrum of phenotypes becomes a/an
    a. multifactorial trait.
    b. threshold liability.
    c. autosomal dominant trait.
    d. X-linked recessive trait.

11. Which is likely not a multifactorial inherited disorder?
    a. cleft palate
    b. hypertension
    c. diabetes mellitus
    d. cystic fibrosis
    e. heart disease

Match the term with the circumstance.

12. recessive disorder
13. multifactorial inheritance
14. aneuploidy
15. chromosomal aberration
16. phenotype
17. pedigree
18. autosomal recessive inheritance

a. due to numerical or structural aberrations
b. many genes are common
c. two or more cell lines with different karyotypes
d. individual homozygous for a gene
e. failure of homologous chromosomes to separate during meiosis or mitosis
f. outward appearance of an individual
g. a probability of .25
h. summarizes family relationships

Match the term with the circumstance.

19. expressivity
20. X-linked
21. inversion
22. dominant trait
23. allele
24. 47 XXY
25. karyotype

a. a probability of .5
b. females unlikely to be affected
c. species chromosomal morphology
d. one pair of alleles permit expression
e. Turner syndrome
f. different version of the same paired gene
g. Klinefelter syndrome
h. no loss or gain of genetic material
i. extent of phenotypic variation of a particular genotype

CHAPTER 5

Genes and Environmental Interaction: Familial Diseases

Prerequisite Objective

a. Relate inheritance and environment.
Review text pages 160-161.

Remember!

- The struggle between nature, or genetic traits, and nurture, or environment, regarding disease causality continues today. However, good epidemiologic data are now making distinctions and establishing relationships. The relative impact of genes and environments varies with disease. For example, an extra chromosome 21 is manifested regardless of environment; it has only a genetic basis. However, an individual genetically lacking the enzyme to metabolize the amino acid phenylalanine could develop brain damage and mental retardation only if exposed to dietary phenylalanine. This, then, is a disease requiring both an inherited defect and an environmental exposure.

Objectives

After successful study of this chapter, the learner will be able to:

1. Relate environmental and genetic causal factors to disease and define multifactorial traits.
Study text pages 167-170.

Factors causing disease can be broadly classified as either genetic or environmental. An individual's age often represents the accumulated effects of genetic and environmental factors over time. Disease expressions because of sex differences may reflect lifestyle, environmental differences, or anatomic and hormonal differences due to genetics. It is difficult to distinguish between the effects of shared environmental factors and the effects of a common genetic background. This is true because dietary customs are shared by ethnic groups, gene traits are shared by racial groups, climate is common to those in shared geographic locations, and health codes are shared by religious groups.

Finding and understanding environmental factors which affect the penetrance of specific genes is important if chronic familial diseases are to be prevented. Studies suggest that genetic makeup predisposes an individual to the disease but environmental factors cause the disease to develop. Therefore, environmental influences enhance an individual's predisposition to disease and produce a **multifactorial** set of causal factors for any given disease. Once environmental influences cause variations in the phenotype for genotypes, a blended spectrum of phenotypes becomes a multifactorial trait.

2. Cite three diseases tending to share environmental factors with a shared gene pool.

Refer to Table 5-2.

Disease	Environmental Factors	Shared Gene Pool
Early coronary heart disease	Animal fat intake	Genes for high blood cholesterol
Early type II diabetes and obesity	Change from scarce food supply to plentiful carbohydrates	Apparent shared gene pool among various Indian tribes
Skin cancers	Ultraviolet light	Inherited level of skin pigmentation

3. Define risk factors and describe two methods to analyze associations between disease and risk.

Study text pages 171-176; refer to Figure 5-2 and Table 5-4 .

Risk factors are indicators of a person's predisposition to develop a disease. A particular risk factor or a set of risk factors predicts increased disease rates within a group of individuals. For example, smokers get more lung cancer than nonsmokers. Risk factors cannot precisely predict whether a specific person will contract or avoid a disease. Notably, many smokers do not get lung cancer.

Although a causal role is suspected for some risk factors, solid evidence establishing a causal relationship is lacking for many. There is a distinction between causal factors and noncausal associations. **Causal risk factors** are those that, when removed or eliminated, delay or prevent the disease. **Noncausal risk factors** may be helpful in predicting a person's chances of developing the disease, but they have no effect on the underlying cause of the disease.

Cigarette smoking, for example, is a causal risk factor leading to lung cancer. Men who drink alcohol are often smokers and are also likely to develop lung cancer. Nonsmoking men and alcohol drinkers do not have an increased risk for lung cancer. Therefore, male gender and alcohol intake are noncausal risk factors for lung cancer.

The association of a disease with a particular risk factor can be evaluated using 2-by-2 **contingency tables.** Any contingency table lists the number of individuals who respectively do or do not have the disease plotted against those who have or have not experienced exposure to a risk factor. The relative risk of developing the disease is then expressed as the ratio of the disease rate among the exposed population to the disease rate in the unexposed population. For lung cancer and cigarette smoking, a relative risk of 13.3 implies a lung cancer rate among smokers that is 13.3 times higher than the rate among nonsmokers. The population-attributable risk indicates the percentage of disease cases in the general population that are attributable to a causal risk factor.

Sometimes, disease can be assessed quantitatively as a group of continuous traits rather than as merely absent or present symptoms. Continuous traits are expressed across a range of severity. Obesity and blood pressure elevation, for example, are related conditions that appear with various degrees of severity.

The statistic commonly used to quantify the degree of association between two continuous traits is called the **correlation coefficient.** If the correlation between two characteristics such as blood and weight plotted on vertical and horizontal axes were perfect, then all plotted points would fall along a single line and the correlation coefficient would be 1.00. A positive number indicates direct relationships and negative numbers indicate inverse relationships. If there were no correlation, there would be a correlation coefficient of 0.00 and plotted points would show a randomly scattered distribution.

4. Identify age as a risk factor for disease.

Refer to Table 5-6.

Age is a risk factor for many diseases; it will be only a matter of time until disease is expressed. Age probably represents the accumulating effects of environmental exposures and inherited characteristics. The general degeneration that accompanies aging can also result from deterioration of genetic material and loss of immunologic defenses. Tissue integrity is also compromised by aging through changes in elastin, bone matrix, and collagen or through loss of neurons.

**5. Identify some major system diseases that
exhibit familial tendencies; suggest possible
contributing environmental factors in these
diseases.**

Study text pages 181-196.

Familial Diseases

Disease	Environmental Factors
Immunologic Disorders	
Rheumatoid arthritis	Viral infections triggering immune responses
Systemic lupus erythematosus	
Hashimoto thyroiditis	
Graves disease	
Type I diabetes	
Gastrointestinal Disorders	
Celiac sprue	Gluten in wheat
Colon cancer	High fat, low fiber
Ulcerative colitis, Crohn disease	Infectious agents
Type II diabetes	Obesity, dietary sugar
Obesity	Excessive caloric intake
Lactose intolerance	Milk products
Peptic ulcer	Stress, diet, microbes
Gallstones, gout	Diet
Hematologic Disorders	
Hemolytic anemia	Aspirin, antibodies, infections
Hemochromatosis	Iron absorption
Cardiovascular Disorders	
Coronary heart disease	Fat intake, exercise, smoking
Hypertension, stroke	Fat intake, exercise, smoking
Rheumatic heart disease	Streptococcal infection
Renal Disorders	
Ureteral stones	Milk, carbonated beverage intake
Neuromuscular Disorders	
Multiple sclerosis	Viruses
Alzheimer disease	Enzyme deficiencies, chemicals (suspected)
Psychiatric disorders	Neurochemicals (suspected)
Alcoholism	Social, environmental intake
Respiratory Disorders	
Lung cancer	Cigarette smoke, environmental pollutants
Asthma, allergies	Allergens - dust, pollen, etc.
Breast Disorders	
Female breast cancer	High fat intake, alcohol consumption

Practice Examination

True/False

____ 1. Hypertension is a form of familial disease.

____ 2. Age is a risk factor for many diseases.

____ 3. A multifactorial trait is expressed when multiple genes and environmental influences blend together.

____ 4. In trisomy 21, the pathology is manifested independent of environment.

____ 5. It is easy to distinguish between the effects of shared environmental factors and the effects of a common pool of genes.

____ 6. Allergies and asthma do not manifest familial patterns.

____ 7. An inherited level of skin pigmentation is a factor in the development of skin cancer.

____ 8. Early type II diabetes may develop when an individual's diet changes to heavy carbohydrate consumption.

____ 9. Finding and understanding environmental factors which affect penetrance of specific genes is important if chronic familial diseases are to be prevented.

____ 10. A variation in the phenotype for different genotypes caused by environmental factors is a threshold liability trait.

____ 11. The frequency of genetic disease in the population depends on phenotypes.

____ 12. Noncausal risk factors, when removed or eliminated, delay or prevent disease.

____ 13. Male gender and alcohol consumption are causal risk factors for lung cancer.

____ 14. A contingency table can evaluate the association of a disease with a particular or specific risk factor.

____ 15. The existence of a particular risk factor indicates an individual will develop a specific disease.

____ 16. The expression of a disease requires both an inherited defect and environmental exposure.

____ 17. The statistic commonly used to quantify association between continuous traits is the correlation coefficient.

____ 18. When plotted points of continuous traits fall along a single line, there is no relationship between the traits.

____ 19. Aging compromises bone matrix, collagen, and neurons.

____ 20. The prevalence rate is the number of individuals living with a disease.

____ 21. The incidence rate is the number of persons who have died from a disease.

Match the disease with the environmental factor(s).

22. rheumatic heart disease	a. wheat gluten
23. Graves disease	b. high fat, low fiber
24. celiac disease	c. milk products
25. ureteral stones	d. iron absorption
	e. streptococcal infection
	f. caloric intake
	g. viral infections
	h. milk, carbonated beverage intake

CHAPTER 6

Immunity

Objectives

After successful study of this chapter, the learner will be able to:

1. **Define immunity, antigen, antibody, and hapten.**
   Review text pages 207 and 210-211.

2. **Distinguish among the HLA complex, the Rh system, and the ABO system.**
   Review text pages 211-212.

3. **Describe the role of the B-cell in humoral immunity.**
   Review text pages 214-216; refer to Figure 6-7.

4. **Identify an important role for each of the five classes of immunoglobulins.**
   Review text pages 216-222; refer to Figures 6-9 through 6-11 and Table 6-3.

5. **Compare and contrast the titer and class of immunoglobulin in the primary and secondary immune response.**
   Review text pages 208-209; refer to Figure 6-2.

6. **Distinguish ways to develop immunity; define active, passive, artificial, and natural.**
   Review text pages 207-208.

7. **Describe the secretory immune system.**
   Review text pages 222-223.

8. **Describe the role of the T-cell in cellular immunity.**
   Review text pages 224-226; refer to Figure 6-14.

9. **Compare fetal and neonatal immune function with immune function in the elderly.**
   Review text pages 230-231.

Practice Examination

Match the term with its definition.

1. phagocytosis
2. specific immunity
3. macrophage
4. nonspecific immunity
5. antigen

a. identical cells having descended from one cell
b. lymphocyte that attacks antibodies directly
c. ingestion and destruction
d. phagocytic, agranular leukocyte of the immune system
e. resists a large variety of antigens
f. macromolecular pattern for antibody production
g. protein produced by T-cells
h. exclusively thymus-dependent

6. Immunogenicity depends on
   a. mass.
   b. foreignness.
   c. complexity.
   d. Both b and c are correct.
   e. a, b, and c are correct.

7. The HLA complex
   a. has both anti-A and anti-B antibodies.
   b. antigens are found on the surfaces of most cells except erythrocytes.
   c. is an antigen system found on erythrocytes.
   d. All of the above are correct.
   e. a, b, and c are incorrect because HLA antigens are involved in rejection of foreign tissue.

8. When antigen binds to its appropriate antibody,
   a. agglutination may occur.
   b. phagocytosis may occur.
   c. antigen neutralization may occur.
   d. All of the above are correct.
   e. None of the above is correct.

9. Antibodies are produced by
   a. B-cells.
   b. T-cells.
   c. helper cells.
   d. plasma cells.
   e. memory cells.

10. An immunoglobulin contains
    a. two heavy and two light polypeptide chains.
    b. four heavy and four light polypeptide chains.
    c. two heavy and four light polypeptide chains.
    d. four heavy and two light polypeptide chains.

11. The antibody class having the highest concentration in the blood is
    a. Ig A.
    b. Ig D.
    c. Ig E.
    d. Ig G.
    e. Ig M.

12. Which antibody is matched with its appropriate role?
    a. Ig A/ allergic reactions
    b. Ig D/ found in respiratory secretions
    c. Ig E/ found in gastric secretions
    d. Ig G/ first to challenge the antigen
    e. Ig M/ first to challenge the antigen
    f. None of the above is correct.

13. The primary immune response involves
    a. a rapid plasma cell response with peak antibody by three days.
    b. macrophage production of antibodies.
    c. T-cell production of antibodies.
    d. a latent period followed by peak antibody production.

14. Which of the following cells is phagocytic?
    a. B-cells
    b. T-cells
    c. T-suppressors
    d. T-killers
    e. macrophages

15. When a child develops measles and acquires an immunity to future subsequent infections, the immunity is
    a. acquired.
    b. active.
    c. natural.
    d. All of the above are correct.

Match the term with its descriptor.

16. antibody combining site
17. epitopes
18. monoclonal antibodies
19. mucous membrane
20. memory cell

a. antigenic determinants
b. useful for diagnosis
c. first line of defense
d. determine the specificity between antibody and antigen
e. secretes antibodies
f. long-term immunity
g. produced after initial contact with an antigen
h. predominant antibody of secondary response

Match the descriptor with the appropriate lymphocytic activity.

21. capable of forming clones
22. produce lymphokines
23. helper and suppressor cells
24. antibody formation
25. cell-mediated response

a. T-cell involvement
b. B-cell involvement
c. both T-cell and B-cell involvement

Inflammation

Objectives

After successful study of this chapter, the learner will be able to:

1. **Define inflammation and contrast it to immunity.**
   Review text pages 235-237.

2. **Indicate the causes of mast cell degranulation and the effects of histamine and serotonin.**
   Review text pages 237-238; refer to Figure 7-4.

3. **State the effects of the long-term synthesis products of the mast cell.**
   Review text pages 238-239.

4. **Identify the plasma protein systems and their interactions in inflammation.**
   Review text pages 239-246; refer to Figure 7-12.

5. **Describe the role of complement in humoral immunity.**
   Review text pages 240-242.

6. **Identify a role for neutrophils, monocytes, macrophages, and eosinophils in the acute and chronic inflammatory process.**
   Review text pages 246-252; refer to Figure 7-15.

7. **State the roles for lymphokines, interferon, and interleukins; note their relationships within the immune system.**
   Review text pages 254-255; refer to Table 7-1.

8. **Name and describe the cardinal (local) and systemic signs of inflammation.**
   Review text pages 255-256 and 258-259.

9. **Define and differentiate the repair and regeneration process; identify factors affecting regeneration.**
   Review text pages 259 and 263-265.

10. **Distinguish first-intention from second-intention healing.**
    Refer to Figure 7-22.

Practice Examination

1. Inflammation
   a. destroys injurious agents.
   b. confines injurious agents.
   c. stimulates and enhances immunity.
   d. promotes healing.
   e. All of the above are correct.

2. Inflammatory microcirculation changes involve all except
   a. vasodilation.
   b. days to develop.
   c. increased vascular permeability.
   d. emigration of leukocytes to injury site.

3. A phagocyte's role begins with an inflammatory response. The sequence for phagocytosis is
   a. margination or pavementing, recognition of the target, adherence or binding, and fusion with lysosomes inside the phagocyte.
   b. diapedesis, margination or pavementing, phagosome formation, recognition of the target, and fusion with lysosomes inside the phagocyte.
   c. recognition of the target, margination or pavementing, and destruction of target by lysosomal enzymes.
   d. margination, diapedesis, recognition, adherence, ingestion, fusion with lysosomes inside the phagocyte, and destruction of target.

4. Chemotactic factors for phagocytes include all except
   a. complement components.
   b. streptolysins.
   c. plasminogen activator.
   d. prostaglandins.
   e. mast cell degranulation products.

5. Which is not a local manifestation of inflammation?
   a. swelling
   b. pain
   c. heat
   d. leukocytosis
   e. redness

6. Complement is
   a. a proenzyme in the blood.
   b. an antibody.
   c. a hormone.
   d. a lymphokine.

7. Diapedesis is a process in which
   a. neutrophils migrate from the bloodstream to an injured tissue site.
   b. phagocytes stick to capillary and venule walls.
   c. bacteria are "coated" with an opsonin.
   d. there is oxygen-dependent killing of cells.

8. Interferon
   a. interferes with the ability of bacteria to cause disease.
   b. prevents viruses from infecting healthy host cells.
   c. inhibits macrophage migration from inflamed sites.
   d. increases the phagocytic activity of macrophages.
   e. increases the number of circulating neutrophils.

9. The complement system can be activated by
    a. the binding of complement 1 to a complement binding site of an antibody.
    b. components of other plasma protein systems.
    c. the binding of complement 3 to bacteria.
    d. Both a and c are correct.
    e. a, b, and c are correct.

10. Which is not a systemic manifestation of inflammation?
    a. leukocytosis
    b. fever
    c. increased acute-phase reactants
    d. exudation

11. The inflammatory response
    a. prevents blood from entering the injured tissue.
    b. elevates body temperature to prevent spread of infection.
    c. prevents formation of abscesses.
    d. minimizes injury and promotes healing.

12. Scar tissue is
    a. non-functional fibrotic tissue.
    b. functional tissue that follows wound healing.
    c. regenerated tissue formed in the area of injury.
    d. fibrinogen which has entrapped phagocytes and neurons.

13. Which cell type is least able to replace itself?
    a. bone and cartilage
    b. nerve and muscle
    c. liver and spleen
    d. skin and blood

14. Swelling during acute inflammation is caused by
    a. collagenase.
    b. the fluid exudate.
    c. lymphocytic margination.
    d. neutrophilic margination.
    e. anaerobic glycolysis.

15. Which is not released from mast cells during degranulation?
    a. chemotactic factors
    b. histamine
    c. complement
    d. serotonin

16. Chronic inflammation is characterized by
    a. hypertrophy.
    b. metaplasia.
    c. neutrophilic infiltration.
    d. lymphocytic and macrophagic infiltration.
    e. All of the above are correct.

17. Which tissue is capable of cellular mitosis after biochemical stimulation?
    a. gastrointestinal epithelium
    b. bone marrow
    c. bone
    d. Both a and b are correct.
    e. a, b, and c are correct.

18. Primary-intention healing
   a. involves collagen synthesis.
   b. requires little wound contraction.
   c. requires little wound epithelization.
   d. Both b and c are correct.
   e. a, b, and c are correct.

19. Which is not true of interleukins?
   a. They provide messages between leukocytes.
   b. They are produced in response to tissue injury.
   c. They stimulate cells to produce antiviral substances.
   d. They increase antibody production and populations of T-cells.
   e. All of the above are true of interleukins.

20. Eosinophils
   a. are agranulocytes.
   b. control the vascular effects of serotonin and histamine by lysosomal mediators.
   c. have a lysosomal protein that can dissolve the surface membranes of parasites.
   d. All of the above are correct.
   e. Both b and c are correct.

Match the term with its definition or characteristic.

21. resolution
22. bradykinin
23. granulation tissue
24. fibroblasts
25. scar

   a. increases the phagocytic activity of macrophages
   b. original structure and physiologic function
   c. inhibits macrophage migration from the inflamed area
   d. increases vascular permeability
   e. new capillaries, fibroblasts, and macrophages
   f. avascular
   g. synthesize and secrete collagen
   h. proliferate antigen-specific clones of B- and T-cells

CHAPTER 8

Alterations in Immunity and Inflammation

Prerequisite Objectives

a. Chart the development and activities of specific immunity.
   Review text pages 214-230.

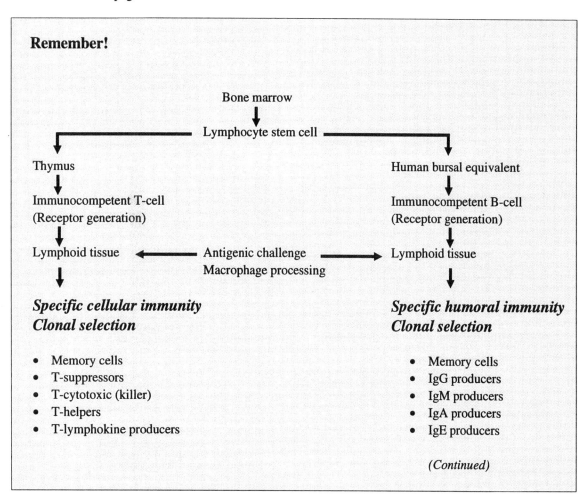

Remember!

Bone marrow
↓
Lymphocyte stem cell

Thymus
↓
Immunocompetent T-cell
(Receptor generation)
↓
Lymphoid tissue ← Antigenic challenge
Macrophage processing

Specific cellular immunity
Clonal selection

- Memory cells
- T-suppressors
- T-cytotoxic (killer)
- T-helpers
- T-lymphokine producers

Human bursal equivalent
↓
Immunocompetent B-cell
(Receptor generation)
↓
→ Lymphoid tissue

Specific humoral immunity
Clonal selection

- Memory cells
- IgG producers
- IgM producers
- IgA producers
- IgE producers

(Continued)

b. Diagram the interrelationships between CMI and HI.
   Review text pages 226-230; refer to Figure 6-16.

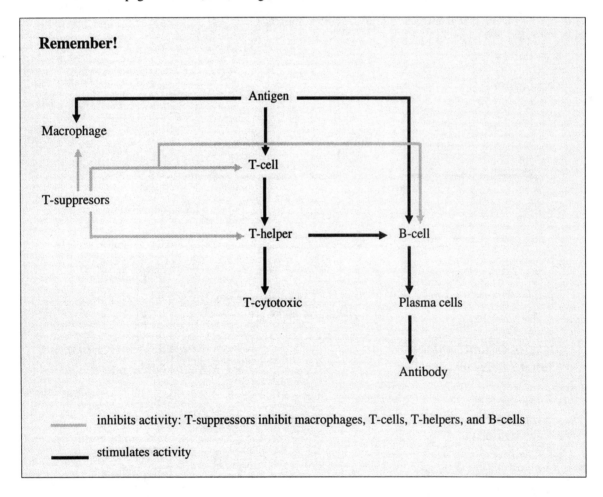

c. Diagram a scheme for complement's role in amplifying the immune response. Relate opsonization, inflammation, and cytolysis to the components of complement.

Review text pages 240-242; refer to Figure 7-6.

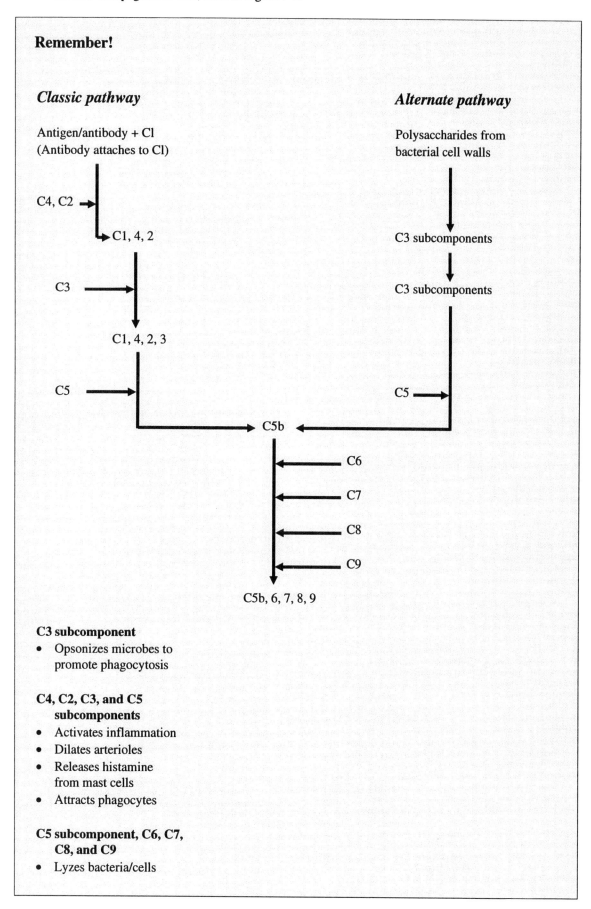

Remember!

Classic pathway

Antigen/antibody + Cl
(Antibody attaches to Cl)

C4, C2 →

C1, 4, 2

C3 →

C1, 4, 2, 3

C5 →

C5b

← C6

← C7

← C8

← C9

C5b, 6, 7, 8, 9

Alternate pathway

Polysaccharides from
bacterial cell walls

C3 subcomponents

C3 subcomponents

C5 →

C3 subcomponent
- Opsonizes microbes to promote phagocytosis

C4, C2, C3, and C5 subcomponents
- Activates inflammation
- Dilates arterioles
- Releases histamine from mast cells
- Attracts phagocytes

C5 subcomponent, C6, C7, C8, and C9
- Lyzes bacteria/cells

d. Diagram the interaction between lymphocytes and phagocytes.
   Review text pages 227-230.

Remember!

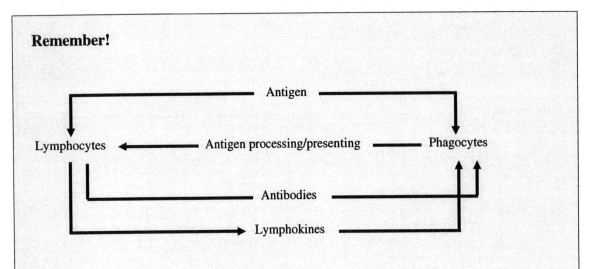

Note: There is interaction between specific and nonspecific areas of the immune system. The phagocytes cannot specifically recognize antigens but process and present them to the lymphocytes. Lymphocytes specifically recognize and produce antibody or lymphokines which help the phagocytes combat the antigen.

Objectives

After successful study of this chapter, the learner will be able to:

1. Define allergy, autoimmunity, and isoimmunity.
   Study text page 269.

Allergy is an inappropriate hypersensitivity response against an innocuous environmental antigen that is harmful to the individual.

Autoimmunity occurs when tolerance to one's self antigens breaks down and antibody is formed against one's own antigens. Self antigens are recognized as foreign in autoimmunity.

Isoimmunity is the development of antibodies against antigens from an individual of the same species. It is observed during immunologic reactions against transfusions, grafted tissue, or a fetus during pregnancy.

2. Compare the four hypersensitivities.

Study text pages 269-280; refer to Figures 8-1, 8-3, 8-4, and 8-5 and Tables 8-1, 8-3, and 8-4.

Comparison of Hypersensitivity Disorders

Hypersensitivity	*Immunity Response Time*	*Effectors*	*Examples*
Type I **IgE mediated** **Anaphylactic**	Humoral Immediate	*Antigen* reacts with IgE bound to *mast cells, histamine* release, histamine effects	Allergic rhinitis, asthma, urticaria, food allergies, anaphylactic shock
Type II **Cytoxic** **Tissue specific**	Humoral Immediate	*IgG or IgM* reacts with *antigen* on cell's membrane, *complement* is activated, lysis or phagocytosis by macrophage of cell, cell mediated cytolysis, antibody binding to receptors	Immediate drug reaction, hemolytic anemia, Graves disease
Type III **Immune complex**	Humoral Immediate	*IgG or IgM* unite with *antigen* to form a complex that is deposited in vessel walls or tissues, neutrophil attraction, *complement* activation, *lysosomal enzymes* injure tissue	Serum sickness, arthus reaction, celiac disease, allergic alveolitis, glomerulonephritis, systemic lupus erythematosus
Type IV **Cell-mediated**	Cellular Delayed	Reaction of sensitized *T-lymphocytes* with *antigen* leads to *lymphokine* release, recruitment of *macrophages* and *lysosomal* release	Contact dermatitis, graft rejection, tuberculin reaction, rheumatoid arthritis, autoimmune thyroiditis

3. Describe the likely causes of autoimmune disease; cite examples.

Study text pages 280-282; refer to Table 8-2.

Self-antigens are usually tolerated by the host's own immune system. This immunologic tolerance develops in humans during the embryonic period. Autoreactive lymphocytes are either eliminated or suppressed. Autoimmunity is a breakdown of tolerance in which the body's immune system begins to recognize self-antigens as foreign. The mechanisms of breakdown are varied and often unknown. Some of the mechanisms implicated in the development of autoimmunity include (1) exposure within the body of a previously sequestered antigen, (2) the development of a neoantigen, (3) the complications of an infectious disease, and (4) an alteration of suppressor T-cells.

To be tolerated after birth, a self-antigen must be present in the fetus and exposed to the developing fetal immune system. Some self-antigens never encounter antigen-processing cells in the draining lymph nodes or other lymphoid organs. They are sequestered or hidden from the immune system. Later, the immune system will recognize these antigens as foreign, if the structure of a site having sequestered antigen is disturbed and the previously **sequestered antigens** are released from the damaged tissue and enter the lymphatics. A primary immune response occurs against these antigens that can inflict extensive immunologic damage to other, similar antigenic, untraumatized sites.

Many **neoantigens** are haptens which become immunogenic after binding to host proteins. The immune reaction against the neoantigen may lead to an immunologic reaction against unaltered host protein.

Foreign antigens from **infectious microorganisms** can initiate autoimmune disease. They do so either by forming immune complexes that precipitate in host tissues which then cause inflammatory disease or by closely resembling a particular self-antigen. The antibodies produced against the similar antigenic sites of the infectious agent also recognize the self-antigen as foreign. Thus, there is an immune response against self. Group A streptococci are capable of initiating both of these mechanisms usually as sequelae to streptococcal pharyngitis.

One of the roles of **suppressor T-cells** is to suppress the immune responses against self antigens. Therefore, suppressor T-cell dysfunction could result in autoimmune disease. If a single antigen-specific population of suppressor cells is affected, a tissue-specific autoimmune disease could result. A generalized autoimmune reaction could occur if many suppressor cell populations were dysfunctional. Systemic lupus erythematosus (SLE) may be caused by a general breakdown in the suppressor cell network.

The cause of some immune diseases is quite apparent. For example, in thrombocytopenia or few platelets, there is likely integration of a drug or its metabolite into the plasma membranes of the platelet. The immune system recognizes the altered plasma membranes as new and foreign. B-cells are stimulated to produce antibody against the drug-cell complex and immune processes destroy the host cells. Viruses can induce autoimmune reactions by altering the plasma membranes of host cells.

Other common immune diseases include rheumatoid arthritis, multiple sclerosis, pernicious anemia, and ulcerative colitis. It is fairly well established that autoimmune diseases are familial. Affected family members may not all develop the same disease but several members may have different disorders characterized by hypersensitivity. An individual with a specific genetic HLA type may have inappropriate or exaggerated immune responses against a microorganism that result in a hypersensitivity reaction.

4. Characterize isoimmune disorders.
Study text pages 282-283.

Isoimmunity occurs when an individual's immune system reacts against antigens of the tissues of other members of the same species. Two examples of this reactivity are transient neonatal diseases and transplant rejection and transfusion reactions. Since a fetus has mother and father antigens, fetal paternal antigens different from maternal antigens can cross the placenta and elicit an immune response in the mother. Maternal antibody may be transported into the fetal circulation to produce isoimmune disease in the fetus. The mother's immune system produces the antibody. Rh isoimmunization or erythroblastosis fetalis wherein maternal antibody against erythrocyte antigens induces anemia in the child is an example of this malady.

Transplantation of organs is commonly complicated by an immune response against donor antigens. The primary mechanism of the rejection of transplanted organs is a type IV, cell-mediated reaction. Because HLA antigens are the principle targets of the rejection reaction, HLA matching of donor and recipient greatly enhances the possibility of a successful graft.

Transplant rejection is classified as hyperacute, acute, or chronic depending on the amount of time that elapses between transplantation and rejection. Hyperacute rejection usually occurs in recipients having pre-existing IgG or IgM antibody to antigens in the graft. As circulation to the graft is reestablished, antibody binds to the grafted tissue and activates the inflammatory response. This response initiates the coagulation or blood clotting cascade which results in cessation of blood flow into the graft. Acute rejection is a cell-mediated immune response that occurs approximately two weeks after the transplantation. The recipient develops an immune response against unmatched HLA antigens and shows an infiltration of lymphocytes and macrophages characteristic of type IV hypersensitivity reaction. Chronic rejection may occur after months or years of normal function. It is characterized by slow, progressive organ failure. Chronic rejection may be caused by inflammatory damage to endothelial cells lining blood vessels. It is likely a result of a weak immunologic reaction against minor histocompatibility antigens on the grafted tissue.

5. Characterize immunodeficiencies; describe examples of congenital or primary diseases.

Study text pages 283-287; refer to Figure 8-8 and Table 8-5.

Immune deficiencies occur because of impaired function of one or more components of the immune or inflammatory response. B-cells, T-cells, phagocytic cells, or complement may be involved. The clinical manifestation of immune deficiency is a tendency to develop unusual or recurrent severe infections. Deficiencies in T-cell immune responses are suspected when recurrent infections are caused by certain viruses, fungi and yeasts, or certain atypical organisms. B-cell deficiencies are suspected if the individual has recurrent infections with encapsulated bacteria or viruses against which humoral immunity is normally effective.

It may be unsafe to administer conventional immunizing agents or blood products to many immunologically compromised individuals because of the risk that the immunizing agent will cause an uncontrolled infection. Uncontrolled infection is particularly a problem when attenuated vaccines that contain live, but weakened, microorganisms are used. Vaccinia virus used for immunization against small pox is an example of such a vaccine. Although the virus is attenuated enough to be destroyed by a normal immune system, it can survive, multiply, and cause severe disease in an immunodeficient recipient.

Individuals with immune deficiencies are also at risk for graft-versus-host disease. This occurs if T-cells in transfused blood are mature and capable of the cell-mediated destruction of tissues in the graft recipient. The grafted T-cells are controlled by normal immune systems and no tissue destruction occurs. If the recipient's immune system is deficient, the grafted T-cells will attack the recipient's tissue.

Congenital or primary immune deficiency occurs if lymphocyte development is disturbed in the fetus or embryo or if there is a genetic anomaly. Some diseases are primarily caused by a defect in one or the other of the cell lines although both T- and B-cell lines may be partially deficient.

Severe combined immune deficiencies (SCID) occur when a common stem cell for all white blood cells is absent. Therefore, T-cells, B-cells, and phagocytic cells never develop. Most children with SCID caused by reticular digenesis, the most severe SCID form, die in utero or very soon after birth. Many individuals with SCID are deficient only in a stem cell for lymphocyte development rather than for all white blood cells, as in reticular dysgenesis, and therefore have normal numbers of all other white cells. T- and B-lymphocytes are few or totally absent in the circulation, the spleen, and lymph nodes. The thymus is usually underdeveloped. IgM and IgA immunoglobulin levels are absent or greatly reduced; however, IgG levels may be almost normal because of the presence of maternal antibodies. Other forms of SCID are caused by autosomal recessive enzymatic defects that result in the accumulation of toxic metabolites to rapidly dividing lymphocytes.

Di George syndrome is the complete lack, or more commonly partial lack, of the thymus. This thymus deficiency causes lymphopenia and greatly decreased T-cell numbers and function. **Bruton agammaglobulinemia** is caused by failure of B-cell precursors to become mature B-cells because of the lack of normal bursal-equivalent tissue. There are few or no circulating B-cells, though T-cell number and function are normal.

Some immune deficiencies involve a defect that results in depressed development of a small portion of the immune system. An example is **Wiskott-Aldrich syndrome**, an X-linked recessive disorder, in which IgM antibody production is greatly depressed. Therefore, antibody responses against polysaccharide antigens from bacterial cell walls are deficient.

Another common defect in which a particular class of antibody is affected is selective IgA deficiency. Individuals with selective **IgA deficiency** are able to produce other classes of immunoglobulin but fail to produce IgA. Individuals with IgA deficiency frequently present with chronic intestinal candidiasis. IgA may normally prevent the uptake of allergens from the environment. Therefore, IgA deficiency may lead to increased allergen uptake and a more intense challenge to the immune system because of prolonged exposure to environmental antigens.

6. Cite causes and consequences of acquired or secondary immune deficiencies.

Study text pages 287-288.

Acquired or secondary immune and inflammatory deficiency develops after birth and is not related to genetic defects. Nutritional deficits in calorie or protein intake can lead to deficiencies in T-cell function and numbers. The humoral immune response is less affected by starvation, although complement activity, neutrophilic chemotaxis, and bacterial killing by neutrophils are frequently depressed. Enzyme cofactors, such as zinc and vitamins, may result in severe depressions of both B- and T-cell function.

Iatrogenic disorders are caused by some form of medical treatment. Cancer chemotherapeutic agents suppress blood cell formation in the bone marrow. Immunosuppressive corticosteroids for treatment of individuals with transplants or autoimmune diseases depress B- and T-cell formation. The consequence of these therapies for cancer and immunosuppression is manifested as a progressive increase in infections with opportunistic microorganisms.

Traumatized burn victims are susceptible to severe bacterial infections because of decreased neutrophil function and complement levels. Burn victims also have increased suppressor cell function which may increase antigen-specific suppression.

A relationship between emotional stress and depressed immune function seems to exist. Many lymphoid organs are innervated and can be affected by nerve stimulation. Also, lymphocytes have receptors for many hormones such as neurotransmitters and can respond to changing levels of these chemicals with increased or decreased function.

7. Describe the best known acquired immune deficiency disorder, AIDS.

Study text pages 288-294; refer to Figures 8-10 through 8-12.

AIDS is caused by a virus currently named human immunodeficiency virus or HIV. The virus was isolated by researchers at the National Institutes of Health as the human T-lymphotropic virus type III or HLV-III and earlier by the Pasteur Institute as the lymphadenopathy/AIDS virus or LAV. At least one other AIDS-virus (HIV-2) has been identified.

HIV is a retrovirus carrying genetic information in RNA rather than DNA. Retroviruses infect cells by binding a target cell through a surface receptor and inserting their RNA into the target cell. A viral enzyme, reverse transcriptase, converts the viral RNA to DNA and inserts that DNA into the infected cell's genetic material. Viral proliferation may occur resulting in the lysis and death of the infected cell. If, however, the cell remains relatively dormant rather than active, the viral genetic material integrated into the infected cell's DNA may remain latent for years, if not for the life of the individual.

CD4 is an antigen on the surface of cells that acts as a receptor for the HIV. The virus primarily infects CD4-positive T-helper lymphocytes but it may also infect and lyze various other cells that express the CD4 antigen.

At the time of diagnosis, the individual may manifest one of four different conditions: serologically negative, serologically positive but asymptomatic, early stages of HIV disease, or AIDS. The currently accepted Centers for Disease Control definition of AIDS relies on both laboratory tests and clinical symptoms. The most common laboratory test is for antibodies against HIV. Without a positive test for antibodies, individuals can be diagnosed as having AIDS if they have a lymphoma of the brain and are less than 60 years of age or if they have lymphoid interstitial pneumonitis and are less than 13 years of age. If they are seropositive, the diagnosis of AIDS is made in association with a variety of clinical symptoms. These include disseminated coccidioidomycosis or histoplasmosis, extrapulmonary tuberculosis, persistent isosporiasis, recurrent salmonella septicemia, recurrent bacterial infections, HIV encephalopathy, HIV wasting syndrome, lymphoma of the brain at any age, non-Hodgkin lymphoma, and uterine cervical cancer. Other clinical symptoms of AIDS include persistent lymphadenopathy, weight loss, recurrent fevers, neurologic abnormalities with dementia in late stages, recurrent pulmonary infiltrates, and the development of opportunistic infections such as *Pneumocystis carinii* pneumonia and other atypical malignances such as Kaposi sarcoma.

The major immunologic finding in AIDS is the striking decrease of T-helper cells or CD4-positive cells. Suppressor cells which have the CD8 antigen are usually normal or slightly elevated. This results in a reversal of the normal helper-to-suppressor T-cell ratio, which is about 1.9. Most individuals with AIDS have ratios much lower than 0.9 and frequently near 0. In contrast, B-cell numbers are usually normal.

The presence of circulating antibody against the AIDS virus apparently indicates infection by the virus. Antibody appears soon after infection through blood products, usually within four to seven weeks. After sexual exposure, the individual can be infected yet seronegative for 6 to 14 months. In the late stages of the disease, some individuals become seronegative because of a deficient immune system. The period between infection and the appearance of antibody is referred to as the window period. Although the patient may not have antibody, he or she may be viremic and infectious to others within two weeks of being infected.

Treatment for AIDS can involve restoration of immune function or prevention of viral replication. Restoration of immune function has been attempted with bone marrow transplants, transfusions of white blood cells from healthy donors, and the injection of interleuken-2 interferon. These attempts have shown little or no success because the virus quickly infects the donor cells. Several agents have been tried to prevent viral replication. Some of these agents are designed to block reverse transcriptase activity, and some have been successful against other viruses or parasites such as acyclovir against herpes simplex virus. Azidothymidine, AZT, and its less toxic analogue cyanothymidine, CNT, have shown remarkable effects in extremely advanced AIDS cases with recurrent *P. carinii* infections.

Drug therapy for AIDS is difficult because the AIDS retrovirus incorporates into the genetic material of the host and may never be removed by antiviral therapy. Therefore, drug administration may have to continue for the lifetime of the individual.

The development of an effective AIDS vaccine has been slowed by several major difficulties. The AIDS virus is genetically and antigenically variable. Thus, a vaccine created against one variant may not provide protection against another variant. This is a real problem since as many as 30 to 40 different genetic variants have been isolated from the same individual during the progression of the disease. Many of these may coexist in the individual. Although AIDS individuals have high levels of circulating antibodies against the virus, these antibodies do not appear to be protective. The AIDS virus is transmitted from cell to cell and may initially enter the body in an infected cell which is not susceptible to circulating antibody. Also, HIV-infected cells tend to fuse with other cells so infection can spread to uninfected cells without viral particles being produced.

Finally, the only good model for AIDS experimentation is the chimpanzee, which is a protected animal species and relatively unavailable for medical research. Thus, efficacy and toxicity of possible vaccines cannot easily be evaluated.

8. Indicate some therapies for immune deficiencies.

Study text pages 294-296.

Individuals with hypogammaglobulinemia or agammaglobulinemia can usually be treated successfully with administration of gamma globulin. Administration of fresh-frozen plasma can be successful in individuals requiring larger amounts of IgM or IgA. Complement deficiencies may also be treated with plasma infusions.

In SCID caused by lack of stem cells, bone marrow can be transplanted from a HLA-matched donor. Graft-versus-host (GVH) disease must be avoided; a HLA match is essential. GVH disease occurs when immunocompetent T-lymphocytes in the grafted material recognize foreign antigens in the recipient thus initiating a type IV hypersensitivity reaction. GVH disease may be prevented by removing mature immunocompetent T-lymphocytes from grafts.

Therapeutic replacement of defective genes may be possible when there is an enzyme immunological deficiency. The normal gene could be cloned and inserted into a retroviral vector. Such a gene replaces some of retroviral genes and results in a virus that carries the normal human gene but will not cause disease. The virus infects defective cells and then inserts the normal gene into the patient's genetic material. The genetically altered cells may then be infused into the individual to reconstitute an immune system.

Practice Examination

Match the immunologic mechanism with the condition.

1. Graves disease
2. serum sickness
3. allergic rhinitis
4. systemic lupus erythematous
5. contact dermatitis
6. hemolytic anemia
7. tuberculin reaction

a. IgE mediated
b. cytotoxic/tissue specific
c. immune complex
d. cell mediated

8. Immunologic response(s) recognized as disease is/are
   a. immediate hypersensitivity.
   b. delayed hypersensitivities.
   c. Both a and b are correct.
   d. Neither a nor b is correct.

9. Which is not characteristic of hypersensitivity?
   a. specificity
   b. immunologic mechanisms
   c. inappropriate or injurious response
   d. prior contact unnecessary to elicit a response

10. When the body produces antibodies against its own tissue, it is a/an
    a. hypersensitivity.
    b. antibody reaction.
    c. cell-mediated immunity.
    d. autoimmune disease.
    e. opsonization.

Match the postulation with the likely mechanism.

11. sequestered antigen
12. neoantigen

a. lymphocytic clones are prevented from maturing
b. suppressor cells become dysfunctional
c. traumatized tissue releases antigens
d. integration of drug into plasma membrane of a cell

13. Which of the following is not an autoimmune disease?
    a. multiple sclerosis
    b. pernicious anemia
    c. transfusion reaction
    d. ulcerative colitis
    e. Goodpasture disease

14. Damage in glomerulonephritis is due to the formation of antigen/antibody complexes mediated by
    a. IgE.
    b. mast cells.
    c. the cell-mediated immune system.
    d. the humoral immune system, complement, and lysosome.
    e. lymphokines.

15. The classical complement cascade begins with
    a. antigen/antibody complexes binding to a component of the complement system.
    b. opsonization.
    c. chemotaxis.
    d. cytolysis.

16. An isoimmune disorder is
    a. erythroblastosis fetalis.
    b. insulin-dependent diabetes.
    c. myxedema.
    d. All of the above are correct.
    e. None of the above is correct.

17. Immunodeficiencies occur because of impaired function of
    a. B- and T-cells.
    b. phagocytic cells.
    c. complement.
    d. All of the above are correct.
    e. Both a and c are correct.

18. The most frequently observed selective antibody-dependent immunodeficiency is a deficit of
    a. IgA.
    b. IgD.
    c. IgE.
    d. IgG.
    e. IgM.

19. Deficiencies in B-cell immune responses are suspected when unusual or recurrent, severe infections are caused by
    a. fungi.
    b. yeasts.
    c. encapsulated bacteria.
    d. Both a and b are correct.
    e. a, b and c are correct.

20. Di George syndrome is a primary immunodeficiency caused by
    a. failure of B-cells to mature.
    b. congenital lack of thymic tissue.
    c. failure of the formed elements of blood to develop.
    d. selective deficiency of IgG.
    e. selective deficiency of IgA.

21. Acquired or secondary immunodeficiencies
    a. develop after birth.
    b. may be caused by viral infections.
    c. may develop following immunosuppressive therapy.
    d. Both a and c are correct.
    e. a, b and c are correct.

22. Rejection of a kidney transplant occurred after two weeks. The reaction was because of
    a. immune response against recipient HLA antigen.
    b. immune response against donor HLA antigens.
    c. a type IV hypersensitivity.
    d. Both a and b are correct.
    e. Both b and c are correct.

23. Zinc and vitamin deficits can depress
    a. only B-cell function.
    b. only T-cell function.
    c. only complement activity.
    d. both B- and T-cell function.

24. A positive HIV antibody test signifies the
    a. individual is infected with HIV and likely so for life.
    b. asymptomatic individual will absolutely progress to AIDS.
    c. individual isn't viremic.
    d. sexually active individual was infected last weekend.

25. Which is incorrect regarding AIDS?
    a. The T_4/T_8 ratio will be less than 1:1.
    b. The patient will be anti-HIV.
    c. The patient will likely develop opportunistic infections and cancer.
    d. The patient will have increased numbers of CD4 cells or T-helper cells.

Stress and Disease

Prerequisite Objective

a. Identify the function of biochemicals that regulate cells in the nervous, endocrine, and immune systems. Review text pages 304-311; refer to Tables 9-2 and 9-3.

Remember!

- There is a relationship between the nervous, endocrine, and immune systems that involves common usage of molecules and receptors in each system. Central nervous system and autonomic nervous system neuropeptides affect immune cells. Endocrine products influence immune and neuro-immune cell function. The immune cell cytokinins affect both nervous and endocrine cell function.

- These intersystem effectors and their actions include the following:

  1. Corticotropin-releasing factor (CRF) is a hypothalamic hormone that stimulates secretion of adrenocorticotropic hormone (ACTH) by the anterior pituitary gland.
  2. Interleukin-1 (IL-1) and interleukin-6 (IL-6) are substances produced by macrophages that stimulate release of ACTH through CRF. These factors affect B- and T-cell proliferation and body temperature.
  3. ACTH controls the production and secretion of glucocorticoids by the cortex of the adrenal glands. ACTH is produced by the anterior pituitary and in small amounts by lymphocytes.
  4. Growth hormone (hGH) is secreted by the anterior pituitary and elevates blood glucose and promotes protein anabolism, tissue repair, and antibody production by plasma cells.
  5. Cortisone is secreted by the adrenal cortex and then circulates in the blood plasma. It elevates blood glucose and is anabolic for liver RNA and protein but catabolic for muscle and lymphoid tissue. It is immunosuppressive for immunoglobulins and reduces eosinophils, macrophages, and lymphocytes; it is generally anti-inflammatory.
  6. Interleukin-2 (IL-2) is produced by T-cells and potentiates B- and T-cell, monocyte, and natural killer cell activity, as well as increasing pituitary ACTH levels.
  7. Interferon (IFN) is produced by lymphocytes, macrophages, and fibroblasts. These proteins are antiviral; they enhance phagocytic activity, suppress neoplastic growth, and stimulate the hypothalamus, pituitary, and adrenal pathway.
  8. Tumor necrosis factor (TNF) is produced mostly by macrophages. It stimulates inflammatory and immune mediators.
  9. Substance P is found in sensory nerves, spinal cord pathways, and parts of the brain; it stimulates the perception of pain.

(Continued)

10. Endorphins are concentrated in the pituitary gland and inhibit pain by blocking release of substance P; they may inhibit CRF secretion.
11. Epinephrine and norepinephrine levels are controlled by sympathetic preganglionic neurons, which stimulate their secretion by the adrenal medulla. Both increase heart rate, blood pressure, and blood glucose. Epinephrine dilates skeletal muscle blood vessels. Lymphoid tissue is innervated and, therefore, influenced by these substances.
12. Histamine and serotonin are both vasoactive amines that participate in inflammation. Serotonin is found in the brain stem and in blood platelets. Histamine is found in basophils, mast cells, and platelets.

Objectives

After successful study of this chapter, the learner will be able to:

1. Define stress, identify stressors, and characterize the stress response.
   Study text pages 300 and 304.

Stress arises when a person interacts or transacts with situations in certain ways. People are not disturbed by situations as they exist but by the ways they individually appraise and react to situations. Stress is a condition in which a demand exceeds a person's coping abilities. Stress reactions may include disturbance of cognition, emotion, and behavior that can adversely affect their well-being. Stressors, such as infection, noise, decreased oxygen supply, pain, heat, cold, trauma, and radiation; prolonged exertional response to life events including anxiety, depression, anger, old age, fear, excitement, and obesity; and disease, drugs, surgery, and medical treatment can all elicit the stress response.

The **stress response** is initiated by the nervous and endocrine systems; specifically, the sympathetic autonomic nervous system, the hypothalamus, the pituitary gland, and the adrenal gland are involved. The activation of these systems redirects adaptive energy to the stressed body sites.

The sympathetic nervous system is aroused during the stress response and causes the medulla of the adrenal gland to release epinephrine, norepinephrine, and dopamine into the bloodstream. Preganglionic fibers from the splanchnic nerve terminate in the medulla where they innervate the cells that produce these hormones. Simultaneously, CRF stimulates the pituitary gland to release a variety of hormones including antidiuretic hormone, growth hormone, and adrenocorticotropin hormone. And, then, ACTH stimulates the cortex of the adrenal gland to release cortisol.

2. Describe Selye historic general adaptation syndrome; cite its stages.
   Study text page 300.

While attempting to discover a new sex hormone, Selye injected crude ovarian extracts into rats. Repeatedly, he found the following triad of structural changes: (1) enlargement of the cortex of the adrenal gland, (2) atrophy of the thymus gland and other lymphoid structures, and (3) development of bleeding ulcers of the stomach and duodenal lining. Selye discovered that this triad of manifestations was not specific for his ovarian extracts but also occurred after he exposed the rats to other noxious stimuli such as cold, surgical injury, and restraint. Selye concluded that this triad or syndrome of manifestations represented a nonspecific response to noxious stimuli. Because many diverse agents caused the same syndrome, Selye suggested that it be called the general adaptation syndrome.

Selye later defined three successive stages in the development of the GAS: (1) the alarm stage, (2) the stage of resistance or adaptation, and (3) the stage of exhaustion. The nonspecific physiologic response identified by Selye consists of interaction among the sympathetic branch of the autonomic nervous system and two glands, the pituitary gland and the adrenal gland. The alarm phase of the GAS begins when a stressor triggers the actions of the pituitary gland and the sympathetic nervous system. The resistance or adaptation phase begins with the actions of cortisol, norepinephrine, and epinephrine. Exhaustion occurs if stress continues and adaptation is not successful. The ultimate signs of exhaustion are impairment of the immune response, heart failure, and kidney failure leading to death.

3. Identify current concepts that modify Selye's work; define homeostasis and cite an example.

Study text page 301.

From the 1950s to the 1970s, studies showed that activation of the adrenal cortex occurred in humans in response to psychologic stressors. Several factors, including degrees of discomfort/unpleasantness or suddenness of the stress, may account for the presence or absence of the physiologic stress response. The triad of adrenal cortical enlargement, thymus and lymphoid shrinkage, and gastrointestinal ulceration may not be as nonspecific as Selye believed it to be. In experiments in which psychologic reactions were minimized, physical stressors did not appear to stimulate the pituitary or adrenal cortex in a nonspecific fashion.

Many physiologists resist Selye's concept of nonspecificity because it appears incompatible with the principles of physiologic homeostasis. Adaptive bodily responses are selective and are organized to counteract the specific bodily changes that elicit them. It is difficult, then, to explain how the body adapts to both cold and heat. Physiologically, the body adapts to cold by peripheral vasoconstriction and shivering and to heat by peripheral vasodilation and sweating while decreasing heat production. To support Selye's concept of nonspecificity, evidence is needed that increased adrenal cortical or medullary activity can promote adaptations to both cold and heat. In fact, no single hormone responds to all stressful stimuli in an absolutely nonspecific fashion.

Selye considered homeostasis the sum of the process by which the body maintains itself at a relatively constant composition. He expanded the definition to mean that the body's need determines body responses and that adaptive responses are necessary to maintain body stability. Research has since demonstrated that homeostasis does not mean "constant composition" but rather a dynamic steady state representing the net effect of all the turnover or synthesis and breakdown of all bodily substances.

Stressors cause a series of reactions that alter the dynamic steady state. This alteration may be either short- or long-term. For example, the normal concentration of glucose in the blood is about 80 mg/100 ml. The concentration of glucose rises with acute stress and then slowly returns to normal as stress subsides. If blood glucose remains high in the absence of a known stressor, it is diagnosed as a sign of disease, probably diabetes mellitus.

4. Summarize the major interactions of the nervous, endocrine, and immune systems in the stress response.

Refer to Figures 9-1 and 9-3.

CRF may be a primary mediator of many stress-induced alterations to immune functions because of its role as an initiator of biologic brain responses to stress. It activates the hypothalamic-pituitary-adrenal (HPA) axis and the autonomic nervous system (ANS). However, direct suppressive effects of CRF have also been reported on two immune cell types processing CRF receptors, namely the monocyte-macrophage and CD4 (T-helper) lymphocyte. The production of CRF is initiated by a high level of IL-1. Production of IL-1 by activated macrophages and monocytes is inhibited by circulating glucocorticoids. The stimulation of CRF production in the hypothalamus by IL-1 demonstrates immune-induced regulation of the CNS and the cytokines (TNF and IFN). The T-cell growth factor IL-2 can increase pituitary ACTH as well.

The following flow chart summarizes interaction of the three systems:

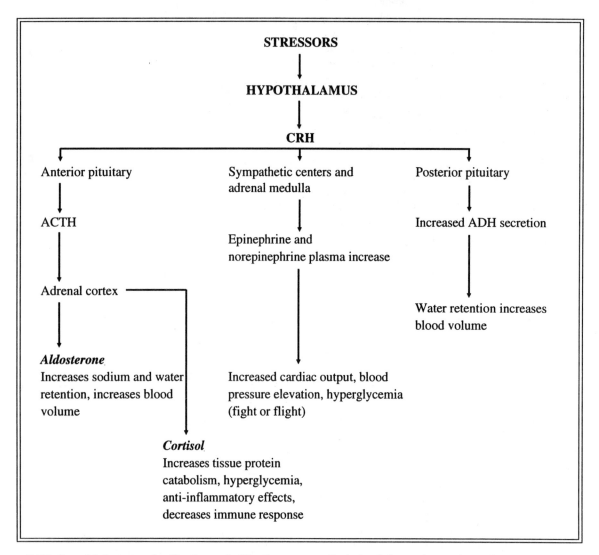

5. Distinguish between ineffective and effective coping for stress.

Study text pages 311-313; refer to Figure 9-4.

Stress is not an independent entity but a system of interdependent processes that are moderated by the nature, intensity, and duration of the stressor. The perception, appraisal, and coping efficacy of the affected individual mediate the psychologic and physiologic responses to stress. Coping is managing stressful demands that exceed the individual's resources.

Periods of depression and emotional upheaval with ineffective coping place the affected individual at risk for immunological deficits. Adverse life events that have the most negative effect on immunity have been characterized as those events that are uncontrollable, undesirable, and which overtax the individual's ability to cope. Those individuals unable to cope may develop immune dysfunction.

Factors that may influence stress susceptibility or resilience include age, socioeconomic status, gender, social support status, personality, self-esteem, genetics, life events, past experiences, and current health status.

Problem-focused and social support coping processes have a beneficial influence during stressful experiences. An individual experiencing distress may draw upon internal and external resources to meet the demands. Social support groups can improve psychologic coping and immune function by increasing natural killer cell activity.

6. Cite examples of stress-related diseases.
Refer to Table 9-4.

Stress-related Diseases

System	Disease or Condition
Cardiovascular	Coronary artery disease, hypertension, stroke, arrhythmia
Muscles	Tension headaches, backache
Connective tissues	Rheumatoid arthritis
Pulmonary	Asthma, hay fever
Immune	Immunosuppression, deficiency, autoimmunity
Gastrointestinal	Ulcer, irritable bowel syndrome, diarrhea, nausea and vomiting, ulcerative colitis
Integumentary	Eczema, neurodermatitis, acne
Endocrine	Diabetes mellitus, amenorrhea
Central nervous	Fatigue and lethargy, type A behavior, overeating, depression, insomnia

Note: The above is an abbreviated grouping of tissues and systems and some stress-related diseases.

Practice Examination

Match the term with its activity.

1. IL-1
2. IL-2
3. melatonin
4. IFN
5. endorphin

a. secreted by the anterior pituitary
b. stimulates the perception of pain
c. produced by macrophages, stimulates release of CRF
d. may augment the immune response
e. stimulates the HPA axis
f. release of CRF potentiates B- and T-cell activity
g. may inhibit CRF secretion
h. released from mast cells, vasoactive

6. Which is not a characteristic of Selye stress syndrome?
    a. adrenal atrophy
    b. shrinkage of the thymus
    c. bleeding gastrointestinal ulcers
    d. shrinkage of lymphatic organs

7. Which characterizes the alarm stage?
    a. increased lymphocytes
    b. increased sympathetic activity
    c. increased parasympathetic activity
    d. increased eosinophils

8. Glucocorticoids would be lowest during the stage of
    a. exhaustion.
    b. alarm.
    c. resistance.

9. Which is a correct sequence for Selye's hypothesis for stress?
    a. increased ACTH secretion, alarm
    b. increased ACTH in the blood, hypertrophy of the adrenal cortex
    c. stimulation of the sympathetic centers, alarm
    d. increased secretion of epinephrine, increased ACTH in the blood

10. Corticotropin-releasing hormone (CRH) is released by the
    a. adrenal medulla.
    b. adrenal cortex.
    c. anterior pituitary.
    d. hypothalamus.

11. Stress may be defined as any factor that
    a. stimulates the posterior pituitary.
    b. stimulates the anterior pituitary.
    c. stimulates the hypothalamus to release CRH.
    d. stimulates the hypothalamus to release ADH.

12. Which is not true?
    a. Stressors are always injurious, unpleasant, or painful stimuli.
    b. Stressors are extreme stimuli.
    c. The emotions of fear, anxiety, and grief can act as stressors.
    d. Stressors differ in different individuals and in one individual at different times.

13. What determines which stimuli are stressors for an individual?
    a. heredity
    b. past experience
    c. diet
    d. All of the above are correct.

14. Which is not true?
    a. Generally, psychological stress is independent of the physiological stress.
    b. Physiological stress is usually accompanied by some degree of psychological stress.
    c. Identical psychological stressors do not induce identical physiological responses.
    d. For any one individual, adaptive responses are selective and counteract specific body changes.

15. The production of cortisol in response to stress can be initiated by
    a. hypothalamus, anterior pituitary, adrenal cortex.
    b. hypothalamus, posterior pituitary, adrenal cortex.
    c. hypothalamus, sympathetic nerve fibers, adrenal cortex.
    d. hypothalamus, sympathetic nerve fibers, adrenal medulla.

16. Cortisol
    a. increases protein catabolism.
    b. decreases blood sugar.
    c. increases immune response.
    d. increases allergic reactions.

17. Which would not occur in response to stress?
    a. increased systolic blood pressure
    b. increased epinephrine
    c. constriction of the pupils
    d. increased adrenocorticoids

18. Which of the following would not be useful to assess stress?
    a. total blood cholesterol
    b. eosinophil count
    c. lymphocyte count
    d. adrenocorticoid levels

19. In response to stress, the adrenal cortex secretes
    a. norepinephrine.
    b. norepinephrine and cortisol.
    c. cortisol and aldosterone.
    d. norepinephrine and aldosterone.

20. Severe stress results in all except
    a. an overactive immune system.
    b. increased heart rate.
    c. a rise in epinephrine levels.
    d. changes in breathing patterns.

Match the term with its definition.

21. corticoids
22. stressors
23. stress response
24. exhaustion stage
25. alarm stage

a. sympathetic activity returns to normal
b. glucocorticoids return to normal
c. secreted by adrenal cortex in response to stress
d. Selye's changes seen in stress
e. stimulates the release of CRH
f. high resistance to stressor
g. bodily changes initiated by stress

Tumor Biology

Prerequisite Objectives

a. Describe the phases of cellular mitosis and cytokinesis.
    Review text pages 34-36; refer to Figure 1-26.

Remember!

- The reproduction or division of somatic cells involves two sequential phases: mitosis, or nuclear, division and cytokinesis, or cytoplasmic, division. These phases occur in close succession with cytokinesis beginning toward the end of mitosis. Before a cell can divide, it must double its mass and duplicate all of its contents. Most of the preparation for division occurs during the growth phase or interphase. The alternation between mitosis and interphase in all tissues having cellular turnover is known as cell cycle.

- There are four designated phases of the cell cycle. They are: (1) the S phase (synthesis), in which DNA is synthesized in the cell nucleus; (2) the G_2 phase, in which RNA and protein synthesis occurs; (3) the M phase (mitosis), which includes both nuclear and cytoplasmic division; and (4) the G_1 phase, which is the period between the M phase and the start of DNA synthesis. Interphase, consisting of the G_1, S, and G_2 phases, is the longest phase of the cell cycle.

- The M phase of the cell cycle, mitosis and cytokinesis, begins with prophase or the first appearance of chromosomes. Each chromosome has two identical halves called chromatids which lie side by side and are attached together at a site called a centromere. The nuclear membrane disappears in this phase. Spindle fibers are microtubules formed in the cytoplasm that radiate from two centrioles located at opposite poles of the cell.

- During metaphase, the next phase of mitosis and cytokinesis, the spindle fibers pull the centromeres till they are aligned in the middle of the spindle or at the equatorial plate.

- Anaphase begins when the centromeres separate and the genetically identical chromatids are pulled apart. The chromatids are pulled, centromeres first, toward opposite sides of the cell. When the identical chromatids are separated, each is considered to be a chromosome. Thus, the cell has 92 chromosomes during this stage. By the end of anaphase, there are 46 chromosomes at each side of the identical cell. Each of the two groups of 46 chromosomes should be identical to the original 46 chromosomes present at the start of the cell cycle.

(Continued)

Remember! *(cont'd)*

- During telophase, a new nuclear membrane is formed around each group of 46 chromosomes, the spindle fibers disappear, and the chromosomes begin to uncoil. Cytokinesis causes the cytoplasm to divide into roughly equal parts during this phase. At the end of telophase, two identical diploid cells, called daughter cells, have been formed from the original cell.

- The difference between slowly and rapidly dividing cells is the length of time spent in the G_1 phase of the cell cycle. Some cells that divide very slowly can remain in the G_1 phase for years. Once the S phase begins, progression through mitosis requires a relatively constant amount of time. Once a cell has progressed out of the G_1 phase, it must complete the S, G_2, and M phases.

b. Identify mechanisms that control cell division.
   Review text pages 35-36; refer to Table 1-4.

Remember!

- Protein growth factors govern the proliferation of different cell types in conjunction with genes involved in the social control or relationship of cells within tissues. It is likely that some genes code for growth factors, some for growth factor receptors, some for intracellular regulatory proteins involved in cell adhesion, and some for proteins that help relay signals for cell division to the cell nucleus.

- Cells require highly specific proteins to stimulate cell division. These growth factors are present in the serum in very low concentrations. For example, platelet-derived growth factor stimulates the production of connective tissue cells. Another important growth factor is interleukin, which stimulates proliferation of T-cells. Cells responding to a particular growth factor have specific receptors for the specific growth factor in their plasma membrane. Some growth factors are also regulators of cellular differentiation.

Objectives

After successful study of this chapter, the learner will be able to:

1. Define neoplasia or cancer.
Study text pages 322-323; refer to Figures 10-1 through 10-3.

Cancerous cells are defined by two heritable properties, autonomy and anaplasia. **Autonomy** is the cancer cell's independence from normal cellular controls. **Anaplasia** is the loss of differentiation or specialization. The cancer cell has lost its ability to function normally and to control its growth and division.

Transformation is the process by which a normal cell becomes a cancer cell. Genes known as proto-oncogenes that were normally turned off during levels of differentiation can be mutated, transformed, or reactivated by carcinogenic agents to become **neoplastic** cells.

Cancer is considered a disorder of growth and differentiation because neoplasms resemble undifferentiated tissue. The less the tumor resembles normal tissue, the more undifferentiated or anaplastic the tumor becomes. As malignant cells grow and divide, they lose their mature characteristics and no longer resemble their tissue of origin.

2. Contrast the properties of benign and malignant tumors.
Refer to Table 10-1.

Properties of Benign/Malignant Tumors

Characteristic	Benign	Malignant
Differentiation	yes	no
Mitotic figures	normal	abnormal
Hormone secretion	yes	no
Growth rate	slow	rapid
Growth mode	expansive	infiltrative
Capsulation	yes	no
Cellular cohesiveness	yes	no
Ulceration/bleeding	no	yes
Surgical effectiveness	yes	no
Metastasis	no	yes
Fatality	usually not	yes, if not treated

3. Cite the method for naming and classifying tumors; provide examples.

Refer to Table 10-2.

Common Benign and Malignant Tumors

Tissue	Benign Tumor	Malignant Tumor
Connective Tissue		
Adult fibrous	Fibroma	Fibrosarcoma
Cartilage	Chondroma	Chondrosarcoma
Bone	Osteoma	Osteosarcoma
Fat	Lipoma	Liposarcoma
Muscle		
Smooth muscle	Leiomyoma	Leiomyosarcoma
Striated muscle	Rhabdomyoma	Rhabdomyosarcoma
Blood Tissue		
Lymph vessels	Lymphangioma	Lymphangiosarcoma
Blood vessels	Hemangioma	Hemangiosarcoma
Lymphoid tissue	Infectious mononucleosis	Lymphosarcoma (Lymphoma)
Bone Marrow	Infectious mononucleosis	Leukemia
Neural Tissue		
Nerve sheath	Neurilemmoma	Neurogenic sarcoma
Glial tissue	Gliosis	Glioma
Epithelium		
Squamous epithelium	Papilloma	Squamous carcinoma
Glandular epithelium	Adenoma	Adenocarcinoma

Tumors are named according to the tissue of origin with the suffix "oma." If the suffix "oma" has no modifiers like "blast" or "multiple", it is likely benign. Malignant neoplasms having an epithelial tissue origin are identified as carcinomas while those with a connective tissue origin are sarcomas.

4. Identify some cellular changes that occur in cancerous cells and their functional significance.

   Study text pages 327-334; refer to Figures 10-4, 10-5, and 10-11 and Tables 10-4 and 10-5.

Cancerous Cell Changes and Their Significance

Change	Significance
Surface loss or alteration of glycoprotein or glycolipid	Receptor alterations change response to growth factors
Reduced fibronectin	Changes cellular organization, decreases adhesion, increases migration
Altered membranes	Increases metabolite transport
Increased plasminogen activator	Increased extracellular proteolysis
Disorganized actin filaments	Cells maintain "rounded-up" nature which is characteristic of mitotic cells
Less anchoring junctions	Encourages proliferation of transformed cells, cells metastasize and grow in new environment
Increased gap junctions	Decreases intercellular communication, causes loss of density-dependent inhibition of growth

5. Postulate a multistep model for the causes of neoplasia or cancer.

   Study text pages 335-345.

Causes of Neoplasia

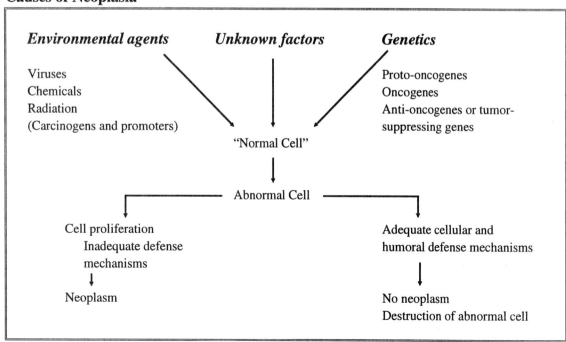

61

Why does a normal cell lose control and become abnormal? There likely are several reasons. First, there are environmental agents — substances in the air we breathe, the water we drink, and the food we eat. A chemical or other environmental agent that produces cancer is called a carcinogen. Examples of carcinogens are cigarette tar, radon gas from the earth, and ultraviolet (UV) radiation in sunlight.

Viruses are another cause of cancer. These tiny packages of nucleic acids, either DNA or RNA, are capable of infecting cells and converting them to transformed cells. Oncogenes are genes that have the ability to transform a normal cell into a cancerous cell when they are inappropriately activated by viruses. Oncogenes develop from normal genes that regulate growth and development. These genes may undergo some change that either causes them to produce an abnormal product or disrupts their control so that they are expressed inappropriately.

Some cancers are not caused by oncogenes but rather by genes called anti-oncogenes or tumor-suppressing genes that have mutated. These genes may produce proteins that normally oppose the action of an oncogene or inhibit cell division.

The multistep process of cancer seems to involve the loss of the cell's ability to terminally differentiate, control growth, travel to distant tissues, and invade and colonize these tissues. Tumors appear to be derived from a single stem cell. In most tumors studied, all the tumor cells have been found to have the same x-chromosome inactivated. This strongly suggests that the tumor cells originated from a single aberrant cell. Tumor development requires several independent accidents to occur together in one cell. If a single mutation were responsible, the chance of developing cancer in any given year would be independent of age. However, the cancerous change increases at a rapid rate with age, so a multistep process is likely.

In most cancers, the cells of the initial mutant clone undergo further mutation that enables them to divide more rapidly before they differentiate. This further supports the model that cancers develop in stages. Because of rapid division, the cancer cells begin to outnumber the normal cells, as well as those having the primary mutation.

6. Describe the initiation-promotion-progression theory of carcinogenesis.
Study text page 345; refer to Figure 10-12 and Table 10-9.

Initiation is an irreversible cellular step requiring exposure to a carcinogen. The affected cell has its DNA irreversibly altered or mutated. However, the initiated cell may not be considered cancerous until a promoting agent acts on that cell to produce an altered cell. **Promotion** accelerates the process by which the initiated cells become cancerous. Initiation and promotion mechanisms have not been experimentally shown for all cancers. However, the process can be applied to chemical agents found in coal tar or cigarette smoke, ionizing and nonionizing radiation, viruses, and hormones.

Initiators cause interruptions in the DNA chain, errors in DNA repair, or an elimination of a base pair or sugar. Promoters may affect cell proliferation by altering cell-to-cell communication, by the production of oxygen radicals, or by interfering with the process of differentiation, usually after division has occurred.

7. Characterize common carcinogens as chemical, physical, or viral.
Study text pages 335-337 and 345-352.

Chemical carcinogens can be grouped as polycyclic aromatic hydrocarbons, aromatic amines, alkylating agents, nitrosamines and other nitrosocompounds, naturally occurring products, drugs, metals, and industrial carcinogens.

Polycyclic aromatic hydrocarbons are present in the condensates of tobacco smoke, automobile exhaust, and other products of combustion. Cancers of the lips, tongue, oral cavity, head, neck, larynx, lungs, and bladder are associated with exposure to polycyclic aromatic hydrocarbons.

Aromatic amines are found in certain foods, coal tars, moth repellents, and insecticides. The aromatic amines have been linked with cancer of the bladder.

Alkylating agents under controlled circumstances are used for therapeutic purposes but can be carcinogenic. Nitrogen mustard and mustard gas are implicated in the causation of leukemia and lymphoid neoplasms.

Nitrosamines and other nitrosocompounds develop from chemical interactions between nitrites and other secondary amines. Numerous drugs and nicotine may supply the amines for the process of converting nitrites to nitrosamine. Nitrites are present in foods as additives. These agents may be contributors to gastric carcinomas.

Aflatoxin, a mold, is found on corn, barley, peas, rice, soybeans, fruit, and some nuts and in milk and cheddar cheese. It has been linked to liver cancer in humans.

Heavy consumption of alcohol is associated with cancer of the mouth, pharynx, esophagus, larynx, and liver. Alcohol apparently enhances the effects of procarcinogens and carcinogens such as nicotine by increasing their solubility, altering liver metabolism, altering the intracellular metabolism of epithelial cells, and causing nutritional deficiencies.

Asbestos, cadmium, chromium, and nickel are some of the metals involved in carcinogenesis. All are associated with cancer of the lung. Asbestos fibers are associated with bronchogenic and gastro-intestinal carcinomas in humans continuously exposed to the substance. The fibers function as promoters for other carcinogens such as cigarette smoke. Chronic injury of the mucosa of the lips and gums from dentures or pipe smoking leads to increased occurrence of oral cancer.

Ionizing radiation is a **physical carcinogen** that causes cellular mutations. Damage to DNA may be direct or indirect. Direct damage results from inter-action of the electron itself with the DNA of the cell. Indirect damage occurs when a secondary elec-tron interacts with a water molecule, giving rise to a free radical, which then damages DNA. Evidence links leukemia to exposure to large doses of irradia-tion. Even low doses of irradiation may cause can-cer in susceptible individuals. The frequency of breast cancer increases with small, widely spread doses of irradiation. Thyroid cancer increases with head and neck radiograms during childhood. Radio-grams of the fetus in utero increase chances of de-veloping childhood cancer. Ultraviolet radiation from the sun is a major cause of skin cancer.

Viruses implicated in human cancers are called oncogenic viruses. Viruses alter the genome of the infected cell which then alters the progeny of the host cell. Oncogenic viruses are either deoxyribonu-cleic acid (DNA) or ribonucleic acid (RNA). The DNA viruses are incorporated into the genes of the host and are then transmitted to subsequent genera-tions. The DNA viruses are implicated in cancers of the cervix and liver and some lymphomas. The RNA viruses involve a synthesis of DNA from an RNA template using an enzyme called reverse tran-scriptase. In this mechanism, genes are expanded and new DNA sequences are developed without the parent structures being altered. As part of the genome of the host cell, the virus is not attacked and destroyed by the immune system. Reverse tran-scriptase acts to accomplish reverse transcription, to degrade RNA in the new DNA-RNA complex, and to form the new DNA double strand. The RNA viruses are implicated in the development of cer-tain types of leukemia and breast cancer.

8. Describe the tumor immune surveillance theory as a defense against neoplasia; ident-ify tumor antigens.

Study text pages 353-357; refer to Figure 10-15.

Cell-mediated cytotoxicity by immunologic cells such as lymphocytes has evolved as a protec-tion against "foreign" structures found on emerg-ing cancer cells. The identification of tumor anti-gens, the increased risk of some cancers in immune-suppressed individuals, the identification of tumor reactive antibodies in some individuals with cancer, and the demonstration of tumor-specific T-cell-mediated cellular immunity — all confirm immune surveillance for neoplastic cells.

Human cancer cells express numerous "foreign" molecules on their surfaces that can be recognized by the immune system as **tumor-specific antigens (TSAs)**. Because cancer is a disease of unregulated cell growth and differentiation, the differences be-tween the molecules expressed on the surfaces of normal and cancer cells may be minor. Thus, the recognition of a molecule as a TSA does not al-ways mean the cell is neoplastic. Serologically de-fined human TSAs include viral antigens, oncofetal antigens, oncogene products, and "mutant" pro-teins and carbohydrates. The **viral antigens** are products expressed by virally transformed cells. Viral antigens are common to all tumors induced by the same virus.

The **oncofetal antigens** are expressed by cells during certain stages of embryonic development but are absent or expressed at very low concentra-tions by normal adult cells. **Alphafetoprotein** (a-FP) and **carcinoembryonic** antigens are com-mon examples of these antigens. Individuals with hepatic, pancreatic, and malignant tumors of epi-thelial cells have high levels of a-FP in their serum. The carcinoembryonic antigen (CEA) is a glycopro-tein that is part of the family of immunoglobulin-re-lated proteins. Seventy percent of colon, 90 percent of pancreas, and 35 percent of breast cancer pa-tients have detectable CEA antibody titers. Because a-FP and CEA antigens are found in large numbers of normal individuals, their use as sole diagnostic markers for cancer screening is not always reliable. Other oncofetal-like antigens include pregnancy-specific human chorionic gonadotropin (HCG), pla-cental lactogen, and haptoglobin-related protein (Hrp). These antigens are expressed by women dur-ing pregnancy and in breast cancers.

Malignancies of hematopoietic tissues express a unique form of oncofetal, or differentiation, anti-gens. The common acute lymphoblastic leukemia-associated antigen referred to as CALLA is a valu-able marker of non-B, non-T acute lymphoblastic leukemia (ALL).

A large number of **oncogene-encoded antigens** are associated with individual tumors; a complex activation of certain oncogenes is required for trans-formation of normal cells. A number of oncogene-encoded antigens are expressed by lung cancers and are associated with cellular growth and differ-entiation. For example, the protein *mcy* binds DNA and regulates transcription. *neu*, another oncogene protein, is likely a growth factor receptor.

Carbohydrate TSAs are transiently expressed in normal tissues during development and re-expressed by neoplasia. These antigens result from blocked synthesis of particular carbohydrate chains, increased synthesis of carbohydrate struc-tures that are absent in normal cells, and changes in membrane organization. These types of antigens are expressed by melanomas and other neuroectodermal cancers.

The major histocompatibility class II antigen, HLA-DR, is not usually expressed by normal epithelial cells. However, HLA-DR as a protein TSA is expressed to varying degrees by melanomas, gastric carcinomas, larynx carcinomas, lung carcinomas, colorectal carcinomas, and breast carcinomas. An example of an enzyme is prostate-specific antigen (PSA) found in prostate tumors. There is a correlation between PSA serum levels and tumor recurrence in individuals undergoing cancer therapy. Recently, a new group of **TSA proteins** has been identified. These are the stress-induced or heat shock proteins. Many of the nonviral TSAs expressed by human cancers are related to proteins. These proteins may bind steroid receptors, immunoglobulin heavy chains, actin, oncogene proteins, and fatty acids.

When a tumor expresses cell surface TSA, the immune system of an immunologically competent host can reject the tumor. B-lymphocytes defend against cancer through the production of TSA-reactive antibodies. Antibodies play a minor role in protecting the individual against tumor emergence and growth. They can prevent cancer growth by activating complement, and thus killing tumor cells, or killing tumors by a mechanism called antibody-dependent cell-mediated cytotoxicity (ADCC).

Lymphoid cells, such as monocytes, neutrophil, B-cells, and killer cells that are capable of killing tumor cells gain the ability to recognize TSA by binding antibodies to their cell surfaces. Once bound to the tumor, ADCC cells deliver a tumor-killing signal for cell lysis of tumor cells. Immune T-lymphocytes release macrophage-activity factors that stimulate macrophages to kill tumor cells. Once activated, macrophages kill tumor cells in a localized, antigen-specific fashion. Activated T-cells cause tumor rejection by secreting lymphokines that directly lyse tumor cells, inhibit the growth of transformed cells, or stimulate noncommitted cells to join in an antitumor response.

9. Indicate the limitations of immune surveillance as a defense against neoplasia.

Study text pages 357-360; refer to Figure 10-16.

Host immunologic potential and the characteristics of growing cancer cells constantly change. Therefore, many cancers can bypass the host's immune surveillance system and escape destruction. Tumors escape immunologic rejection by (1) antigenic modulation; (2) secretion of immunosuppressive substances; (3) escape and sneaking through; (4) blocking factor; (5) immunostimulation; and (6) TSA-reactive suppressor T-lymphocytes.

Cancer cells can alter their expression of TSA. A number of agents such as cyclic-AMP, interferons, interleukins, growth factors, and tumor promoters can modulate tumor antigens. Some cancer cells can also mask surface antigens with a hyaluronic acid-rich glycosaminoglycan coat. These modulated and masked TSAs can't be recognized by the antibodies or cells that cause antitumor immune responses.

Some tumors secrete soluble **immunosuppressive substances** like prostaglandins which block lymphocyte proliferation and clonal expansion of TSA-reactive T-lymphocytes. The overall immune response to the tumor is thus weakened.

Tumors arise from a single transformed cell. As cancer cells actively divide and increase the tumor mass, there are changes in the original transformed cell. As a tumor grows, the cells within it become a heterogenous mixture of subclones. This is especially true if daughter cells lose or modify their TSA. Such a process can facilitate escape from earlier host defense mechanisms.

Since tumors originate from a single transformed cell, it is possible that some or small amounts of TSA are not immunogenic. As a tumor develops enough mass so that antigen is present in sufficient amounts to stimulate an immune response, it may have too many rapidly growing cells for elimination by the immune system.

Tumor rejection may be inhibited by the presence of **blocking antibodies** that bind TSA but do not activate complement function in ADCC responses. These antibodies might also form antigen-antibody complexes that cannot be processed by antigen-presenting cells or inhibit T-cell interaction with the tumor.

Progressively growing tumors increase the population of **suppressor T-lymphocytes**. T_s cells block other types of immune response, switch off ongoing immune responses, or modify the magnitude or type of immune response. Because most cell surface molecules or antigens present on tumor cells are also present on normal cells, the immune system may be unable to determine if a rapidly dividing cell is detrimental or beneficial. T-cell suppression activity that avoids destruction of normal cells is likely increased in the tumor response. Thus, the immune response is slowed.

In conclusion, transformation processes may select for cancer cells that escape the host's tumor surveillance system. It is likely that many carcinogenic agents cause immune suppression; this makes individuals more susceptible to the growth of neoplasia or cancers.

Practice Examination

Match the term with its definition.

1. neoplasia
2. anaplasia
3. transformation

a. variation in size, shape, arrangement of cells
b. differentiation of dividing cells into cellular types not ordinarily found in a given area
c. abnormal, proliferating cells possessing a higher degree of autonomy
d. increase in absolute number of cells
e. lack of cellular differentiation or specialization, primitive cells
f. normal cell becomes cancerous

4. Which characterizes benign tumors?
   a. poorly differentiated
   b. metastasis
   c. capsulation
   d. poor cellular cohesiveness
   e. embryonic nature

5. Which is false regarding neoplasms?
   a. Benign neoplasms develop capsules.
   b. Benign neoplasms cause complications by local obstruction or expansion.
   c. Malignant neoplasms more often secrete hormones than benign tumors.
   d. Malignant neoplasms lack cellular differentiation.

6. The group of individuals most susceptible to cancer often
   a. are immunodeficient.
   b. are anemic.
   c. have hypercalcemia.
   d. have chronic joint disturbance.
   e. have neurologic dysfunction.

7. Metastasis is
   a. an alteration in normal cellular growth.
   b. growth of benign or malignant neoplastic cells.
   c. mutational.
   d. the ability to establish a secondary neoplasm at a new site.

8. An adenoma is
   a. benign.
   b. a glandular epithelial neoplasm.
   c. a teratoma.
   d. a malignant epithelial tumor.
   e. Both a and b are correct.

Match the cellular change with its functional significance.

9. fewer anchoring junctions
10. reduced fibronectin
11. loss of surface glycolipid
12. increased gap junctions

a. increased metabolite transport
b. proliferation of transformed cell encouraged
c. altered response to growth factors
d. loss of density-dependent inhibition of growth
e. "rounded-up" cells
f. increased migration, decreased adhesion
g. increased extracellular proteolysis

13. Which are carcinogens or promoters?
    a. viruses
    b. chemicals
    c. radiation
    d. Both b and c are correct.
    e. a, b, and c are correct.

14. Anti-oncogenes are
    a. genes having the ability to transform a normal cell into a cancerous cell.
    b. normal genes that regulate growth and development.
    c. genes that produce proteins that inhibit cellular division.
    d. Both b and c are correct.

15. In a theory of carcinogenesis, promotion
    a. precedes initiation.
    b. accelerates the process by which initiated cells become cancerous.
    c. interrupts DNA chain sequence.
    d. may alter cell-to-cell communication.
    e. Both b and d are correct.

16. The polycyclic aromatic hydrocarbon carcinogens include
    a. insecticides.
    b. tobacco smoke condensates.
    c. nitrates, food additives.
    d. aflatoxin.
    e. All of the above are correct.

17. Oncogenic viruses are
    a. DNA viruses.
    b. RNA viruses.
    c. capable of incorporation into host genes.
    d. capable of establishing new DNA sequences.
    e. All of the above are correct.

18. Ionizing radiation
    a. injures the DNA of a cell as DNA interacts with an electron.
    b. causes cellular mutations.
    c. damages DNA because of interaction of DNA with a free radical.
    d. Both a and b are correct.
    e. a, b, and c are correct.

19. Which serum TSA is an example of an oncofetal antigen?
    a. carcinoembryonic antigen
    b. prostate-specific antigen
    c. HLA-DR antigen
    d. Both a and b are correct.
    e. None of the above is correct.

20. The postulate in the immune surveillance theory is
    a. cancerous cells do not express "nonself" antigens.
    b. neoplastic "nonself" antigens are tolerated.
    c. TSAs are very similar to those of normal cells.
    d. neoplastic cells express antigens recognized as "nonself" which are then rejected.
    e. Both b and c are correct.

21. Neoplasms may "escape" immunological rejection by
    a. producing blocking antibodies.
    b. stimulating suppressor cells.
    c. secreting immunosuppressive substances.
    d. Both a and c are correct.
    e. a, b, and c are correct.

Match the cancer with the carcinogen.

22. liver cancer
23. uterine cervical cancer
24. lung cancer
25. melanoma

a. asbestos
b. estrogen
c. aflatoxin
d. human papillomavirus
e. ionizing radiation

Tumor Metastasis in Adults and Cancer in Children

Prerequisite Objective

a. Describe mechanisms that confine cells and tissues to a specific anatomical site.
Review text pages 36-37; refer to Figure 1-27.

Remember!

- All cells are within a network of extracellular macromolecules known as the extracellular matrix. The extracellular matrix holds cells and tissues together and provides an organized framework in which cells can interact with each other.

- To confine themselves and form tissues, cells must have intercellular recognition and adhesion. Specialized cells likely form a tissue in one of two ways. The first way is mitosis of one or more founder cells. Founder cells, basic precursor cells, are prevented from "wandering away" by macromolecules in the extracellular matrix and by adherence to one another at specialized junctions on their plasma membranes. The second way specialized cells form tissues involves their migration to and subsequent accumulation at the site of tissue formation. Migrant cells are thought to arrive at the specific site of tissue formation through chemotaxis or contact guidance. Cells at the migrant cells' destination secrete a chemical known as chemotactic factor that attracts specific migrant cells. Contact guidance is movement along a pathway or "pavement" within the extracellular matrix. In order to stay together in groups, cells must recognize each other and remain distinct from the cells of surrounding tissues.

- Cells in direct physical contact with neighboring cells are often linked together at specialized regions of their plasma membranes. These regions are known as cell junctions. Cell junctions hold cells together and allow small molecules to pass from cell to cell. This coordinates the activities of cells that form tissues. There are three main types of cell junctions: (1) desmosomes, (2) tight junctions, and (3) gap junctions. Desmosomes hold cells together by forming either continuous bands of epithelial sheets or buttonlike points of contact. Desmosomes also provide a system of braces to maintain structural stability. Tight junctions act as a barrier to diffusion, prevent movement of substances through transport proteins of the plasma membrane, and prevent the leakage of small molecules between the plasma membranes of adjacent cells. Gap junctions are clusters of protein channels that allow small ions and molecules to pass directly from the inside of one cell to the inside of another. Cells connected by gap junctions are considered ionically and metabolically joined. Gap junctions coordinate the activities of adjacent cells. For example, these junctions synchronize contractions of heart muscle cells through ionic coupling. The junctions permit action potentials to spread rapidly from cell to cell in neural tissues.

Objectives

After successful study of this chapter, the learner will be able to:

1. Describe prerequisites for metastasis to occur.

Study text pages 367-368; refer to Figure 11-1.

Invasion or local spread is a prerequisite for metastasis and is the first step in the metastatic process. In early stages, local invasion may occur by direct tumor extension. Eventually, cells or clumps of cells become detached from the primary tumor and invade the surrounding interstitial spaces. Possible important factors in local invasion include (1) cellular multiplication, (2) mechanical pressure, (3) release of lytic enzymes, (4) decreased cell-to-cell adhesion, and (5) increased motility of individual tumor cells. These mechanisms are not mutually exclusive, and it is likely that in a given neoplasm any combination of the five may be involved. The rate of cellular multiplication depends on the cell generation time, the number of cells that are dividing, and the cell loss from the tumor. Malignant cells can divide rapidly, but the tumor may not grow because cells are rapidly dying. Mechanical pressure generates pressure that forces cellular sheets or fingerlike projections along the lines of least mechanical resistance; spread is enhanced. Growing mass blocks local blood vessels and leads to local tissue death. This reduces mechanical resistance and further aids the spread. Many tumors have higher levels of protease and collagenases, plasminogen activators, and lysosomal enzymes than corresponding normal tissue. These lytic enzymes destroy normal tissue which increases tumor invasion.

Cancer cells do not adhere to one another as well as normal cells. This trait has partially been attributed to fibronectin. Cancer cells may either make a defective type of fibronectin or break down fibronectin as they make it. Low levels or loss of this anchoring molecule may help cancer cells "slip" between normal cells and allow more invasion. Cell movement is essential for tumor cells to invade and travel. The neoplastic cell must detach and infiltrate into adjacent tissue, migrate through the vascular wall into the circulation, and then migrate out of the vascular wall into a secondary site. Tumor cells may actually move by means of their own chemotactic factors known as "autocrine motility factors." If these mechanisms are valid, the tumor cell would secrete a factor that binds to a specific receptor on the cell surface to stimulate motility. Thus, the neoplastic cell acquires independent and continuous stimulation for its motile and invasive behavior.

2. Describe the proposed sequence of events during tumor cell invasion of extracellular matrix.

Study text pages 368-370; refer to Figure 11-2.

Once the tumor cell is in the blood circulation, a three-step theory likely describes the events during tumor cell invasion of the extracellular matrix. These steps involve tumor cell attachment to the basement membrane of vascular matrix, degradation or dissolution of the matrix, and locomotion or movement into the interstitial matrix. **Laminin** is a complex glycoprotein and a major constituent of all basement membranes. Since membrane vesicles of tumor cells are rich in **laminin receptors**, the first step is complete when binding occurs between the vascular basement membrane laminin and its receptors. Once anchored, the tumor either secretes **collagenase** or induces host cells to produce proteolytic enzymes. Degradation of the matrix constitutes the second step. Such enzymes may degrade both the attachment proteins and the structural collagenous proteins of the vascular basement membrane matrix. The third step is tumor cell locomotion. Fingerlike projections, called pseudopodia, extend from the tumor cell and attach to blood vessel walls. Thus, the tumor cells leave the vasculature and enter the interstitial stroma. The direction of locomotion to a distant site is likely influenced by chemotactic factors.

3. Describe the avenues for metastatic spread.

Study text pages 370-371.

Three routes for metastasis exist: direct or continuous extension, lymphatic spread, and bloodstream dissemination. These routes are not mutually exclusive. Tumor dissemination through one route often facilitates metastasis through others because tumor cells move through numerous microscopic anatomic connections. Direct tumor extension is thought to be initiated by a complex sequence of events. These events, noted in Objective 1, are initiated by loss of intracellular adhesion enabling cells to "slip" past one another. Movement of cells through tissue barriers is further influenced by protease and autocrine motility factors.

The process of metastasis involves invasion and penetration of tumor cells into blood vessels as described in Objective 2 or via lymphatics or both. The most common route for distant metastases is through the lymphatics. Tumors generally lack a well-formed lymphatic network; rather, lymphatic channels occur at the periphery of the tumor and not within the tumor mass. Tumor cells entering the lymphatic vessels from interstitial sites are carried to regional lymph nodes. Initially, regional lymph nodes may prevent the further spread of tumor cells into the lymphatic. A cancer cell that becomes lodged in lymph nodes may die as a result of local inflammatory reaction or because of an incompatible local environment, grow into a discernable lump, remain dormant for unknown reasons, or detach and enter the efferent lymphatics.

If tumor cell emboli are released into efferent lymphatic vessels, lymphatic metastasis occurs. The shedding of emboli may be caused by changes in vessel pressure, by turbulent alterations in lymphatic flow, or by manipulation of the tumor during diagnostic tests or surgery. Tumor cells eventually move into the venous drainage because of numerous veno-lymphatic communications.

Hematogenous spread requires tumor cells to penetrate and detach from blood vessels and spread to distant organs. To establish a metastatic site, tumor cells must "escape" host defenses, survive mechanical trauma in the bloodstream, and lodge in the vascular bed of the target organ. Tumor cells circulate and attach directly to the endothelial surface of the basement membrane as indicated earlier. The formation of a leukocyte-fibrin-platelet complex around tumor cells is thought to protect tumor cells within these complexes from host defenses and to assist successful attachment to the vascular epithelium. After invading the vascular wall, these neoplastic cells leave the vascular bed and enter the interstitial stroma preparatory to invading the parenchyma of the target organ.

4. Describe angiogenesis; identify factors that may determine metastatic sites.
Study text pages 371-372; refer to Table 11-2.

Tumors likely cannot grow more than a few millimeters in diameter without developing new blood vessels. This new vascular network development is called **angiogenesis**. Development of blood vessels is the result of diffusible substances secreted by the tumor. These secreted substances are known as **tumor-angiogenesis factors** (TAF). Heparin-binding endothelial mitogen and angiogenin may be factors that induce and regulate the growth of new blood vessels in neoplasms.

The ability of metastatic cells to grow and develop requires not only the development of a vascular network but evasion of host defenses and a compatible new environment. The metastatic potential of many common carcinomas is related to the size of the primary tumor. Larger tumors may overwhelm host defenses thus favoring survival of disseminated malignant cells.

Distant metastatic sites may or may not be the first capillary bed encountered by the circulating cells. Several mechanisms have been proposed to explain preferential growth in specific organs. This feature is collectively called "organ tropism." These mechanisms include local growth factors or hormones present in the target organ, preferential adherence by tumor receptors to the surface of certain target organs, and the presence of chemotactic factors diffusing from the target organ, causing circulating tumor cells to extravasate from the vessels and accumulate in the target organ. Evidence exists that organ tropism is genetically determined.

5. Describe the clinical manifestations of cancer.
Study text pages 372-374.

Usually little or no **pain** is associated with the early stages of malignant disease, but pain will affect 60 to 80 percent of individuals terminally ill with cancer. The pain may or may not be directly related to the malignancy but might be the result of inflammation and infection. A very common cause of pain is bone metastasis caused by periosteal irritation, medullary pressure, or pathologic fractures. Abdominal pain is often caused by stretching, obstructions, or surgical adhesions of the hollow visceral organs. An enlarged liver from hepatic malignancies results in a dull pain or fullness over the right upper quadrant of the abdomen. Any tumor having very little space to grow without compressing blood vessels and nerve endings against bone will elicit pain. Tissue destruction from infection and necrosis can cause pain.

Cachexia is a wasting, emaciation, and decreased quality of life seen in malignancy. Anorexia, or loss of appetite, contributes to the syndrome of cachexia. Reductions in sensitivities to sweet, sour, and salty tastes make ordinary seasoned foods seem bland. Also, aversions to food likely develop because of poor use of glucose and increased mobilization of protein. Elevated glucose and amino acid levels in the blood stimulate the satiety center resulting in reduced appetite.

Anemia is commonly associated with malignancy. The majority of individuals with cancer usually have a mild anemia, although 20 percent may have hemoglobin concentrations which are depressed by more than 40 percent. Chronic bleeding, severe malnutrition, medical therapies, or malignancy in blood-forming organs may cause anemia by depleting erythrocyte building blocks or destroying the site for synthesis of erythrocytes.

Direct tumor invasion into the bone marrow causes decreased leukocyte counts and decreased numbers of platelets. Chemotherapy and radiotherapy of areas of the bone marrow also cause **leukopenia** and **thrombocytopenia**.

Infection is the most significant cause of complications and death in individuals with malignant disease. Individuals with cancer are very susceptible to infection because of reductions in immunologic functions, debility from advanced disease, and immunosuppression from radiotherapy and chemotherapy. Surgery can create favorable sites for infection. The incidence of hospital-related or nosocomial infections for cancer patients is increased because of indwelling medical devices, compromised wound care, and the introduction of microorganisms from visitors and other patients.

6. Compare the modalities for the treatment of neoplasms; identify the advantages of immune therapy.

Study text pages 374-383; refer to Tables 11-4 through 11-7.

Cancer is treated with chemotherapy, radiotherapy, surgery, immunotherapy, and combinations of these modalities. The mechanism by which **chemotherapy** acts to eradicate tumor cells depends largely on its effect on the cell cycle. Chemotherapy hopes to kill cells undergoing mitosis and cytokinesis and those in interphase. To be effective, chemotherapy must eliminate enough neoplastic cells so that the body's own defenses can eradicate the remaining cells. Faster growing neoplasms are generally more sensitive to chemotherapy.

Radiation or ionizing radiation is a common approach to the treatment of malignant disease. To eradicate neoplastic cells without producing excessive toxicity and to avoid damage to normal structures is the challenge of radiation therapy. Ionizing radiation damages important macromolecules, especially DNA. Rapidly renewing and dividing cells are generally more radiosensitive than other cells.

Surgical therapy is useful when the neoplasm is accessible and has not yet spread beyond the limits of surgical excision. If there is any chance of regional lymph node involvement and no evidence of distant disease, the lymph nodes also should be removed. Palliative surgery, alleviation without cure, may be used to relieve or avoid symptoms of malignancy. Surgery is also indicated for benign tumors and those that could become malignant tumors.

Immunotherapy is promising in the treatment of cancer. Chemotherapy and radiation treatments act by eliminating both normal and neoplastic mitotically or metabolically active cells. However, some inactive or nondividing cells may not be affected by either radiation or metabolic inhibitors or mitotic poisons. Because the transformed cells in a tumor mass can adapt to changes in their environment, no single form of cancer therapy may be effective against all types of cancer. A specific method, like immunotherapy, may eliminate transformed cells without damaging normal tissues. The immune system has specificity for antigen recognition and is highly regulated, thus capable of sparing normal tissues. Also, immune memory cells are long-lived and capable of providing extended protection against the emergence of recurrent primary tumor cells and metastatic cancer cells.

Immunotherapies for the treatment of cancer are known as **biological response modifiers** (BRM). These BRMs can have a direct cytotoxic effect on cancer cells, initiate or augment the host's tumor-immune rejection response, or modify cancer cells' susceptibility to the lytic or tumor-arresting effects of the immune system. The BRMs include immunomodulating agents, interferons, antigens, effector cells, and monoclonal antibodies.

The use of immunomodulating agents involves nonspecific stimulation of the immune system by an **adjuvant**. An adjuvant is a substance, such as bacteria, that enhances the immune response. Retardation of tumor growth is due to activation of macrophages, augmentation of natural killer cells, or some degree of antigenic cross-reactivity between the microbe and the antigen produced by the tumor cell.

In addition to its antiviral activity, **interferon** inhibits tumor growth, enhances natural killer cell activity, and increases cancer cell expression of tumor antigens thus eliciting stronger tumor-immune rejection responses.

Tumor regression may be induced by creating a contact hypersensitivity response to an **antigen material**. Tumor cells are probably killed because this antigen has become incorporated within their cell surface and functions as an antigen, which elicits an immune response.

An effective form of cellular immunotherapy could occur by the transfer or augmentation of effector cytotoxic T-cells specific for the antigens expressed by the individual's tumor cells. The principle is to establish **tumor-specific cytotoxic cell lines** in tissue culture that can mediate tumor lysis or rejection when injected back into the cancer patient.

Monoclonal antibodies may be used both to detect developing cancer and to treat the neoplasm. These antibodies would be specific for tumor antigens and would reject neoplastic lesions without affecting normal tissue.

7. Compare childhood neoplasms with adult neoplasms.

Study text pages 385-388; refer to Table 11-8.

Comparison of Usual Childhood and Adult Cancers

Characteristic	Childhood Cancers	Adult Cancers
Incidence	< 1% of all cancers	> 99% of all cancers
Environmental causation	Weak relationship to environmental exposures and lifestyle	Strong relationship to environmental exposures and lifestyle
Latency (from initiation to diagnosis)	Short	Long
Sites involved	Tissue	Organs
Cells involved	Nonepithelial: sarcomas, embryonal, leukemia, lymphoma	Epithelial: carcinomas
Prevention	Few strategies to prevent	80% may be preventable
Early detection	Generally accidental	Possible by early detection screening tests/exams
Stage at diagnosis	80% have metastasized	Local or regional spread
Treatment/side effects	Less difficulty with acute toxicity but more significant long-term consequences	More difficult with acute toxicity but fewer long-term consequences
Response to treatment	Very responsive to chemotherapy	Less responsive to chemotherapy
Prognosis	> 60% cure	< 60% cure

Practice Examination

1. Tumor spread depends on
   a. growth rate of tumor and its degree of differentiation.
   b. unknown factors.
   c. the presence or absence of anatomical barriers.
   d. Both a and c are correct.
   e. a, b, and c are correct.

2. Which of the following is the correct sequence during the process of metastasis?
   a. vascularization, adherence of neoplastic cells, invasion into lymph and vascular systems
   b. transport, vascularization, adherence of neoplastic cells
   c. vascularization, invasion into lymph and vascular systems, transport
   d. vascularization, extravasation, transport

3. In order for metastasis to occur, local invasive factors include all except
   a. cellular multiplication.
   b. mechanical pressure.
   c. lytic enzyme release.
   d. increased cellular adhesion.
   e. increased individual tumor cells.

4. Known routes for metastasis of malignant cells include all except
   a. continuous extension.
   b. lymphatic spread.
   c. bloodstream dissemination.
   d. Both b and c are correct.
   e. a, b, and c are correct.

5. Common sites for metastatic cells include all except
   a. lung.
   b. liver.
   c. brain.
   d. bone.
   e. heart.

6. A malignant cell that becomes lodged in a lymph node may
   a. die.
   b. divide.
   c. become dormant.
   d. enter efferent lymphatics.
   e. All of the above are correct.

7. The process by which tumors develop new vascular networks is
   a. heparinization.
   b. angiogenesis.
   c. anaplasia.
   d. autonomy.
   e. differentiation.

8. Organ tropism involves
   a. local growth factors.
   b. chemotactic factors.
   c. tumor receptors.
   d. genetic determinants.
   e. All of the above are correct.

9. Routes for metastasis include all except
   a. blood vessels.
   b. lymph channels.
   c. ducts.
   d. skin-to-skin contact.

10. Neoplasms may cause all except
    a. obstruction of passageways.
    b. hormonal imbalances.
    c. viral infections.
    d. nutrient depletion.

11. Metastatic behavior may be due to _____ in neoplastic cells.
    a. altered cytoplasm
    b. altered ribosomes
    c. altered genetic code
    d. chromosomal breakage

12. The pain experienced with cancer
    a. affects individual in the early stages of malignancy.
    b. occurs in bone metastasis.
    c. results from tissue necrosis.
    d. Both b and c are correct.
    e. a, b, and c are correct.

13. The anorexia or loss of appetite seen in the syndrome of cancer cachexia may occur because of
    a. elevated blood serum levels of glucose and amino acids.
    b. hyperinsulinism.
    c. late satiety.
    d. hypoproteinemia.

14. The anemia associated with malignancy can be
    a. due to depletion of hemoglobin building blocks.
    b. severe in the majority of cases.
    c. caused by destruction of bone marrow.
    d. All of the above are correct.
    e. Both a and c are correct.

15. Chemotherapy for cancer hopes to kill cancerous cells
    a. in interphase.
    b. undergoing mitosis and cytokinesis.
    c. Both a and b are correct.
    d. Neither a nor b is correct.

16. Immunotherapy for cancer
    a. is a nonspecific treatment.
    b. injures both transformed and normal cells.
    c. suppresses tumor-immune response.
    d. is augmented by memory cells.
    e. None of the above is correct.

17. Interferons
    a. inhibit tumor growth.
    b. possess antiviral activity.
    c. increase neoplastic cell expression of tumor antigens.
    d. All of the above are correct.
    e. None of the above is correct.

18. Childhood cancers
    a. most often involve nonepithilial tissue.
    b. most often involve epithelial tissue.
    c. have a strong relationship to environmental exposure.
    d. are less responsive to chemotherapy than adult cancers.
    e. None of the above is correct.

19. Adult cancers have
    a. a better cure rate than childhood cancers.
    b. a short latency period.
    c. mostly metastasized at time of diagnosis.
    d. organ involvement more often than tissue involvement.
    e. None of the above is correct.

20. Which is not involved in metastasis?
    a. initial establishment
    b. interference
    c. invasion
    d. dissemination
    e. proliferation

Match the cancer treatment with its characteristic.

21. radiation
22. monoclonal antibodies
23. immunomodulating agents
24. surgery
25. antigens

    a. hypersensitivity response
    b. T-cell transfer
    c. specific antibodies for tumor antigen
    d. cancerous cells attacked in cell cycle
    e. nonspecific stimulation of immune system
    f. tumor removal
    g. direct ionization

CHAPTER 12

Structure and Function of the Neurologic System

Objectives

After successful study of this chapter, the learner will be able to:

1. **Identify the structural and functional subdivisions of the nervous system.**
   Review text page 398.

2. **Compare the functions of neurons and neuroglia; identify the parts and configurations of neurons.**
   Review text pages 398-401; refer to Figures 12-1 through 12-3 and Table 12-1.

3. **Describe the circumstances under which nervous tissue can regenerate.**
   Review text page 402.

4. **Describe synaptic transmission of impulses by neurotransmitters.**
   Review text pages 402-404; refer to Table 12-2.

5. **Identify the three main regions of the brain; characterize their associated structures and functions.**
   Review text pages 404-410; refer to Table 12-3.

6. **Identify the significance of decussation of motor fibers.**
   Review text page 410; refer to Figure 12-9.

7. **Describe the location and structure of the spinal cord; define a reflex arc.**
   Review text pages 410-412; refer to Figures 12-10 through 12-13.

8. **Identify the structures responsible for maintaining and protecting the central nervous system.**
   Review text pages 412-415.

9. **Identify the route of blood circulation within the central nervous system; note the significance of the circle of Willis.**
   Review text pages 416-420; refer to Figures 12-18 through 12-20.

10. **Describe the structure of a spinal nerve; locate plexuses.**
    Review text page 420; refer to Figure 12-23.

11. **Name the cranial nerves and state functions of each.**
    Refer to Table 12-6.

12. **Identify the subdivisions of the autonomic nervous system, their origins, and general functions.**
    Review text pages 420-425; refer to Figures 12-24 and 12-25.

13. **Identify the type of neurotransmitter secreted by preganglionic and postganglionic fibers in the autonomic nervous system.**
    Review text pages 425-427; refer to Figure 12-26 and Table 12-7.

Practice Examination

1. One function of the somatic nervous system which is not performed by the autonomic nervous system is
   a. conduction of impulses to involuntary muscles and glands.
   b. conduction of impulses to the central nervous system.
   c. conduction of impulses to skeletal muscles.
   d. conduction of impulses between the brain and spinal cord.

2. A neuron with a single dendrite at one end of the cell body and a single axon at the other end of the cell body would be classified as
   a. unipolar.
   b. multipolar.
   c. monopolar.
   d. bipolar.

3. Neurons which carry impulses away from the CNS are called
   a. afferent neurons.
   b. sensory neurons.
   c. efferent neurons.
   d. association neurons.

Match the structure with the most appropriate function/description.

4. Schwann cell
5. dendrite

   a. the outer, nucleated layer of a certain cell type
   b. produces myelin sheath
   c. carries impulses away from perikaryon
   d. a covering over neuron fibers
   e. conducts impulses to cell body

6. Neurons are specialized for the conduction of impulses; whereas neuroglia
   a. support and protect nerve tissue.
   b. serve as motor end plates.
   c. synthesize acetylcholine and cholinesterase.
   d. All of the above are correct.

7. There is one-way conduction at a synapse because
   a. only postsynaptic neurons contain synaptic vesicles.
   b. acetylcholine prevents nerve impulses from traveling in both directions.
   c. only the presynaptic neuron contains neurotransmitters.
   d. only dendrites release neurotransmitters.

8. Which contains the thalamus and hypothalamus?
   a. diencephalon
   b. cerebrum
   c. medulla oblongata
   d. brain stem

9. The reticular activating system
   a. programs for fine repetitive motor movements.
   b. maintains wakefulness.
   c. maintains constant internal environments.
   d. affects the positioning of the head to improve hearing.

10. Which phrases best describe the spinal cord?
    1. descends inferior to the lumbar vertebrae
    2. conducts motor impulses from the brain
    3. descends to the fourth lumbar vertebra
    4. conducts sensory impulses to the brain
    5. inferior includes gray horns

    a. 1, 3, 4
    b. 1, 3, 5
    c. 2, 3, 5
    d. 2, 4, 5
    e. 2, 3, 4

Match the component of a reflex arc with its descriptor.

11. sensory neuron
12. effector

a. carries impulses to the CNS
b. carries impulses to a responding organ
c. responds to motor impulse
d. stimulated by one neuron and passes impulse on to another neuron
e. responds directly to changes in environment

13. Which is not a protective covering of the CNS?
    a. cauda equine
    b. dura mater
    c. arachnoid
    d. cranial bone

14. The composition of cerebrospinal fluid is
    a. the same as blood.
    b. distilled H_2O with dissolved salts.
    c. a plasma-like liquid with glucose, salts, proteins, and urea.
    d. a heavy mucous solution with dissolved salts, glucose and urea.

Match the function with the cranial nerve.

15. tasting
16. balance maintenance

a. facial
b. olfactory
c. vestibulocochlear
d. hypoglossal
e. optic

17. An autonomic ganglion can be described as
    a. the site of synapses between visceral efferent neurons.
    b. a site where spinal reflexes occur.
    c. a point of synapse between parasympathetic and sympathetic neurons.
    d. the place where unconscious sensations occur.

18. Clusters of nerve cell bodies and dendrites located within the CNS are called
    a. nuclei.
    b. tract.
    c. nerves.
    d. ganglia.

19. A mass of nerve cell bodies and dendrites located within the CNS is a
    a. sulcus.
    b. ganglion.
    c. nucleus.
    d. tract.

Match the characteristic with the appropriate division of the autonomic nervous system.

20. more extensive use of norepinephrine as a transmitter substance
21. effects more widespread and long-lasting
22. elicits rest-response

a. sympathetic
b. parasympathetic

Classify the effect of sympathetic nerve stimulation on the structures.

23. breathing passageways
24. intestines
25. liver

a. increases diameter
b. decreases diameter
c. increases metabolic activity
d. decreases metabolic activity

78

CHAPTER 13

Pain, Temperature Regulation, Sleep, and Sensory Function

Prerequisite Objectives

a. Identify receptors, pathways, and perceptions of pain.
   Review text pages 399, 410, and 438-442;
   refer to Table 13-2.

Remember!

- Pain receptors, also known as nociceptors, are naked nerve endings found in nearly every tissue in the body. Sensory nerves transmit the stimuli from pain receptors into the dorsal root ganglia. The impulses travel to the spinal cord synapse, cross the cord, and ascend by either the neospino-thalamic tracts or the paleospinothalamic tract. The paleospinothalamic tract ascends and branches into the brain stem reticular formations, the pons, and the medulla. The neospinotha-lamic tract ascends with fibers synapsing in the thalamus where the sensation of pain occurs and then proceeds into the cortex where precision and discrimination occur.

---

b. Describe thermoregulation.
   Review text pages 255-256 and 447-448; refer to Figure 13-7.

Remember!

- The control of body temperature is a function of centers located in the hypothalamus. Thermore-ceptors provide the hypothalamus with information about peripheral and core temperatures. If the temperature is low, the body initiates heat-conservation measures by a series of hormonal mechanisms which release epinephrine into the bloodstream. Epinephrine causes vasoconstric-tion, glycolysis, and increased metabolic rates which establish a new set-point within the hypo-thalamus. Warmer peripheral and core temperatures reverse the process. The sympathetic path-way produces vasodilation, decreased muscle tone, and increased perspiration.

- When interleukin-1 (IL-1), a product of monocytes or macrophages (and probably eosinophils), engages thermosensitive centers in the hypothalamus, the thermostat set-point is elevated and heat-generating and conserving mechanisms are initiated. In response to IL-1, the synthesis of prostaglandins of the series is increased and the hypothalamic set-point is further increased.

---

c. Identify the normal sleep stages; describe nervous system control of sleep.
    Review text pages 454-455; refer to Figure 13-9.

Remember!

- Normal sleep has two phases that can be documented by electroencephalography (EEG): rapid eye movement (REM) sleep and non-REM, or slow wave, sleep. Non-REM sleep is divided into four stages based on changes in the EEG pattern. Non-REM sleep is initiated by the withdrawal of neurotransmitters from the reticular formation and by the inhibition of arousal mechanisms in the cerebral cortex. During non-REM sleep, respiration is controlled by metabolic processes. The basal metabolic rate, temperature, heart rate, blood pressure, and muscle tone all decrease. Knee-jerk reflexes are absent. Pupils are constricted. During stages I and II, cerebral blood flow to the brain stem and cerebellum decreases; during stages III and IV, cerebral blood flow to the cortex is decreased. Growth hormone is released during stage IV, and levels of corticosteroids and catecholamines are depressed.

- REM sleep occurs about every 90 minutes beginning after 1 or 2 hours of non-REM sleep. The EEG pattern of REM sleep is similar to the normal awake pattern. Alternating periods of REM and non-REM sleep occur throughout the night, with lengthening intervals of REM sleep and fewer intervals of the deeper stages of non-REM sleep toward morning. REM sleep is characterized by bursts of rapid eye movement; atonia of antigravity muscles; loss of temperature regulation; alteration in heart rate, blood pressure, and respiration; penile erection in men and clitoral engorgement in women; and a high rate of memorable dreams. Steroids are released in short bursts and cerebral blood flow to both hemispheres is increased. REM sleep is controlled by the pontine reticular formation.

- The reticular formation is primarily responsible for generating REM sleep. Projections from the reticular formation and other areas of the mesencephalon and brain stem produce non-REM sleep. The first cycle of the night begins with stage I. The individual then progresses through stages II, III, IV, III, II, and REM sleep. A new cycle, beginning with stage II, follows each REM sleep. With each successive cycle, the amount of time spent in stage IV decreases and the amount of time spent in REM increases. The individual who is awakened begins the next cycle with stage I.

---

d. Characterize the cranial and spinal nerves.
    Review text page 420; refer to Figure 12-10 and Table 12-6.

Remember!

- A cranial or spinal nerve is composed of individual axons wrapped in a myelin sheath. The coverings provide structural support, a blood supply, and interstitial compartments holding essential electrolytes that support nerve impulse conduction. Thirty-one pairs of spinal nerves contain both sensory and motor neurons and arise from the ventral and dorsal horn cells of the spinal cord. These two spinal nerve roots converge in the region of the intervertebral foramen to form the spinal nerve trunk. Shortly after converging, the spinal nerve divides into anterior and posterior rami. The anterior rami, except the thoracic, initially form plexuses which then branch into the peripheral nerves. Instead of forming plexuses, the thoracic nerves pass through the intercostal spaces to innervate regions of the thorax.

- The posterior rami of each spinal nerve are distributed to specific areas in the body. Sensory signals, therefore, arise from specific sites associated with a specific spinal cord segment. The area of skin supplied with afferent fibers from a single spinal ramus are called dermatomes. Most cranial nerves are mixed nerves like the spinal nerves, although some are purely sensory or purely motor. Cranial nerves arise from nuclei in the brain and brain stem.

Objectives

After successful study of this chapter, the learner will be able to:

1. Compare the theories of pain.
>   Study text pages 443-444; refer to Figure 13-4.

Theories proposed to describe the mechanism of pain include the specificity theory, the intensity theory, the pattern theory, and the gate control theory. The **specificity theory** identifies cutaneous sensation as (1) touch, (2) warmth, (3) cold, or (4) pain. Each cutaneous sensation results from stimulation of specific receptor sites on the skin. Stimulation of the pain receptors causes transmission of the painful stimuli to the spinal cord. The pain neurons form synapses and cross to the opposite side of the spinal cord to ascend to the brain through the spinothalamic tract. The perception of pain occurs in special areas of the thalamus and cerebral cortex. This theory fails to account for adaptation to pain and effects of psychosocial factors on pain perception.

The **intensity theory** proposes that pain results from excessive stimulation of sensory receptors. Pain occurs if the stimulus is of sufficient intensity. This theory does not explain the intense stimulation of some sites that produce no pain.

The **pattern theory** suggests that pain perception is the result of the length of time, the amount of tissue involved, and the summation of the afferent impulses. Summation may occur in the spinal cord or in the brain. Although pattern theories do not account for adaptation to pain, they do allow for multiple pain perception factors.

According to the **gate control theory**, nociceptive impulses are transmitted from specialized skin receptors to the spinal cord through large A and small C fibers. These fibers terminate in the dorsal horn of the spinal cord. Cells in the substantia gelatinosa of the dorsal horn function as a gate and permit some impulses to reach the central nervous system for interpretation. Stimulation of larger, faster transmitting fibers causes the cells in the substantia gelatinosa to "close the gate." A closed gate decreases stimulation of trigger cells, decreases transmission impulses, and diminishes pain perception. Persistent stimulation of the large fibers, however, allows adaptation. When adaptation to impulses from large fibers occurs, the result is a relative increase in small neuron activity. With time, adaptation by larger fibers may thus "open the gate," as will small fiber transmission. Slower transmitting small fiber input inhibits cells in the substantia gelatinosa and opens the gate. An open gate increases the stimulation of trigger cells, increases

transmission of impulses, and enhances pain perception. In addition to gate control through large and small fiber stimulation, the central nervous system through efferent pathways may close, partially close, or open the gate.

Cognitive functioning may thus modulate pain perception. Interaction of the cognitive/evaluative, motivational/affective, and sensory/discriminative systems determine each individual's pain response.

2. Identify chemicals that modulate pain.
>   Study text page 444; refer to Figure 13-5.

Tissue injury results in the release of prostaglandins, bradykinins, and histamine that depolarize adjacent nociceptors. **Lymphokines** released from lymphocytes in chronic inflammatory lesions may contribute to some chronic pain. **Substance** P, **neurokinin** A, and **calcitonin-gene-related peptide** are released from peripheral pain receptors to permit the spread of pain locally. **Norepinephrine** and **5-hydroxytryptamine** contribute to pain inhibition in the medulla and pons.

Endorphins are neuropeptides that inhibit transmission of pain impulses in the spinal cord and brain. All endorphins attach to opiate receptors on the plasma membrane of the afferent neuron. The combination of the opiate receptor and endorphin inhibits the release of excitatory neurotransmitters, thereby blocking the transmission of the painful stimulus. Stress, excessive physical exertion, acupuncture, and intercourse are factors that increase the level of circulating endorphins.

3. Differentiate between acute and chronic pain.
>   Study text pages 444-447; refer to Figure 13-6.

Acute pain may be somatic, visceral, or referred. **Somatic pain** comes from the skin or close to the surface of the body. **Visceral pain** occurs in internal organs, the abdomen, or skeleton. It is poorly localized because of fewer mechano-receptors in the visceral structures. It is associated with nausea and vomiting, hypotension, restlessness, and possible shock. Visceral pain often radiates or is referred. **Referred pain** is present in an area removed or distant from its point of origin. The area of referred pain is supplied by the same spinal segment as the actual site of injury. Impulses from many cutaneous and visceral neurons converge on the same ascending neuron and the brain cannot distinguish between the the origin of the two.

Acute pain is a warning of actual or impending tissue injury. Physiologic responses include increased heart rate, increased respiratory rate, elevated blood pressure, pallor or flushing, dilated pupils, and diaphoresis. The response is basically one of sympathetic nervous stimulation. Psychologically, individuals often respond to acute pain with fear, anxiety, and a general sense of unpleasantness or uneasiness. The stress of fear may subsequently contribute to the physiologic signs of pain.

Chronic pain is prolonged; it may last longer than six months and may either persist or be intermittent. Physiologic responses to chronic pain depend on the persistent or intermittent nature of the pain. **Intermittent pain** produces physiologic response similar to acute pain; whereas **persistent pain** permits physiologic adaptation. Individuals with chronic pain often are depressed, have difficulty sleeping and eating, and may become preoccupied with their pain.

Common chronic pain conditions include low back pain, neuralgias, hyperesthesia, myofascial pain syndrome, hemiageusias, and phantom limb pain. Sometimes, chronic pain is associated with cancer. **Low back pain** results from poor muscular tone, inactivity, muscle strain, or sudden vigorous activity. **Neuralgias** are painful conditions that result from infections or damaged peripheral nerves. **Hyperesthesias** are characterized by increased sensitivity and decreased pain threshold to tactile and painful stimuli that usually do not produce pain. **Myofascial pain syndromes** are common causes of chronic pain. These conditions involve injury to the muscles and fascia. The pain results from muscle spasm, tenderness, and stiffness. **Hemiagnosia** is an inability to identify the source of pain on the affected side of the body. Application of painful stimuli to the affected side produces discomfort, anxiety, moaning, agitation, and distress, but there is no attempt to withdraw from or push aside the offending stimulus. Hemiagnosia is associated with stroke. **Phantom limb pain** is pain that an individual feels in an amputated limb after the residual stump has completely healed. If the neuronal pathway from the amputated limb is stimulated at any point along its pathway, action potentials are transmitted toward the cortex where CNS integration results in the perception of pain. The pain experienced in cancer is attributed to the advance of the disease, associated with treatment of the disease, and attributed to coexisting entities such as osteoarthritis. As cancer advances, pain can be caused by infection and inflammation, increasing pressure of a growing tumor on nerve endings, stretching of visceral surfaces, and/or obstruction of ducts and intestines. Damage from radiation, chemotherapy, or surgical sectioning of the nerve produces another form of chronic pain referred to as deafferntion pain. Deafferntion is loss of sensory input from a portion of the body.

4. Describe the alternations occurring in fever, hyperthermia, and hypothermia.

Study text pages 450-454; refer to Figure 13-7.

Fever is not the failure of the normal thermoregulatory mechanism. Instead, it is considered a "a resetting of the hypothalamic thermostat" to a higher level. The normal thermoregulatory mechanisms are raised so that the thermoregulatory center adjusts heat production, conservation, and loss to maintain the core temperature at a new, higher set-point temperature.

The pathophysiology of fever begins with the introduction of exogenous pyrogens or endotoxins. The production and release of interleukin-1 (IL-1) occur as exogenous bacteria are destroyed and absorbed by phagocytic cells within the host. Tumor necrosis factor, interleukin-6, and interferons are known to be involved in fever. As the set-point is raised, the hypothalamus signals an increase in heat production and conservation to raise body temperature to the new level as described in Prerequisite b.

During fever, arginine vasopressin (AVP), alpha-melanocyte-stimulating hormone, and corticotropin-releasing factor are released, which act as endogenous antipyretics to help diminish the febrile response. During this antipyretic effect, as fever breaks, the set-point is returned to normal. The hypothalamus signals a decrease in heat production and an increase in heat reduction.

Fever can be beneficial. Elevated body temperature kills many microorganisms and has adverse effects on the growth and replication of others. Increased temperature causes lysosomal breakdown with autodestruction of cells; this prevents viral replication in infected cells. Heat increases lymphocytic transformation and motility of polymorphonuclear neutrophils, which facilitates the immune response. The elderly may have decreased or no fever response to infection. The absence of beneficial aspects of fever production may explain the increase in morbidity and mortality seen in the very elderly. In contrast to the very elderly, children develop higher fevers than adults from relatively minor infections. Febrile seizures may occur in children with temperatures above 39° C (102.2° F). Febrile seizures are generally brief and self-limiting, lasting less than five minutes in 40 percent of children and less than 20 minutes in 75 percent of children. There appears to be no long-term effect on the child; however, a very few children may develop epilepsy.

Hyperthermia can produce nerve damage, coagulation of cell proteins, and death. At 41° C (106° F), nerve damage produces convulsions in the adult. At 43° C (109° F), death follows. In hyperthermia, there is no resetting of the hypothalamic set-point. Forms of accidental hyperthermia are heat cramps, heat exhaustion, and heat-stroke.

Heat cramps are severe, spasmodic cramps in the abdomen and extremities subsequent to prolonged sweating and associated sodium loss. Heat cramps usually appear in individuals who are unaccustomed to heat or in those who are performing strenuous work in very warm climates. Fever, rapid pulse, and increased blood pressure often accompany the cramps.

Heat exhaustion or collapse results from prolonged high body core or environmental temperatures. These high temperatures cause hypothalamic inducement of profound vasodilation and profuse sweating. Over a prolonged period of elevated temperatures, the hypothalamic responses produce dehydration, decreased plasma volumes, hypotension, decreased cardiac output, and tachycardia.

Heatstroke is a potentially lethal consequence of a breakdown in control of an overstressed thermoregulatory center. The brain cannot tolerate temperatures over 40.5° C (105° F). In cases of very high core temperatures, the regulatory center may cease to function appropriately. Sweating ceases, and the skin becomes dry and flushed. The individual may become irritable, confused, stuporous, or comatose.

As evaporation of perspiration ceases, core temperatures rise rapidly. High core temperatures and vascular collapse produce cerebral edema, degeneration of the central nervous system, and renal tubular necrosis. Death results unless immediate, effective treatment is initiated. Treatment requires more than the fluid and electrolyte replacement required in heat cramps and exhaustion. Removing the person from the warm environment, if possible, and surface cooling are required. Too rapid surface cooling may cause peripheral vasoconstriction which would prevent core cooling. Children are more susceptible to heat stroke than adults because they produce more metabolic heat when exercising, they have a greater surface area-to-mass ratio, and their perspiring capacity is less than that of adults.

Malignant hyperthermia is a potentially lethal complication of an inherited muscle disorder. The condition is precipitated by the administration of volatile anesthetics and neuromuscular blocking agents. The risk for this muscle disorder may be about 1 in 200 individuals. Malignant hyperthermia causes intracellular calcium levels to rise, producing sustained, uncoordinated muscle contractions. As a result of these contractions, acidosis develops and body temperature may rise 1° C (1.8° F) every five minutes. Approximately 20 percent of those who develop malignant hyperthermia do not survive. Treatment includes withdrawal of the provoking agents and administration of skeletal muscle relaxants to inhibit calcium release during muscle contraction, treatment of cardiac arrhythmias, so-dium bicarbonate administration, and cooling of the body.

Hypothermia slows chemical reactions, increases blood viscosity, slows blood flow, facilitates blood coagulation, and stimulates profound vasoconstriction. Accidental hypothermia, temperature below 35° C (95° F), is generally the result of sudden immersion in cold water or prolonged exposure to cold environments. The young and the elderly are at risk because of their less effective thermoregulatory mechanisms. Individuals with conditions that diminish their ability to generate heat, such as hypothyroidism, hypopituitarism, malnutrition, Parkinson disease, and rheumatoid arthritis, are also at risk.

The hypothalamic center stimulates shivering in an effort to increase heat production at core temperatures of 35° C and continues until core temperature drops between 30° and 32° C. Thinking becomes sluggish and coordination is decreased at 34° C. At 30° C, the individual becomes stuporous, heart rate and respiratory rates decline, and cardiac output is diminished. In severe hypothermia, core temperature of 20° to 28° C, pulse and respirations may be undetectable. Acidosis becomes moderate to severe. Ventricular fibrillation and asystole are common. Depending on the severity of the hypothermia, rewarming of the peripheral tissues may be the only treatment required. Core rewarming is performed when core temperatures have dropped below 30° C or when severe cardiovascular abnormalities appear. Core rewarming may require administration of warm intravenous solutions, gastric or peritoneal lavage, or inhalation of warmed gases. Rewarming generally should proceed at no faster than a few degrees per hour.

5. Describe sleep disorders; cite examples.
Study text pages 456-458.

Sleep disorders are classified by signs and symptoms rather than by their etiology. Sleep disorders can be classified as (1) disorders of initiating sleep, (2) disorders of excessive somnolence, (3) disorders of the sleep-wake schedule, and (4) dysfunctions of sleep, sleep stages, or partial arousals.

Disorders of initiating sleep are classified as **insomnia**, the inability to fall or stay asleep. Insomnia may be transient and related to travel across time zones or due to acute stress. Long-term insomnia is associated with drug or alcohol abuse, chronic pain disorders, or chronic depression. Two disorders of excessive **somnolence** or excessive daytime sleepiness are **Pickwickian syndrome** and **hypersomnia sleep apnea** (HSA) syndrome. Both Pickwickian syndrome and HSA syndrome are associated with periodic breathing and episodes of apnea during stages I, II, and REM sleep.

In Pickwickian syndrome, the apneic periods are generally due to obesity, decreased chemosensitivity to carbon dioxide and oxygen tensions, or upper airway obstruction occurring while sleeping. The sleep apnea reduces oxygen saturation and eventually produces polycythemia, pulmonary hypertension, right-sided congestive heart failure, liver congestion, cyanosis, and peripheral edema. Because the apnea may be due to alteration of central nervous control of respiration, daytime hypercapnia also occurs. Treatment requires weight loss, controlled oxygen therapy, administration of a respiratory stimulant, and congestive heart failure therapy.

HSA syndrome is primarily a result of upper airway obstruction occurring during sleep. Persons with HSA syndrome may experience hundreds of apneic episodes each night and excessive daytime sleepiness. Their spouses often observe excessive snoring, snorting, and thrashing about during sleep. Pathologic changes include polycythemia and right-sided heart failure. Treatment involves relief of the upper airway obstruction during sleep.

Common **disorders of the sleep-wake schedule** include rapid time-zone change or "jet-lag syndrome," an altered sleep schedule with an advance or a delay of three hours or more in sleep time, or a change in total sleep time from day to day. Vigilance of psychomotor performance and arousal are markedly depressed after alterations in the sleep-wake schedule. Individuals affected by disorders of the sleep-wake schedule require several days to synchronize circadian rhythm, to adjust the body temperature cycle, and to adjust cortisol secretion.

Dysfunctions of sleep, **sleep stages**, or **partial arousals** are common in children. They are somnambulism, night terrors, and enuresis. **Somnambulism**, or sleepwalking, appears to resolve itself within several years after the onset of the sleepwalking episodes. Sleepwalking occurs in stages III and IV. During the sleepwalking episode, the child functions at a very low level of arousal and has no memory of the event upon awakening. **Night terrors** are characterized by "sudden apparent arousals in which the child expresses intense fear or emotion." However, the child is not awake and is very difficult to arouse. Once awakened, the child has no memory of the night terror event. Night terrors occur during stage IV. Neither somnambulism nor night terrors are associated with the dreams of REM sleep.

Enuresis, or bed wetting, occurs when the child is dreaming and during the first third of the night, when the child is most difficult to arouse. Children do eventually "outgrow" the enuretic episodes.

6. Identify common diseases, their etiology, and manifestations that are associated with the special senses.

Study text pages 458-470.

Vision

Blepharitis is an inflammation of the eyelids caused by staphylococcal infections or seborrheic dermatitis. Redness, edema, and itching occur.

Conjunctivitis is an inflammation of the conjunctiva, or the mucous membrane covering the front part of the eyeball. It may be caused by bacteria, viruses, allergies, or chemical irritations. The inflammatory response produces redness, pain, and lacrimation.

Keratitis is an infection of the cornea usually caused by bacteria or viruses. Bacterial infections often cause corneal ulceration and require extensive antibiotic treatment. Type I herpes virus usually infects the cornea and conjunctiva. Common symptoms include photophobia, pain, and lacrimation.

Strabismus is the deviation of one eye from the other when the person is looking directly at an object. It is due to a weak or hypertonic muscle in one of the eyes. The deviation may be upward, downward, inward, or outward. The primary symptom of strabismus is diplopia or double vision.

Amblyopia is a vision reduction or dimness for unknown reasons. Amblyopia is associated with diabetes mellitus, renal failure, malaria, and toxic substances such as alcohol and tobacco.

A *scotoma* is a circumscribed defect of the central field of vision. It is most often a sequel to an inflammatory lesion of the optic nerve and is frequently associated with multiple sclerosis.

A *cataract* is a cloudy or opaque ocular lens. Although the most common form of cataract is degenerative, cataracts may also occur as a result of infection, radiation, trauma, drugs, or diabetes mellitus. Cataracts cause decreased visual acuity, blurred vision, glare, and decreased color perception.

Papilledema is edema and inflammation of the optic nerve at its point of entrance into the eyeball. Generally, papilledema is caused by obstruction to the venous return from the retina. An early symptom is distention of the retinal vein.

Dark adaptation affects visual acuity. An average 80-year-old individual needs over 200 times as much light as a 20-year-old to see equally well. Changes in rhodopsin, a substance found in the rods and responsible for low-light vision, are likely responsible for reduced dark adaptation in older adults. Vitamin A deficiencies can cause the same disorder in individuals of any age.

Glaucoma is characterized by intraocular pressures above the normal range of 12 to 20 mm Hg maintained by the aqueous fluid in homeostasis. Intraocular fluid accumulation involves obstruction to aqueous humor outflow. Chronic increased intraocular pressure first causes loss of peripheral vision which is followed by central vision impairment and blindness.

Loss of accommodation in the elderly is termed *presbyopia,* a condition in which the ocular lens becomes larger, firmer, and less elastic. The major symptom is reduced near vision, causing reading material to be held at arm's length.

In *myopia,* or nearsightedness, light rays are focused in front of the retina when the person is looking at a distant object. In *hyperopia,* or farsightedness, light rays are focused behind the retina when the person is looking at a near object. *Astigmatism* is caused by an unequal curvature of the cornea; light rays are bent unevenly and do not come to a single focus on the retina. Blurred vision and headache develop in all three of the above conditions.

Hearing

A *conductive hearing loss* occurs when a change in the outer and/or middle ear impairs sound conduction from the outer to the inner ear. Conditions that commonly cause a conductive hearing loss include impacted cerumen, foreign bodies lodged in the ear canal, neoplasms of the external auditory canal and/or middle ear, eustachian tube dysfunction, otitis media, cholesteatoma, and otosclerosis. Symptoms of conductive hearing loss include diminished hearing and soft speaking voice. The voice is soft because the individual may hear his or her voice conducted by bone ossicles.

A *sensorineural hearing loss* is due to impairment of the organ of Corti and its hearing receptors or its central connections. Conditions that commonly cause sensorineural hearing loss include congenital and hereditary factors, noise exposure, aging, ototoxicity, and systemic diseases. Congenital and neonatal sensorineural hearing loss may be caused by maternal rubella, infant prematurity, traumatic delivery, or erythroblastosis fetalis.

Olfaction

Hyposmia is impaired sense of smell; *anosmia* is complete loss of smell. When hyposmia or anosmia occurs bilaterally, it is usually the result of inflammation of the nasal mucosa, severe head colds, or excessive smoking. Unilateral hyposmia or anosmia may indicate tumor compression of one olfactory bulb or nerve tract. *Olfactory hallucinations* arise from hyperactivity in cortical neurons and involve the smelling of odors that are not actually present. They are mostly associated with temporal lobe seizures. *Parosmia,* abnormal or perverted sense of smell, may occur in severely depressed individuals.

Taste

Hypogeusia is decreased taste sensation; *ageusia* is the absence of taste. Ageusia affecting the entire tongue may follow head injury. Damage to the glossopharyngeal nerve causes inability to detect bitterness; damage to the facial nerve causes inability to detect sour, sweet, and salty tastes. *Parageusia* is a perversion of taste in which substances possess an unpleasant flavor. Parageusia is common in individuals receiving chemotherapy for cancer. Parageusia often leads to anorexia.

Touch

Any impairment of reception, transmission, perception, or interpretation of touch alters tactile sensation. Trauma, tumor, infection, metabolic changes, vascular changes, and degenerative disease may cause tactile dysfunction. Sedative drugs and prefrontal injury which interrupt connections between the prefrontal cortex and subcortical centers diminish the interpretation of the sensations.

Proprioception

Proprioception is the perception and awareness of the position of the body and its parts. It depends on impulses from the inner ear and from receptors in joints and ligaments. *Proprioceptive dysfunction* may be caused by alterations at any level of the nervous system, similar to that observed in tactile dysfunction.

Vestibular nystagmus is the constant, involuntary movement of the eyeball caused when the semicircular canal system is overstimulated. *Vertigo* is the sensation of spinning that occurs with inflammation of the semicircular canals in the ear. *Ménière disease* is a vestibular disorder that can cause proprioceptive dysfunction. The pathologic basis of this disease is unclear. The individual with acute Ménière disease may experience loss of proprioception and become unable to stand or walk.

Peripheral neuropathies are probably caused by metabolic disturbances of the neuron itself. The result is a diminished or absent sense of body position or position of body parts. Gait changes often occur.

Practice Examination

Match the nervous system component with the pain characteristic for which it is responsible.

1. basic sensation of pain
2. initiation of pain stimulus
3. discrimination and precision given
   to painful stimulus

a. nociceptive receptors
b. thalamus
c. brain stem
d. A fibers
e. cortex

4. Endorphins are found in the brain stem and
   a. increase pain sensations.
   b. decrease pain sensations.
   c. may increase or decrease pain sensations.
   d. have no effect on pain sensations.

5. Referred pain is either projected from the spine into areas of the lumbar and upper sacral dermatomes or projected from pelvic and abdominal visceral to the spine. Referred pain from upper abdominal diseases involve
   a. the sacral region.
   b. L2 to L4.
   c. T8, L1, L2.
   d. the gluteal regions, posterior thighs, and calves.

6. In the gate control theory of pain,
   a. a "closed gate" increases pain perception.
   b. stimulation of large A fibers "close the gate."
   c. Both a and b are correct.
   d. Neither a nor b is correct.

7. Which is not a neuromodulator of pain?
   a. prostaglandins
   b. bradykinins
   c. norepinephrine
   d. lymphokines
   e. heparin

8. Interleukin-1
   a. activates helper/inducer T-cells to synthesize interleukin-2.
   b. is released by monocytes during inflammation.
   c. activates fibroblasts to synthesize collagen which facilitates tissue repair.
   d. None of the above is correct.
   e. a, b, and c are correct.

9. Increased serum levels of epinephrine increase body temperature by
   a. increasing shivering.
   b. increasing muscle tone.
   c. increasing heat production.
   d. decreasing basal metabolic rate.

10. In heat stroke,
   a. core temperature usually reaches 101° F.
   b. facial perspiration occurs even during dehydration.
   c. core temperature decreases rapidly as perspiration ceases.
   d. adults are more susceptible than children.

11. Which is not involved in fever?
    a. tumor necrosis factor
    b. interferons
    c. elevation of a higher "set-point" in the hypothalamus
    d. Only a is involved in fever.
    e. a, b, and c are involved in fever.

12. In hypothermia,
    a. the viscosity of blood is decreased.
    b. core temperatures of 26° to 28° C result in acidosis.
    c. the hypothalamic center prevents shivering.
    d. All of the above are correct.

13. Although Non-REM and REM sleep are defined by electrical recordings, they are characterized by physiological events. Which of the following does not occur?
    a. The sleep sequence is I, II, III, IV, III, II, and REM sleep.
    b. Non-REM is initiated by withdrawal of neurotransmitters from the reticular formation.
    c. During stages III and IV, cerebral blood flow to the cortex is decreased.
    d. During stage IV, levels of corticosteroids are increased.

Match the abnormality with the sleep stage.

14. Pickwickian syndrome
15. somnambulism or sleepwalking
16. enuresis
17. dreaming

   a. REM
   b. Non-REM
   c. both REM and Non-REM

18. Sleep apnea
    a. is lack of breathing during sleep.
    b. results from airway obstruction during sleep.
    c. is associated with "jet-lag syndrome."
    d. All of the above are correct.
    e. Both a and b are correct.

19. Individuals affected by disorders of the sleep-wake schedule
    a. show increased accident proneness.
    b. require days to adjust body temperature cycle.
    c. require days to adjust cortisol secretions.
    d. All of the above are correct.

Match the term with its defining characteristic.

20. blepharitis
21. strabismus
22. anosmia
23. hypogeusia
24. vertigo
25. neuropathy

   a. inflammation of mucous membrane covering the eyeball
   b. infection of the cornea
   c. weak muscle in one of the eyes
   d. reduction or dimness of vision
   e. inflammation of the eyelids
   f. high intraocular pressures
   g. metabolic disturbance of the neuron
   h. inflammation of the semicircular canals
   i. decreased taste sensation

Case Study

Mrs. D. is a 45-year-old female who sought care for chronic insomnia of 15 months' duration. Various hypnotics had been unsuccessful. She was pleasant and well-informed and responded appropriately during the recording of the health history.

Her history revealed that about 18 months earlier some important life changes occurred. Her only child, a daughter, left for an out-of-state university. A lifelong friend, who was a confidante, moved to another community. Her husband, a successful dentist, had become more involved in various men's organizations than in the past. She stated that she awakes 15 to 20 times a night and rarely sleeps more than four hours. A sedating antidepressant was prescribed and a second appointment was made for 10 days later.

On the second appointment, which lasted one hour, she noted her sleep pattern had improved. She was able to articulate that she felt unneeded, incompetent, and old.

As an allied health caregiver, how do you assess Mrs. D.'s case?

Concepts of Neurologic Dysfunction

Prerequisite Objectives

a. Identify the structural modulators of consciousness.
   Review text page 404; refer to Figure 12-5.

Remember !

- The reticular activating system (RAS) affects many CNS activities including sleep and wakefulness. It ascends from the lower brain stem through the midbrain and thalamus and projects throughout the cerebral cortex. Following prolonged wakefulness, the neurons in the RAS gradually fatigue and become less excitable. In this circumstance, neuronal mechanisms revert to lower level functioning and sleep. The ability to respond to stimuli or arousal depends on an intact RAS in the brain stem and the ability to respond to the environment. Cognition relies on an intact cerebral cortex. Therefore, consciousness or responsiveness to impressions made by the senses requires functioning along the reticular formation in the brain stem to the cerebral cortex.

---

b. Identify the structure and functional components of the brain.
   Review text pages 404-410.

Remember!

- The central nervous system (CNS) consists of the brain and spinal cord encased within the meninges and bathed in cerebrospinal fluid (CSF). The brain is divided into several areas, including the cerebrum, midbrain, cerebellum, and medulla oblongata. The midbrain, the medulla, and pons comprise the brain stem.

- The outer covering of the cerebrum is the cortex. The entire cerebrum is divided into two halves or hemispheres connected by a neural bridge, the corpus callosum. The cortex is concerned with thinking and sensory perception. Emotional responses and control of body temperature, water and food intake, and sex drive have their origin in the midbrain area. The cerebellum primarily integrates muscular movements to produce coordination in walking, talking, and other complex muscular activities. The medulla oblongata controls vital functions such as respiration, heart rate, and blood pressure, although these are modified by higher brain centers.

(Continued)

---

c. Identify the parts of the CNS that control voluntary muscle movement.
Review text page 407; refer to Figure 12-9.

Objectives

After successful study of this chapter, the learner will be able to:

1. Define terms describing levels of consciousness.
Refer to Table 14-3.

Consciousness is alertness with orientation to person, place, and time. The individual has normal speech, voluntary movement, and oculomotor activity. **Confusion** is an alteration in perception of stimuli. First, there is disorientation to time, then to place, and eventually to person. The attention span is shortened. **Lethargy** exhibits orientation to person, place, and time. However, slow vocalization, decreased motor skills, and oculomotor activity are present. **Obtundation** is awakening in response to stimulation. Continuous stimulation is needed for arousal. Eyes are usually closed. **Stupor** is vocalization only, in response to painful stimuli. Markedly decreased spontaneous movement with eyes closed is seen. **Coma** displays no vocalization, no spontaneous eye movement, and no arousal to any stimulus; however, brain stem reflexes are intact.

2. Identify sites and causes for alterations in arousal.
Study text page 478; refer to Tables 14-1 and 14-2.

Possible causes of an **altered level of arousal** may be separated into three major groups: structural, metabolic, and psychogenic. Structural causes are divided according to five locations of the pathology: (1) supratentorial, meaning above the tentorium cerebelli; (2) infratentorial, meaning below the tentorium cerebelli; (3) subdural; (4) extracerebral; and (5) intracerebral.

Supratentorial processes produce a decreased level of consciousness because of encephalitis, brain stem trauma, or cerebral vascular accident or by impairing function of the thalamic or hypothalamic activating systems. **Infratentorial processes** produce a reduction in arousal by cerebrovascular disease, demyelinating diseases, neoplasms, granulomas, abscesses, and head injuries which destroy the brain stem. Decreased level of consciousness may also be caused by compression of the reticular activating system. Specific causes of compression of the brain stem include hematoma, hemorrhage, and aneurysm; cerebellar hemorrhage, infarcts, abscesses and neoplasms; and demyelinating disorders. **Extracerebral disorders** include neoplasms, closed-head trauma with subsequent bleeding, and subdural accumulation of pus. **Intracerebral disorders** manifest as masses. These disorders include bleeding, infarcts and emboli, and tumors.

A wide spectrum of diseases may produce a metabolically induced alteration in arousal. In these disorders, there is widespread direct or indirect interference with neuronal metabolism throughout much of the brain.

Psychogenic unresponsiveness may develop in general psychiatric disorders. Despite apparent unconsciousness, the person is actually physiologically awake.

3. **Summarize the changes in levels of consciousness, pupillary response, muscle tone, and respiratory activity as the diencephalon through the medulla is affected.**
   Study text pages 478-487; refer to Figures 14-1 through 14-5 and Tables 14-4 through 14-6.

Rostral-Caudal Progression of Nonresponsiveness

Area Involved	Level of Consciousness	Pupils	Muscle Tone	Respiration
Diencephalon (thalamus/ hypothalamus)	Decreased concentration, agitation, dullness, lethargy, obtundation	Respond to light briskly; Full-range eye movements only on "doll's eyes" — none in direction of rotation or after injection of hot or cold water in ear canal (caloric posturing)	Some purposeful movement in response to pain, combative movement Decorticate — flexion in upper extremities and extension in lower extremities	Yawning and sighing to Cheyne-Stokes
Midbrain	Stupor to coma	Midposition fixed (MPF)	Decerebrate— arms rigid, palms turned away from body	Neurogenic hyperventilation
Pons	Coma	MPF	Decerebrate	Apneustic— prolonged inspiration and expiration
Medulla	Coma	MPF	Flaccid	Atactic— uncoordinated and irregular

4. Distinguish between cerebral death and brain death.

Study text page 486.

Cerebral death, or irreversible coma, is death of the cerebral hemispheres, exclusive of the brain stem and cerebellum. The individual is permanently unable to respond in any significant way to the environment. The brain may continue to maintain normal respiratory and cardiovascular functions, normal temperature control, and normal gastrointestinal function.

Brain death occurs when irreversible brain damage is so extensive that the brain can no longer maintain the body's internal respiratory and cardiac vascular functions. There is destruction of the brain stem and cerebellum.

5. Define seizure and cite conditions associated with seizure disorders.

Study text pages 487-490; refer to Tables 14-7 and 14-9.

A **seizure** is a sudden, explosive disorderly discharge of cerebral neurons and is characterized by a sudden, transient alteration in brain function, usually involving motor, sensory, autonomic, or psychic clinical manifestations and an alteration in levels of arousal. The alteration in level of arousal is temporary. Among the causes of seizure activity are:

Metabolic defects
    hyperthermia
    hypoglycemia
    uremia
Congenital malformation
Genetic predisposition
Perinatal injury
Postnatal trauma
Motor syndromes
Epilepsy
Infection
    meningitis
Brain tumor
Vascular disease
    stroke
Overhydration

An **epileptogenic focus** appears to be a group of neurons having lost their afferent stimulation. The plasma membranes of these neuronal cells appear to be more permeable. This makes them more easily activated by hyperthermia, hypoxia, hypoglycemia, hyponatremia, repeated sensory stimulation, and certain sleep phases. These neurons are hypersensitive and may even remain in a chronic, partially depolarized state. The neural excitation spreads to the subcortical, thalamic, and brain stem areas to initiate the phase of muscle contraction which is followed by increased muscle tone and loss of consciousness.

The phase of alternating contraction and relaxation of muscles begins as inhibitory neurons in the cortex, anterior thalamus, and basal ganglia begin to inhibit the cortical excitation. This inhibition interrupts seizure discharge and produces an intermittent contract-relax pattern of muscle contractions.

Status epilepticus is the occurrence of a second, a third, or multiple seizures before the person has fully regained consciousness from the preceding seizure. Status epilepticus most frequently results from abrupt discontinuation of antiseizure medications but may also occur in untreated or inadequately treated persons with seizure disorders. The situation is serious because of developing cerebral hypoxia.

6. Differentiate between partial and generalized seizures.

Refer to Tables 14-8 and 14-10.

Common Epileptic Seizure Types

Disorder	Areas Involved	Change in Consciousness	Impaired Capacities/ Symptoms
Partial			
Jacksonian	Unilateral — motor strip on precentral gyrus in frontal lobe	Unilateral — no change in consciousness; bilateral — loss of consciousness	Disturbance in motor capacity, seizure activity marches along limb or side of body in orderly progression
Psychomotor	Unilateral — temporal lobe	No loss of consciousness; confusion, amnesia	Hallucinations, dyscognitive states, automatism, loss of awareness
Generalized			
Generalized clonic (grand mal)	Bilateral — multifocal subcortical or deeper	Loss of consciousness with postictal sleeping	Aura of odor, taste, or light; major tonic muscular contraction followed by longer phase of contractions; possible bowel and bladder control loss; weakness; injury; learning disorders
Absence (petit mal)	Bilateral — multifocal subcortical or deeper	Transient losses of consciousness, no postictal state	Interference with conscious response to environment; possible learning disorders; a triad: blank spells, akinetic seizures, myoclonic jerks

7. Define descriptive terms of cognitive deficits.

Refer to Table 14-11.

Selective attention deficit refers to the inability to select appropriately from available, competing environmental and internal stimuli for conscious processing.

Dysmnesia/amnesia is a disorder of recent memory. Retrograde amnesia is the loss of past memories. Anterograde amnesia is an inability to form new memories.

A **remote memory deficit** manifests as an agnosia, or an inability to recognize sensory input as sounds, sight, or touch.

A **concept-formation deficit** is the inability to analyze the relationships between objects and their properties in order to reach a generalization; individual cannot abstract.

A **vigilance deficit** is the inability to concentrate over time or to maintain sustained attention; individual cannot concentrate.

A **reasoning deficit** is the inability to understand relationships, identify essential parts, synthesize the parts, and arrive at a common theme.

Executive function deficit prevents overseer functions, systems of programming, verification, and correction.

Generally, the primary pathophysiological mechanism that operates in cognitive system disorders is direct destruction of the hippocampus, located in the lateral ventricle of the brain. The disorders are due directly to ischemia and hypoxia or indirectly to compression, toxins, and chemicals.

8. Characterize dementing processes; describe Alzheimer disease.

Study text pages 504-506; refer to Table 14-16.

Intellectual function is impaired in the **dementing process.** The result may be a decrease in orientation, general knowledge and information, vigilance, recent memory, remote memory, concept formation, abstraction, reasoning, executive functions, judgment, insight, and interpretation. Because of declining intellectual ability, the individual exhibits alterations in behavior. The culmination of a progressive dementing process is nerve cell degeneration and brain atrophy.

Mechanisms in dementing processes include tissue destruction, compression, inflammation, and biochemical imbalances. Acetylcholine is needed for recent memory at the biochemical level. As the level of acetylcholine is reduced, the individual stores less and less information until all recent memory is lost. Slow-growing viruses are likely associated with some unexplained dementias. A genetic predisposition is probably a contributing factor to the dementing process.

If a specific treatable cause is identified, the appropriate treatment is initiated. For example, an infectious process requires the appropriate antibiotic and a potentially resectable mass may require neurosurgery. Nutritional deficiencies should be corrected. If the cause is metabolic, the imbalance requires correction and/or the metabolic disorder is treated.

Unfortunately, most progressive dementias have no specific treatment or cure for the process. In such instances, therapy is directed at maintaining and maximizing use of the remaining capacities, restoring functions, if possible, and accommodating lost abilities.

Alzheimer disease is one of the most common causes of severe cognitive dysfunction in older persons. The exact cause of Alzheimer disease is unknown. Several possible theories are notable, including loss of neurotransmitter stimulation by choline acetyltransferase, mutation for encoding amyloid precursor protein, and alteration in apolipoprotein E which binds beta amyloid. Early-onset familial Alzheimer disease (FAD) includes gene defects on chromosomes 14, 19, and possibly 21. Late-onset FAD is linked to a defect on chromosome 19. Each of these mechanisms may be linked to aggregation and precipitation of insoluble amyloid or senile plaques in brain tissue and blood vessels. Alzheimer disease has also been linked to a lysosomal pathway in the breakdown of amyloid precursor protein to yield beta amyloid, a neurotoxic substance. A reduction in protein kinase C (PKC) and the scavenging of phospholipid from the cell membrane are being studied as the cause of the lysosomal pathway mechanisms.

Antibrain antibodies may account for Alzheimer disease; an autoimmune etiology is also being investigated. Aging and injury decrease oxygen and glucose transport, impair the blood-brain barrier, and cause mitochondrial defects that alter cell metabolism and processing of amyloid proteins. Familial risk appears to be greatest in families affected by the classic early onset of Alzheimer disease. The risk when a sibling develops Alzheimer disease after age 70 does not differ from that of the general population.

Microscopically, the protein in the neurons becomes distorted and twisted, forming a tangle called a **neurofibrillary tangle**. These abnormal protein fibers accumulate within the neurons. Groups of nerve cells, especially terminal axons, degenerate and coalesce around an amyloid core. These areas appear like plaques and are called **senile plaques**. These plaques disrupt nerve impulse transmission. Senile plaques and neurofibrillary tangles are more concentrated in the cerebral cortex and hippocampus. The greater the number of senile plaques and neurofibrillary tangles, the more dysfunction. Essentially, the dementing process noted earlier will develop.

Dyspraxias, or the inability to perform coordinated acts, may appear. Motor changes may occur if the posterior frontal lobes are involved. The individual may exhibit rigidity with flexion posturing, propulsion, and retropulsion. There is great variability in age of onset, intensity and sequence of symptoms and in location and extent of brain pathology among individuals with the disease.

9. Characterize the stages of increased intracranial pressure; describe herniation syndrome.

Study text pages 506-508; refer to Figure 14-9.

Increased intracranial pressure may result from an increase in intracranial content which occurs with tumor growth, edema, excess cerebrospinal fluid, or hemorrhage. Since the cranial vault is a nonflexible encasement around the brain and its extracellular fluid, a rise in intracranial pressure from one component requires an equal reduction in volume of other components. The most readily displaced content of the cranial vault is cerebrospinal fluid (CSF). In Stage 1 of intracranial hypertension, vasoconstriction and external compression of the venous system occurs in an attempt to decrease further the intracranial pressure following CSF displacement from the cranial vault. Clinical manifestations at this stage are subtle and transient and include confusion, drowsiness, and slight pupillary and breathing changes.

With continued expansion of the intracranial content, the resulting increase in intracranial pressure may exceed the brain's compensatory capacity to adjust to the increasing pressure. In this state, Stage 2, the pressure begins to compromise neuronal oxygenation. Systemic arterial vasoconstriction occurs to elevate the systemic blood pressure sufficiently to overcome the increased intracranial pressure.

Intracranial pressure begins to approach arterial pressure and the brain tissues begin to experience hypoxia and hypercapnia. Cheyne-Stokes respiration occurs, pupils become sluggish and dilated, pulse pressure widens, and bradycardia develops. Accumulating CO_2 causes vasodilation at the local tissue level. The hydrostatic pressure in the vessels drops, and blood volume increases. The brain volume increases, and intracranial pressure continues to rise. This is Stage 3 of intracranial hypertension. Cerebral perfusion pressure falls and cerebral perfusion slows dramatically; the brain tissues experience severe hypoxia and acidosis.

In the last stage of intracranial hypertension, Stage 4, brain tissue shifts or **herniates** from the compartment of greater pressure to a compartment of lesser pressure. The herniated brain tissues increase the content volume within the lower pressure compartment, exerting pressure on the brain tissue that normally occupies that compartment; now, both the herniated and lower tissue's blood supply is impaired. Mean systolic arterial pressure soon equals intracranial pressure, and cerebral blood flow ceases.

Two types of herniation syndromes exist, supratentorial and infratentorial, based on whether they are located above or below the tentorium. The tentorium divides the cerebrum from the cerebellum.

Supratentorial herniation occurs when brain tissue shifts through the tentorial notch into the posterior fossa and presses on the third cranial nerve. Infratentorial herniation occurs as cerebellar tonsils shift inferiorly through the foramen magnum because of increased pressure within the posterior fossa. The clinical manifestations of supratentorial and infratentorial herniation syndromes vary and may be manifested as identified in Objective 3.

10. Describe the pathogenesis of cerebral edema.

Study text pages 508-509; refer to Figure 14-10.

Cerebral edema is an increase of extracellular or intracellular fluid within the brain after brain insult from trauma, infection, hemorrhage, tumor, ischemia, infarct, or hypoxia. Cerebral edema will distort blood vessels, displace brain tissues, and eventually herniate brain tissue from one brain compartment to another. The four types of cerebral edema are (1) vasogenic edema, (2) cytotoxic (metabolic) edema, (3) ischemic edema, and (4) interstitial edema.

Vasogenic edema is clinically the most important type. It is caused by the increased permeability of the capillary endothelium of the brain after injury to the vascular structure. Plasma proteins leak into the extracellular spaces, drawing water to them, and the water content of the brain parenchyma increases. Vasogenic edema starts in the area of injury and spreads with preferential accumulation in the white matter of the ipsilateral side because the parallel myelinated fibers separate more easily.

In **cytotoxic (metabolic) edema,** toxic factors directly affect the neuronal, glial, and endothelial cells, causing failure of the active transport systems. The cells lose their potassium and gain larger amounts of sodium. Water follows by osmosis into the cell, causing the cells to swell. Cytotoxic edema principally occurs in the gray matter.

Ischemic edema follows cerebral infarction. Soon after the onset of ischemia, the initial edema is confined to the intracellular compartment. Later in the process, brain cells begin to undergo necrosis and die. The released lysosomes increase the blood-brain barrier's permeability by lyzing it.

Interstitial edema is caused by movement of cerebrospinal fluid from the ventricles into the extracellular spaces of the brain tissues. The brain fluid volume is mostly increased around the ventricles.

11. Define common terms that describe alterations in motor functions.

Refer to Tables 14-17, 14-18, 14-20, 14-21, and 14-23.

Movements are influenced by the cerebral cortex, the pyramidal system, the extrapyramidal system, and the motor units. Dysfunction in any of these areas may cause motor dysfunction.

Hypotonia is decreased muscle tone shown by passive movement of a muscle against resistance. It is thought to be due to decreased muscle spindle activity secondary to decreased excitability of neurons. Hypotonia is caused by cerebellar damage or in rare cases by pyramidal tract damage.

Hypertonia is increased muscle tone shown by passive movement of a muscle with resistance. Spasticity, a type of hypertonia, results from hyperexcitability of the stretch reflexes and is associated with damage to the motor, premotor, and supplementary motor areas and lateral corticospinal tracts. Rigidity, another hypertonic, is produced by tonic reflex activity. The involved muscles are firm and tense; the increase in muscle movement is even and uniform throughout the range of passive movement.

Hyperkinesia is excessive movement; whereas **dyskinesias** are abnormal, involuntary movements.

Hypokinesia, or decreased movement, is a loss of voluntary movement despite consciousness and normal peripheral nerve and muscle function. Types of hypokinesia include paresis/paralysis, akinesia, bradykinesia, and loss of associated movement.

Hemiparesis/hemiplegia is paresis/paralysis of the upper and lower extremity on one side. **Diplegia** is the paralysis of both upper and lower extremities due to cerebral hemisphere injuries. **Paraparesis/paraplegia** refers to weakness/paralysis of the lower extremities. **Quadriparesis/quadriplegia** refers to paresis/paralysis of all four extremities. Both paraparesis/paraplegia and quadriparesis/quadriplegia may be caused by dysfunction of the spinal cord.

When the pyramidal system is destroyed below the level of the pons, **spinal shock** occurs. It is the complete cessation of spinal cord functions below the lesion. It is characterized by complete flaccid paralysis, absence of reflexes, and marked disturbances in bowel and bladder function.

Lower motor syndrome originating in the anterior horn cells or the motor nuclei of the cranial nerves are called **amyotrophies.** Paralytic poliomyelitis is the prototype of these disorders. In the amyotrophies, muscle strength, muscle tone, and muscle bulk are affected in the muscles innervated by the involved motor neurons. Several brain stem syndromes involve damage to one or more of the cranial nerve nuclei. These are called **nuclear palsies** and may be caused by vascular occlusion, tumor, aneurysm, tuberculosis, or hemorrhage.

Akinesia is a decrease in associated and voluntary movements. It is related to dysfunction of the extrapyramidal system. Pathogenesis is related to either a deficiency of dopamine or a defect of the postsynaptic dopamine receptors. **Bradykinesia** is

slowness of voluntary movements. In **hypokinesia,** the normal, habitually associated movements that provide skill, grace, and balance to voluntary movements are lost. An expressionless face, a statuesque posture, absence of speech inflection, and absence of spontaneous gestures are exhibited as well.

Dystonia is the maintenance of abnormal posture through muscular contractions. **Decorticate posture** is characterized by upper extremities flexed at the elbows and held closely to the body and lower extremities that are externally rotated and extended. Decorticate posture is thought to occur when the brain stem, which facilitates the antigravity position, is not inhibited by the motor function of the cerebral cortex. **Decerebrate posture** refers to increased tone in extensor muscles and trunk muscles with active tonic neck reflexes. The decerebrate posture is caused by severe injury to the brain and brain stem. **Basal ganglion posture** refers to a stooped, hyperflexed posture with a narrow-based, short-stepped gait. **Senile posture** is characterized by an increasingly flexed posture similar to a basal ganglion posture. The posture is associated with frontal lobe dysfunction.

A **spastic gait** is associated with unilateral, pyramidal injury and is manifested by a shuffling gait with the leg extended and held stiff. This gait causes a scraping over the walking surface. A **scissors gait** is associated with bilateral pyramidal injury and spasticity. The legs are abducted, so the legs touch each other. A **cerebellar gait** manifests as a wide-based gait with the feet apart and often turned outward and inward for greater stability. Cerebellar dysfunction accounts for this particular gait. A **basal ganglion gait** is a broad-based gait. Small steps are taken, and there is a decreased arm swing when walking. The individual's head and body are flexed, the arms are semiflexed and abducted, whereas the legs are flexed and rigid in more advanced states. Basal ganglion and frontal lobe dysfunction, respectively, account for these two gaits.

Hypermimesia is most commonly manifested as pathological laughter or crying. Pathological laughter is associated with right hemisphere injury, whereas pathological crying is associated with left hemisphere injury. **Hypomimesia** is manifested as aprosodias, or the loss of emotional language. Aprosodias involve an inability to understand emotion in speech and facial expression. Aprosodias are associated with right hemisphere damage.

Dyspraxia/apraxia is the inability to perform purposeful or skilled motor acts in the absence of paralysis, sensory loss, abnormal posture and tone, abnormal involuntary movement, incoordination, or inattentiveness. Dyspraxias arise when the connecting pathways between the left and right cortical areas are interrupted; conceptualization and execution of a complex motor act is impaired.

12. Differentiate between pyramidal and extrapyramidal motor syndromes, and upper motor neuron and lower motor neuron or motor unit syndromes.

Refer to Tables 14-19 and 14-22.

Pyramidal and Extrapyramidal Motor Syndromes

	Pyramidal motor syndrome	*Extrapyramidal motor syndrome*
Unilateral movement	Paralysis	Little or no paralysis
Tendon reflexes	Increased	Normal or slightly increased
Involuntary movements	Absent	Presence of tremor, chorea, or dystonia
Muscle tone	General spasticity in muscles; hypertonia present in flexors of arms and extensors of legs	Possible rigidity or intermittent rigidity

Motor Neuron Syndromes

	Upper motor neuron syndrome	*Lower motor neuron and motor unit syndromes*
Affected muscles	Muscle groups; when movement is possible, relationship among agonists, antagonists, synergists, and fixators is preserved	Individual muscles
Muscle tone	Hypertonia, spasticity	Hypotonia, flaccidity
Tendon reflexes	Hyperreflexia	Hyporeflexia
Atrophy	Slight, due to disuse	Pronounced
Fasciculations	Absent	May be present

97

Practice Examination

Match the term with its characteristic.

1. confusion
2. coma

    a. orientation to person, time, and place
    b. slow vocalization, decreased oculomotor activity
    c. altered stimuli perception
    d. vocalization in response to pain stimuli
    e. no arousal

3. Supratentorial processes produce reductions in arousal by
    a. developing the reticular activating system.
    b. encephalitis.
    c. destroying the brain stem.
    d. Both a and c are correct.
    e. None of the above is correct.

4. An individual shows flexion in upper extremities and extensions in lower extremities. This is
    a. decorticate posturing.
    b. decerebate posturing.
    c. excitation posturing.
    d. caloric posturing.

5. Cerebral death
    a. is death of the cerebellum.
    b. maintains normal respiratory and cardiovascular functions.
    c. no longer maintains respiratory and cardiovascular functions.
    d. is death of the brain stem.

6. Precipitating causes of seizure include all except
    a. meningitis.
    b. stroke.
    c. hyperglycemia.
    d. hyperthermia.
    e. All of the above are correct.

7. Which epileptic seizure is characterized by temporal lobe spikes in the EEG?
    a. autonomic
    b. status epilepticus
    c. absence
    d. Jacksonian
    e. psychomotor

8. Postictal sleeping can be seen in _____ seizures.
    a. partial
    b. unilateral
    c. absence
    d. grand mal
    e. psychomotor

Match the term with its chacteristic.

9. amnesia
10. agnosia
11. vigilance deficit

    a. inability to understand relationships
    b. inability to verify and correct input
    c. inability to concentrate
    d. inability to recognize sound
    e. inability to form new memories

12. Late-onset familial Alzheimer disease is linked to a deficit on chromosome
    a. 14.
    b. 19.
    c. 21.
    d. 23.
    e. All of the above are likely.

13. The senile plagues and neurofibrillary tangles of Alzheimer disease are mostly concentrated in the
    a. cerebral cortex and hippocampus.
    b. thalamus.
    c. cerebellum.
    d. basal ganglia.

14. An individual with increased intracranial pressure from a head injury shows dilated and sluggish pupils, widened pulse pressure, and bradycardia. What stage of ICP exists?
    a. stage 1
    b. stage 2
    c. stage 3
    d. stage 4

15. Infratentorial herniation occurs in
    a. shifting of the mesencephalon.
    b. shifting of the diencephalon.
    c. shifting of the cerebellum.
    d. Both a and b are correct.
    e. None of the above is correct.

16. In cerebral vasogenic edema,
    a. active transport fails.
    b. there is autodigestion.
    c. plasma proteins leak into extracellular spaces.
    d. cerebrospinal fluid leaves the ventricles.

17. Which is not true of increasing intracranial pressures?
    a. Accumulating CO_2 causes vasoconstriction.
    b. Hydrostatic pressure in the vessels drops.
    c. The blood volume in the vessels increases.
    d. Brain tissue shifts from the compartment of greater pressure to one of lesser pressure.
    e. Both b and c are correct.

18. Intellectual function is impaired in the dementing process. Which intellectual function is not impaired?
    a. recent memory
    b. remote memory
    c. abstraction
    d. interpretation
    e. All of the above functions are impaired.

Match the term with its definition or characteristic.

19. hypotonia
20. rigidity
21. hemiparesis
22. akinesia
23. senile posture
24. dyspraxia
25. lower motor neuron syndrome

a. paralysis of both upper and lower extremities
b. difficult initiation of spontaneous and voluntary movements
c. absence of spontaneous gestures
d. abnormal posture maintained through muscular contractions
e. frontal lobe dysfunction
f. impaired conceptualization and execution of complex acts
g. individual muscles affected
h. involuntary writing movements
i. organically caused impairment of intellectual functions
j. cerebellar damage
k. toxic reflex activity
l. upper and lower extremity paralysis on same side

Case Study

A 12-year-old male complained of strange odors prior to loss of consciousness and major tonic-clonic seizure. During the seizure he lost bladder and bowel control, and his parents rushed him to an emergency room of a local hospital. On arrival at the hospital, he appeared to be asleep. No neurological signs associated with focal areas of the brain were found.

Studies at the hospital showed routine laboratory work within normal limits (WNL), lumbar puncture (CSF) was WNL, no evidence of skull fracture on x-ray study was revealed, and an electroencephalograph (EEG) showed no increase or decrease in the size and frequency of voltage function.

How would you interpret the episode and findings?

CHAPTER 15

Alterations of Neurological Functions

Prerequisite Objectives

a. Identify the protective structures of the central nervous system.
   Review text pages 412-415.

Remember!

- The cranium is composed of eight bones that fuse early in childhood. The cranial vault encloses and protects the brain and its associated structures. The floor of the cranial vault is irregular and contains many foramina or openings for cranial nerves, blood vessels, and the spinal cord to exit. The foramen magnum is large enough for the spinal cord to exit. Surrounding the brain and spinal cord are three protective membranes called the meninges: the dura mater, the arachnoid membrane, and the pia mater.

- The dura mater is composed of two layers and has venous sinuses between the layers. The outermost dural layer forms the periosteum of the skull. The inner dural meningeal layer forms the rigid plates that support and separate various brain structures.

- One of these membranous plates, the falx cerebri, transverses between the two cerebral hemispheres and anchors the base of the brain to the ethmoid bone. The tentorium cerebelli is a membrane that surrounds the brain stem and separates the cerebellum from the cerebral structures.

- Below the dura mater lies the arachnoid membrane, that is characterized by its spongy weblike structure. The space between the dura and arachnoid membrane is the subdural space. Many small bridging veins traverse the subdural space. The subarachnoid space between the arachnoid membrane and the pia mater contains cerebrospinal fluid. The delicate pia mater provides support for blood vessels serving brain tissue. The choroid plexuses, structures that produce cerebrospinal fluid, arise from the pial membrane. The spinal cord is anchored to the vertebrae by extension of the meninges. Between the dura mater and skull is a potential space, the epidural space.

- Cerebrospinal fluid (CSF) is a clear, colorless fluid similar to blood plasma and interstitial fluid. It cushions the CNS's soft tissues from traumatic jolts and blows because of the CSF's buoyant properties. The choroid plexuses in the lateral, third, and fourth ventricles produce the major portion of CSF.

b. Describe the blood supply to the brain.
   Review text pages 416-420; refer to Figures 12-18, 12-19, and 12-21.

Remember!

- The brain receives approximately 20 percent of the cardiac output, or 800 to 1000 ml of blood flow per minute. Carbon dioxide is a potent vasodilator in the CNS and ensures an adequate cerebral blood supply. The brain derives its arterial supply from two systems: the internal carotid arteries and the vertebral arteries.

- The internal carotid arteries originate from the common carotid arteries, enter the cranium through the base of the skull, and pass through the cavernous sinus. After giving off some small branches, they divide into the anterior and middle cerebral arteries. The vertebral arteries originate at the subclavian arteries and pass through the transverse foramina of the cervical vertebrae and enter the cranium through the foramen magnum. They join to form the basilar artery. The basilar artery divides at the level of the midbrain to form paired posterior cerebral arteries. Superficial arteries supply small branches that project into the brain. The circle of Willis is a structure having the ability to provide collateral blood flow. It is formed by many communicating arteries that extend to various brain structures.

- The venous drainage of the brain stem and cerebellum parallels the arterial supply; the venous drainage of the cerebrum does not. The cerebral veins are classified as superficial and deep. The veins drain into venous plexuses and dural sinuses and eventually drain into the internal jugular veins at the base of the skull. The blood-brain barrier selectively inhibits certain substances in the blood from entering the interstitial spaces of the brain or CSF. It is believed that the supporting cells and tight junctions between endothelial cells are involved in the formation of the blood-brain barrier and are responsible for its impermeability.

---

c. State the functions of the parts and associated structures of the brain.
   Review text pages 404-410.

Remember!

Structural Functions of the Brain

Structure	Function
Brain stem	Performs sensory, motor, and reflex functions; controls cardiac, vasomotor, and respiratory centers; cranial nerve reflex
Cerebellum	Coordinates the activities of groups of muscles, maintains equilibrium, controls posture
Diencephalon	
Thalamus	Conscious recognition of crude pain, temperature, and touch; relays sensory impulses except smell to cerebrum, emotions, arousal mechanism, complex reflex movements
Hypothalamus	Links nervous system to endocrine system; coordinates ANS; controls body temperature, hunger, thirst, and sleep

(Continued)

Remember! *(cont'd)*

Structure	Function
Cerebrum	
Cerebral cortex lobes	
Frontal	Voluntary control of skeletal muscles, unconscious skeletal muscle movement, speaking and writing
Temporal	Interpretation of odor and sound
Parietal	General body sensations
Occipital	Interpretation of sight
All lobes	Memory, emotions, reasoning, and intelligence
Left hemisphere	Language, numerical skills, controls right side of body
Right hemisphere	Musical and artistic awareness, space and pattern perception, insight, controls left side of body

d. Cite some examples of neurotransmitters.
    Review text pages 402-404.

Remember!

Neurotransmitters

Neurotransmitter	Location	Function
Acetylcholine	Junctions with motor effectors, many parts of brain	Excitatory or inhibitory memory
Amines		
Serotonin	CNS	Mostly inhibitory, moods and emotions, sleep
Histamine	Brain	Most excitatory, emotions, body temperature, water balance
Dopamine	Brain in autonomic system	Mostly inhibitory emotions/moods, motor control
Epinephrine	CNS, sympathetic division of ANS	Excitatory or inhibitory
Norepinephrine	CNS, sympathetic division of ANS	Excitatory or inhibitory

(Continued)

Neurotransmitter	Location	Function
Amino acids		
Glutamate (glutamic acid)	CNS	Excitatory
Gamma-aminobutyric acid (GABA)	Brain	Inhibitory
Glycine	Spinal cord	Inhibitory
Neuropeptides		
Substance P	Brain, spinal cord, sensory pain pathways, gastrointestinal tract	Mostly excitatory, transmits pain information
Enkephalins	Several regions of CNS, retina, intestinal tract	Mostly inhibitory, blocks pain
Endorphins	Several regions of CNS, retina, intestinal tract	Mostly inhibitory, blocks pain

Note: These are examples only; most of the neurotransmitters are also found in other locations and many have additional functions.

Objectives

After successful study of this chapter, the learner will be able to:

1. Differentiate between concussion and contusion, and epidural, subdural, and intracerebral hematomas.

Study text pages 527-536; refer to Figures 15-1 through 15-7 and Tables 15-1 and 15-2.

Traumatic brain injuries are broadly categorized into blunt or closed trauma and open or penetrating trauma. In blunt trauma, the head strikes a hard surface or a rapidly moving object strikes the head. The dura remains intact and brain tissues are not exposed to the environment. Blunt trauma may result in both focal brain injuries and diffuse axonal injuries. When a break in the dura exposes the cranial contents to the environment, open trauma has occurred. Open trauma results in focal brain injuries.

Diffuse brain injury or diffuse axonal injury (DAI) results from the inertial force to the head; it is associated with high levels of acceleration and deceleration. Severity of the diffuse injury correlates with how much shearing force is applied to the brain stem. In DAI, increased intravascular blood within the brain, vasodilation, and increased cerebral blood volume are frequently seen. Several categories of diffuse brain injury exist: mild concussion, classical concussion, mild DAI, moderate DAI, and severe DAI.

Mild concussion involves temporary axonal disturbances. Cerebral cortical dysfunction related to attentional and memory systems result and consciousness is not lost.

Classical cerebral concussion causes diffuse cerebral disconnection from the brain stem reticular activating system; it is neurologic dysfunction without substantial anatomical disruption. This disconnection results in the immediate loss of consciousness which lasts more than six hours.

In **mild DAI**, post-traumatic coma lasts six to 24 hours. Death is uncommon but residual cognitive, psychological, and sensorimotor deficits may persist.

In **moderate DAI**, widespread physiological impairment exists throughout the cerebral cortex and diencephalon. Actual tearing of some axons in both hemispheres occurs. Basal skull fracture is commonly associated with moderate DAI. Prolonged coma lasting more than 24 hours is present and recovery is often incomplete in surviving individuals.

Severe DAI, formally called primary brain stem injury or brain stem contusion, involves severe mechanical disruption of many axons in both cerebral hemispheres and those extending to the diencephalon and brain stem.

Focal brain injury involves specific, grossly observable brain lesions seen in cortical contusions, epidural hemorrhage, subdural hematoma, and intracerebral hematoma. The force of impact typically produces **contusions** or bruises on the brain. The contusion, in turn, produces epidural hemorrhage, subdural, and intracerebral hematomas. Contusion and bleeding occur because of small tears in blood vessels resulting from these forces. The smaller the area of impact, the greater the severity of injury because the force is concentrated into a smaller area. The focal injury may be coup or contrecoup. **Coup** is the direct impact area. **Contrecoup** lies opposite the line of force; the lesions occur where the brain strikes hard tissue on the opposite side.

DAI is associated with physical, cognitive, psychological/behavioral, and social consequences. Spastic paralysis, peripheral nerve injury, swallowing disorders, dysarthria, visual and hearing impairments, and taste and smell deficits are some of the physical consequences. Common cognitive deficits include disorientation and confusion, short attention span, memory deficits, learning difficulties, dysphasia, poor judgment, and perceptual deficits. Behavioral disorders that emerge include agitation, impulsivity, blunted affect, social withdrawal, and depression.

The clinical manifestations of a contusion may include immediate loss of consciousness, loss of reflexes, transient cessation of respiration, brief period of bradycardia, and fall in blood pressure. Vital signs may stabilize in a few seconds. Reflexes return next and the person begins to regain consciousness. Returning to full alertness takes variable periods of time from minutes to days. Large contusions and lacerations with hemorrhage may be surgically excised. Otherwise treatment is directed at controlling intracranial pressure and managing symptoms.

Extradural hematomas, also epidural hematomas or epidural hemorrhages, most often have an artery as the source of bleeding. Extradural hemorrhages may result in herniation of the posterior fossa contents through the foramen magnum.

Tearing of the bridging veins is the major cause of rapidly developing and subacutely developing **subdural hematomas**. However, torn cortical veins or venous sinuses and contused tissue may be the source of the bleeding. The subdural space gradually fills with blood, and herniation can result.

In **intracerebral hematomas,** small blood vessels are traumatized by shearing forces. The intracerebral hematoma expands and increases intracranial pressure with compression of brain tissues.

Individuals with classic temporal extradural hematomas lose consciousness at the time of injury; some lucid periods follow. As the hematoma mass accumulates, a headache of increasing severity, vomiting, drowsiness, confusion, seizure, and hemiparesis may develop. Level of consciousness declines rapidly as the temporal lobe herniation begins. Clinical manifestations of temporal lobe herniation also include ipsilateral pupillary dilation and contralateral hemiparesis. Surgical therapy evacuates the hematoma through burr holes followed by ligation of the bleeding vessel(s).

An acute subdural hematoma classically begins with headache, drowsiness, restlessness or agitation, slowed cognition, and confusion. These symptoms worsen over time and progress to loss of consciousness, respiratory pattern changes, and pupillary dilatation. Most persons with chronic subdural hematomas appear to have a progressive dementia accompanied by generalized rigidity. Chronic subdural hematomas require a craniotomy to evacuate the gelatinous blood.

In intracerebral hematomas, as the intracranial pressure rises, clinical manifestations of temporal lobe herniation may appear. Delayed intracerebral hematoma results in the following: sudden, rapidly progressive decreased levels of consciousness with pupillary dilatation, breathing pattern changes, hemiplegia, and bilateral positive Babinski reflexes. Evacuation of a singular intracerebral hematoma is occasionally helpful for subcortical white matter hematomas. Otherwise treatment is directed at reducing the intracranial pressure and allowing the hematoma to reabsorb slowly.

2. Discuss pathogenesis and manifestations of spinal cord injuries.

Study text pages 536-542; refer to Figures 15-8 through 15-12 and Tables 15-3 through 15-6.

Spinal cord injuries mostly occur because of vertebral injuries. Traumatic forces injure the vertebral and/or neural tissues by compressing the tissue, pulling or exerting a traction on the tissues, or shearing tissues so that they slide into one another.

Vertebral injuries occur mostly at the first to second cervical, fourth to seventh cervical, and twelfth thoracic to second lumbar vertebrae. These are the most mobile portions of the vertebral column. The cord occupies most of the vertebral canal in these areas and its size makes it more easily injured. Within a few minutes following injury, microscopic hemorrhages appear in the central gray matter and pia-arachnoid. Edema progresses into the white matter impairing the microcirculation of the cord with reduced vascular perfusion and development of metabolic changes in spinal cord tissues including lactate and increasing concentrations of norepinephrine. The elevated norepinephrine levels may produce further ischemia, vascular damage, and necrosis of tissue. Cord swelling increases the individual's degree of dysfunction. In the cervical region cord, swelling may be life-threatening because of impairment of diaphragm function. The traumatized cord is replaced by acellular collagenous tissue usually in three to four weeks. Meninges thicken as part of the scarring process.

Normal activity of the spinal cord cells at and below the level of injury ceases because of the lack of continuous tonic discharges from the brain or brain stem and inhibition of suprasegmental impulses immediately after cord injury. This causes **spinal shock** which is characterized by a complete loss of reflex function in all segments below the level of the lesion. This condition involves all skeletal muscles; bladder, bowel, and sexual function; and autonomic control.

Spinal shock may last for 7 to 20 days following onset; it may persist as long as 3 months. Indications that spinal shock is terminating include the reappearance of reflex activity, hyperreflexia, spasticity, and reflex emptying of the bladder. Loss of motor function and sensory function depends upon the level and degree of injury. Paraplegia or quadriplegia can result. Return of spinal neuron excitability occurs slowly. Either motor, sensory, reflex, and autonomic functions return to normal, or autonomic neural activity in the isolated segment develops.

Autonomic hyperreflexia is a syndrome that may occur at any time after spinal shock resolves. The syndrome is associated with a massive, uncompensated cardiovascular response to stimulation of the sympathetic nervous system. Individuals most likely to be affected have lesions at the T6 level or above. Hyperreflexia involves the stimulation of sensory receptors below the level of the cord injury. The intact autonomic nervous system reflexively responds with an arteriolar spasm that increases blood pressure. Baroreceptors in the cerebral vessels, the carotid sinus, and the aorta sense the hypertension and stimulate the parasympathetic system. The heart rate decreases, but the visceral and peripheral vessels do not dilate because efferent impulses cannot pass through the cord and cardiovascular compensation is incomplete. The most common precipitating cause is a distended bladder or rectum but any sensory stimulation can elicit autonomic hyperreflexia.

For a suspected or confirmed vertebral fracture or dislocation, the immediate intervention is immobilization of the spine to prevent further injury. De-

compression and surgical fixation may be necessary. Corticosteroids are given to decrease secondary cord injury. In cases of autonomic hyperreflexia, intervention must be prompt because cerebrovascular accident is possible. The head of the bed should be elevated and the injurious stimulus should be found and removed. Medications may be used if these measures do not effectively reduce blood pressure.

3. Cite the causes of low back pain; describe a herniated disk.
Study pages 543-546; refer to Figures 15-13 and 15-14.

The local processes involved in **low back pain** range from tension caused by tumors or disk prolapse, bursitis, synovitis, degenerative joint disease, abnormal bone pressures, spinal immobility, and inflammation caused by osteomyelitis, bony fractures, or ligamentous strains. Pain may be referred from viscera or the posterior peritoneum. General processes resulting in low back pain include bone diseases such as osteoporosis or osteomalacia seen in hyperparathyroidism.

The etiology for **degenerative disk disease** includes biochemical and biomechanical alterations of tissue comprising the intervertebral disk. Fibrocartilage replaces the gelatinous mucoid material of the nucleus pulposus as the disk changes with aging; the narrowing disk results in variable segmental instability. The process seems to stabilize when segmental fibrosis results; often, the incidence of back pain decreases also.

Spondylolysis is a structural defect involving the lamia or neural arch of the vertebra. The most common site is the lumbar spine. Heredity plays a significant role and spondylolysis is associated with other congenital spinal defects. As a result of torsional and rotational stress, microfractures occur at the affected site and eventually cause dissolution of the pars interarticularis. **Spondylolisthesis** is caused when a vertebra slides forward in relation to an inferior vertebra. **Spinal stenosis** may represent several conditions ranging from entrapment of a single nerve root in the lateral recess to diffuse central stenosis involving many roots.

Most individuals having acute low back pain benefit from bed rest, analgesic medications, exercises, physical therapy, and education. Surgical treatments include diskectomy and spinal fusions. Individuals with chronic low back pain can be treated with anti-inflammatory and muscle relaxant medications and exercise programs. Spinal surgery has a limited role in curing chronic low back pain.

Herniation of an intervertebral disk is a protrusion of part of the nucleus pulposus through a tear in the fibrous capsule enclosing the gelatinous center of the disk. Rupture of intervertebral disks is usually caused by trauma, degenerative disease, or both. Lifting with the trunk flexed and sudden straining when the back is in an unstable position are the most common causes; males are more affected than females. Most commonly affected are the lumbosacral disks; disk herniation occasionally occurs in the cervical area. The symptoms may be immediate or occur within a few hours or they may take months to years to develop. The pain of a herniated disk in the lumbosacral area radiates along the sciatic nerve over the buttock and into the calf or ankle. With the herniation of a lower cervical disk, paresthesia and pain are present in the upper arm, forearm, and hand according to the affected nerve root distribution.

The conservative therapeutic approach comprises traction, bed rest, heat, and ice to the affected areas and an effective analgesic regimen. The surgical approach is indicated if there is weakness, decreased deep tendon reflexes and bladder/bowel reflexes or if the conservative approach is unsuccessful.

4. Compare and contrast cerebrovascular accidents.

Study text pages 547-553.

Cerebrovascular accidents are classified as thrombotic, embolic, or hemorrhagic. The accidents are vascular in origin but are manifested neurologically. **Thrombotic strokes** arise from arterial occlusions caused by thrombi formed in the intracranial vessels or the arteries supplying the brain.

The risk factors for cerebrovascular occlusive disease are:

hypertension
cigarette smoking
elevated blood cholesterol
elevated triglyceride levels
diabetes mellitus
sedentary lifestyle
hypothyroidism
use of oral contraceptives
sickle cell disease
coagulation disorders
polycythemia vera
arteritis
subclavian steal syndrome
chronic hypoxia
dehydration

The development of a cerebral thrombosis is most frequently attributed to atherosclerosis and inflammatory disease processes that damage arterial walls. Atheromatous plaques tend to form at branchings and curves in the cerebral circulation. Degeneration or bleeding into the vessel wall may cause endothelial damage. Platelets and fibrin adhere to the damaged wall and delicate thrombi form. Small thrombi collect over time; gradual occlusion of the artery occurs. Once the artery is occluded, the thrombus may enlarge lengthwise in the vessel.

Thrombotic strokes may be further subdivided on the basis of clinical manifestations into transient ischemic attacks, strokes-in-evolution, and completed strokes. **Transient ischemic attacks** (TIA) represent thrombotic particles which cause an intermittent blockage of circulation. In a true transient ischemic attack, all neurologic deficits must completely clear within 24 hours and leave no residual dysfunction. The typical development of thrombotic stroke causes the clinical syndrome known as a **stroke-in-evolution.** An intermittent progression of a neurologic deficit over hours to days is characteristic of thrombotic stroke or slow intracranial hemorrhage. The **completed stroke** has reached its maximum destructiveness in producing deficits, although cerebral edema may not have reached its maximum.

An **embolic stroke** involves fragments that break from a thrombus formed outside the brain. Common sites are in the heart, aorta, common carotid, or thorax. The embolus usually involves small vessels and obstructs a bifurcation or other narrowing to cause ischemia. Conditions associated with an embolic stroke include atrial fibrillation, myocardial infarction, endocarditis, rheumatic heart disease, valvular prostheses, atrial-septal defects, and disorders of the aorta, carotids, or vertebral-basilar circulation. In persons who experience an embolic stroke, usually a second stroke follows at some point because the source of emboli continues to exist. Emboli usually lodge in the distribution of the middle cerebral artery.

Hemorrhagic stroke or intracranial hemorrhage is a frequent cause of cerebrovascular accidents. The most common causes of hemorrhagic stroke are hypertension, ruptured aneurysms or arteriovenous malformation, and hemorrhage associated with bleeding disorders.

Hypertensive hemorrhage is associated with a significant increase in systolic-diastolic pressure over several years and usually occurs within the brain tissue. A mass of blood forms as its volume increases; adjacent brain tissue is displaced and compressed. Rupture or seepage into the ventricular system occurs in many of the cases. The most common sites for hypertensive hemorrhages are in the putamen of the basal ganglia.

Lacunar strokes, or lacunar infarcts, are very small and involve the small arteries predominantly in the basal ganglia, internal capsules, and brain stem. Because of the subcortical location and small area of infarction, these strokes may have limited motor and sensory deficits.

Cerebrovascular Accidents

	Thrombotic	*Embolic*	*Hemorrhagic*
Presence of earlier transient ischemia attacks (TIAs)	Frequent	Occasional	Infrequent
Onset	Acute, hours to days	Acute	Acute, progressing, worsening
Associated headache	Occasional, not severe	Often moderately severe	Frequent, severe
Stiff neck	Rare	Rare	Frequent
Loss of consciousness	Occasional, not at onset	Occasional, brief	Frequent
Blood in CSF	Rare	Rare	Frequent

Cerebral infarction results when an area of the brain loses blood supply due to vascular occlusion. In ischemic infarcts, neuronal cell bodies change, myelin sheaths and axis cylinders are interrupted and disintegrate, and there is loss of function.

The symptoms depend on the blood vessel involved. Essentially, if the internal carotid artery branches are involved, there is confusion, inability to plan, aphasia, perception disorders, paralysis or blindness. If the vertebral artery branches are involved, there is diplopia, ataxia, vertigo, dysphagia, and dysphonia. If a TIA is the cause of the thrombotic lesion, the neurological deficit will usually clear within 24 hours. Other CVA usually have permanent neurological deficits.

In thrombotic strokes, treatment is directed at supportive management to control cerebral edema and increased intracranial pressure. Intervention to restore blood supply may be indicated. Arresting the disease process by controlling risk factors is critical. In embolic strokes, treatment is directed at preventing further embolization by instituting anticoagulation therapy and correcting the primary problem. Rehabilitation is indicated in both thrombotic and embolic stroke. Treatment of an intracranial stroke, regardless of cause, is focused on stopping or reducing the bleeding, controlling the increased intracranial pressure, preventing another hemorrhagic episode, and preventing vasospasm. At times, an attempt is made to evacuate or aspirate the blood.

5. **Describe the pathophysiology, manifestations, and treatment of CNS tumors; classify common brain tumors.**
   Study text pages 553-561; refer to Figures 15-18 and 15-19 and Table 15-7.

Cranial tumors can be either primary or metastatic. Primary intracerebral tumors originate from brain substance, neuroglia, neurons, cells of the blood vessels, and connective tissue. Primary extracerebral tumors originate outside the substance of the brain and include meningiomas, acoustic nerve tumors, and tumors of the pituitary and pineal glands. Metastatic tumors can be found inside and/or outside the brain substance.

Cranial tumors cause local and generalized clinical manifestations. The local effects are due to the destructive action of a particular site in the brain and to compression that reduces cerebral blood flow. The effects are varied and include seizures, visual disturbances, unstable gait, and cranial nerve dysfunction. The generalized effects result from increased ICP. Intracranial brain tumors do not metastasize as readily as tumors in other organs because there are no lymphatic channels within the brain substance. If metastasis does occur, it is usually through seeding of cerebral blood or cerebrospinal fluid, during cranial surgery, or through artificial shunts.

The principal treatment for cerebral neoplasms is surgical or radiosurgical excision or surgical decompression if total excision is not possible. Chemotherapy and radiotherapy also may be used. Supportive treatment is directed at reducing edema.

Classification of Common Primary Brain Tumors

Type	Frequency	Age Group
Astrocytoma	30 percent	Adults
Meningioma	15 percent	All ages
Oligodendroglioma	7 percent	Adults
Ependymoma	5 percent	All ages

An estimated 25 percent of persons with cancer develop metastasis to the brain. One-third of metastatic brain tumors arise from the lung, approximately one-sixth from the breast, and a lesser number from the gastrointestinal tract and kidney. Other tumors metastasize less frequently. Carcinomas are disseminated to the brain by the circulation. Metastatic brain tumors carry a poor prognosis. If a solitary tumor is found, surgery and/or radiation therapy is used; but if multiple tumors exist, symptomatic relief only is pursued.

Spinal cord tumors are classified as **intramedullary tumors**, those originating within the neural tissues, or **extramedullary tumors**, those originating from tissues outside the spinal cord. Intramedullary tumors have the same cellular origins as brain tumors. Extramedullary tumors arise from the meninges, epidural tissue, or vertebral structure. The most common primary extramedullary spinal cord tumors are neurofibromas and meningiomos. Metastatic spinal cord tumors are usually carcinomas, lymphomas, or myelomas. Their location is often extradural.

The acute onset of clinical manifestations suggests a vascular insult caused by thrombosis of vessels supplying the spinal cord. Clinical manifestations fall into three major categories: a compressive syndrome, an irritative syndrome, or rarely, a syringomyelic syndrome. In the **compressive syndrome**, the motor dysfunction is paresis and spasticity depending on the level of involvement. The sensory manifestations of tingling paresthesias have a similar pattern to that of the motor signs. Pain and temperature dysfunctions are more commonly found than touch, vibration, and proprioceptive changes. Bladder and bowel deficits usually appear when paresis develops in the legs.

The **irritative syndrome** combines the clinical manifestations of a cord compression with radicular pain. This pain is in the sensory root distribution and indicates root irritation. Sensory changes include paresthesia and impaired pain and touch perception; motor disturbances include cramps,

atrophy, fasciculation, and decreased or absent deep tendon reflexes.

Intradural-extramedullary tumors are surgically removed or decompressed by excision of the posterior vertebral arch or laminectomy. Laminectomy with decompression and excision is used for gliomas and is followed by radiotherapy. Extradural metastatic tumors are often managed by radiotherapy, chemotherapy, hormonal therapy, or pain management protocols.

6. Compare meningitis with encephalitis.

Study text pages 561-562 and 564-565; refer to Table 15-9.

	Bacterial Meningitis	*Aseptic Meningitis*	*Encephalitis*
Site	Pia mater, arachnoid, subarachnoid space, CSF, ventricles	Meninges	Meninges, white and gray matter
Infectious agents	Neisseria, pneumococci haemophilus	Enteroviral viruses, herpes simplex I	Arthropod-borne viruses, herpes simplex I, complications of systemic viral infection
Lesion	Meningeal vessels become hyperemic and permeable	Similar to bacterial	Nerve cell degeneration
Manifestations	Throbbing headache, flexion of legs and thighs, neck stiffens, projectile vomiting, confusion	Mild symptoms compared with bacterial meningitis but similar	Fever, delirium, confusion, coma, seizure, cranial nerve palsies, paresis and paralysis
CSF	Internal pressure, bacteria, elevated protein levels, decreased glucose levels, neutrophils and monocytes	Increased pressure, normal glucose levels, lymphocytes	Same as aseptic meningitis

7. Characterize CNS abscesses.

Study text pages 562-564.

Abscesses are localized collections of pus within the parenchyma or functioning cells of the brain and spinal cord. Abscesses occur following open trauma and during neurosurgery; with foci of infection such as the middle ear, mastoid cells, nasal cavity, and nasal sinuses; and through metastatic or hematogenous spread from distant foci. Streptococci, staphylococci, and bacteroides in combination with anaerobes are the most common bacteria that cause abscesses. However, yeast and fungi have also been found in CNS abscess.

Initially, a localized inflammatory process leads to edema, hyperemia, softening, and petechial hemorrhage. After a few days, fibroblasts from capillaries deposit collagen fibers which contain and encapsulate the purulent focus. The infection becomes limited with a center of pus and a wall of granular tissue.

Clinical manifestations of **brain abscesses** include fever, headache, nausea, vomiting, decreasing cognitive abilities, paresis, and seizures. These signs and symptoms develop because of the infection and expanding mass. Clinical manifestations of **spinal cord abscesses** are spinal discomfort; root pain accompanied by spasms of the back muscles and limited vertebral movement due to pain and spasm; weakness due to progressive cord compression; and paralysis.

Aspiration or excision accompanied by antibiotic therapy is the recommended but somewhat controversial treatment for brain abscesses. Intracranial pressure must be managed. Spinal cord abscesses are treated with surgical excision or aspiration because decompression is necessary. Antibiotic and supportive therapy is also required.

8. Identify the neurologic complications of AIDS.

Study text pages 565-567; refer to Table 15-10.

Approximately 40 to 60 percent of all persons with AIDS develop neurologic complications. The most common neurologic disorder is HIV encephalopathy. Other common neurologic disorders are peripheral neuropathies, vacuolar myelopathy, opportunistic infection of the CNS, and neoplasms.

HIV encephalopathy is characterized by progressive cognitive dysfunction in conjunction with motor and behavioral alterations. HIV encephalopathy is likely the result of direct brain tissue infection by the virus. HIV is mostly found in white matter subcortical areas.

Vacuolar myelopathy involving diffuse degeneration of the spinal cord may occur in persons with AIDS. A progressive spastic paraparesis with ataxia is the predominant clinical manifestation. Leg weakness, upper motor neuron signs, incontinence, and posterior column sensory loss may be present.

Peripheral neuropathy is a sensory neuropathy. Individuals experience painful dysthesias and paresthesias in the extremities. Weakness and decreased - or absent distal reflexes may be present.

Some individuals develop an acute **aseptic meningitis** at approximately the time of positive seroconversion. Headache, fever, and meningismus with cranial nerve involvement, especially V and VII, may appear.

Opportunistic viral infections may cause nervous system disease. Persons with cytomegalovirus encephalitis may experience altered cognitive functions, tremor, focal neurologic deficits, and sensory deficits.

Opportunistic nonviral infections are the most common CNS disorders associated with AIDS. Clinical manifestations of CNS toxoplasmosis, a common AIDS disorder, are highly variable and include clumsiness to hemiplegia, aphasia, seizures, ataxia, and cognitive changes.

CNS neoplasms associated with AIDS include CNS lymphoma, systemic non-Hodgkin lymphoma, and metastatic Kaposi sarcoma.

9. **Distinguish between the degenerative diseases of Parkinson, Huntington, multiple sclerosis, and amyotrophic lateral sclerosis (ALS).**

Study text pages 567-576; refer to Figures 15-27 through 15-32.

Degenerative CNS Diseases

	Parkinson	*Huntington*	*Multiple Sclerosis*	*ALS*
Lesion site	Basal ganglia, degeneration of dopamineric receptors	Basal ganglia frontal cortex, depletion of GABA	CNS demyelination	Scarring of corticospinal tract in lateral column of spinal cord — upper and lower motor neurons
Etiology	Dopamine insufficiency, trauma, infection, neoplasms, drugs, toxins	Autosomal dominant	Immunogenetic-viral cause genetic/ environmental	Viral-immune
Onset	> age 40, peak 60s	40s and 50s	Between 20 and 40 years of age	40s, peaks in early 50s
Manifestations	Resting tremor, muscle stiffness, poverty of movement or akinesia, flexed or forward leaning, possible late-stage dementia	Dementia, delusions and depression, chorea movements beginning in face and arms and finally the entire body	Remissions and exacerbations but progressive paresthesia, diplopia, cerebellar incoordination, urinary dysfunction	Muscle weakness and atrophy, progress to paralysis, normal intellectual and sensory function until death
Treatment	Symptomatic, dopaminergic drugs	No known treatment	Steroids to shorten exacerbations, supportive and rehabilitative management	No known treatment

10. Describe peripheral nervous system disorders; characterize myasthenia gravis.
Study text pages 577-581.

As spinal roots emerge from or enter into the vertebral canal, they may be injured or damaged by compression, inflammation, or direct trauma that stretches or tears the roots. **Radiculopathies** and **radiculitis** are disorders of the spinal nerve roots. Roots may be injured by a forceful tearing of a nerve whenever there are injuries to the head and shoulders. A herniated disk or a tumor may compress nerve roots. Chronic meningitis, neurosyphilis, sarcoidosis, and arachnoiditis also are causes of spinal root injury.

Diseases that involve spinal roots typically produce pain and paresthesia in the sensory root distribution. Treatment is directed at the cause of the injury and may include surgery, antibiotics, removal of the injurious agent, steroids, and radiotherapy and chemotherapy.

Plexus injuries involve the nerve plexus distal to the spinal roots but proximal to the the peripheral nerves. Such injuries may be caused by trauma, compression, infiltration, or iatrogenically by positioning during surgery or by intramuscular injections. Clinical manifestations include motor weakness, muscle atrophy, and sensory loss in affected areas. Paralysis can occur with complete plexus lesions. Treatment is directed at removal of the cause, repair and approximation of nervous tissue, prevention of further injury, discomfort control, and rehabilitation where appropriate.

Where the peripheral nerves themselves are affected, **neuropathy** develops. Sensory neuropathies are mostly caused by leprosy, some industrial solvents, chloramphenicol, and heredity. Motor neuropathies are predominantly caused by Guillain-Barré syndrome, infectious mononucleosis, viral hepatitis, acute porphyria, lead, mercury, and triorthocresylphosphates (TCP).

Tenderness of the nerve trunks and sensory alterations are seen in sensory neuropathy. These include paresthesia and dysthesia, as well as decreased or absent primary sensations such as temperature, touch, light pain, position sense, or vibratory sense. Ataxia of gait or limb may arise from proprioceptive loss. When motor axons are affected, muscle strength, muscle tone, and muscle bulk are diminished. Whole muscles or groups of muscles may become paralyzed. Atrophy of muscles is manifested according to the peripheral nerves involved.

Axonal regrowth and recovery of function may take months. This is possible if the cell body survives. The therapeutic management is directed at elimination of the cause, if possible. Further damage to the axon must be prevented by avoiding too-early reuse of the nerve.

The neurologic dysfunctions observed in **Guillain-Barré syndrome** are caused by a cell-mediated immunologic reaction directed at the peripheral nerves. Lymphocytes migrate into the areas adjacent to the nerve and attack the myelin sheath surrounding the nerve fibers; this causes demyelination of nerve segments. The muscle innervated by the damaged peripheral nerves undergoes denervation and atrophy. Clinical manifestations vary. The individual may have a symmetrical weakness or paralysis involving the legs, the trunk, and possibly the neck and face. Any paresthesia ascends upward. Individuals may experience respiratory arrest or cardiovascular collapse.

If the cell body survives, regeneration of the peripheral nerve takes place with recovery of motor function. If the cell body dies from intense ventral root involvement in the inflammatory–degenerative process, then regeneration is impossible. If collateral reinnervation from surviving axons exists, some motor function recovery occurs.

Ventilatory support is a dominant aspect of therapeutic management. During the acute phase, steroid therapy may be used. After the disorder begins to remit, aggressive rehabilitation is required.

Any disorder that interferes with the synthesis or packaging of a neurotransmitter or its release into the synaptic cleft or any interference with the binding of a neurotransmitter to the receptor may cause muscular weakness. **Myasthenia gravis** is a disorder of voluntary or striated muscles characterized by muscle weakness and fatigability because of a defect in nerve impulse transmission at the neuromuscular junction. Between 75 and 80 percent of persons with myasthenia gravis have pathological changes in the thymus; this disorder is an autoimmune disease. Different types of myasthenia gravis exist. **Ocular myasthenia**, which is more common in males, involves muscle weakness confined to the eye muscles. **Generalized myasthenia** involves the proximal musculature throughout the body and exhibits varying rates of progression with possible remissions. **Bulbar myasthenia** involves the muscles innervated by cranial nerves IX through XII and tends to be rapidly progressive or severe.

In myasthenia gravis, postsynaptic acetylcholine receptors on the muscle cell's plasma membrane are no longer recognized as "self." Therefore, IgG antibody is secreted against the acetylcholine receptors. These antibodies fix onto the receptor sites and block the binding of acetylcholine. Eventually, the antibody action causes the destruction of receptor sites and the diminished transmission of the nerve impulse across the neuromuscular junction.

The muscles of the eyes, face, mouth, throat, and neck are usually affected first. Manifestations include diplopia, ptosis, and ocular palsies; facial droop and an expressionless face; difficulty chewing and swallowing; drooling, episodes of choking and aspirations; and a nasal, low-volume but high-pitched monotonous speech pattern. The muscles of the neck, shoulder girdle, and hip flexor are less frequently affected.

Myasthenic crisis occurs when severe muscle weakness causes extreme quadriparesis or quadriplegia, respiratory insufficiency that can lead to respiratory arrest, and extreme difficulty in swallowing. **Cholinergic crisis** is caused by the muscle hyperactivity secondary to excessive accumulation of acetylcholine at the neuromuscular junctions and excessive parasympathetic activity. As in myasthenic crisis, the individual is in danger of respiratory arrest.

Anticholinesterase drugs, steroids, and immunosuppressant drugs are used to treat myasthenia gravis and myasthenic crisis. Treatment of individuals with cholinergic crisis involves withholding anticholinergic drugs until blood levels fall out of the toxic range while providing ventilatory support.

Practice Examination

1. Following a head injury, which is a significant indicator of CNS damage?
   a. frontal headache
   b. swelling of head surface at the site of injury
   c. increased pulse and respiratory rate
   d. lack of pupillary light reflex

2. In an automobile accident, an individual's forehead struck the windshield. The coup/contrecoup injury would be in the
   a. frontal/parietal region.
   b. frontal/occipital region.
   c. parietal/occipital region.
   d. occipital/frontal region.

3. In moderate diffuse axonal injury,
   a. coma lasts more than 24 hours.
   b. coma lasts less than 24 hours.
   c. disruption of axons occurs in cerebral hemispheres and those extending into the diencephalon and brain stem.
   d. tearing of axons in the cerebral hemisphere occurs.
   e. Both a and d are correct.

Match the term with its definition.

4. concussion
5. contusion
6. extradural hematoma
7. subdural hematoma
8. intracerebral hematoma

   a. bleeding into the brain's parenchyma
   b. bruising of part of the brain
   c. violent displacement of brain tissue due to acceleration or deceleration
   d. arterial bleeding
   e. venous bleeding

9. The regions where most spinal cord injuries occur are the
   a. cervical and thoracic regions.
   b. cervical and lumbar regions.
   c. thoracic and lumbar regions.
   d. lumbar and sacral regions.

10. Injury of the cervical cord may be life-threatening because of
    a. increased intracranial pressure.
    b. disrupted reflexes.
    c. spinal shock.
    d. loss of bladder and rectal control.
    e. diaphragmatic impairment.

11. Autonomic hyperreflexia is characterized by all except
    a. hypotension.
    b. slower heart rate.
    c. stimulation of sensory receptors below the level of the cord lesion.
    d. precipitation because of a distended bladder or rectum.

12. Intervertebral disk herniation
    a. usually occurs at the thoracic level.
    b. in the lumbosacral area causes pain over the gluteal region and into the calf or ankle.
    c. is infrequent in the lumbosacral disks.
    d. Both b and c are correct.
    e. a, b, and c are correct.

13. Transient ischemic attacks (TIAs) are
    a. unilateral neurological deficits that slowly resolve.
    b. generalized neurological deficits that occur a few seconds every hour.
    c. focal neurological defects that develop suddenly, last for several minutes, and clear in 24 hours.
    d. neurological deficits that slowly evolve or develop.

14. Which of the following is a risk factor for the development of CVA?
    a. polycythemia vera
    b. hypertension
    c. diabetes mellitus
    d. elevated blood cholesterol
    e. All of the above are risk factors.

15. Which most typically characterizes the victims of a cerebral embolic stroke?
    a. Individuals older than 65 years of age with a history of hypertension.
    b. Individuals with a long history of TIA.
    c. Middle-aged individuals with a history of heart disease.
    d. Individuals with gradually occurring symptoms which then rapidly disappear.

16. Blood in the CSF of an individual is mostly likely in _____ cardiovascular accidents.
    a. TIA
    b. thrombotic
    c. embolic
    d. hemorrhagic

17. Which is not a primary intracerebral neoplasm?
    a. astrocytoma
    b. meningioma
    c. oligodendroglioma
    d. glaucoma

18. In bacterial meningitis, the CSF has
    a. normal glucose levels.
    b. an elevated number of lymphocytes.
    c. neutrophilic infiltration.
    d. None of the above is correct.
    e. a, b, and c are correct.

19. Chorea-type movements are
    a. slow and rhythmic.
    b. brief, rapid, and explosive.
    c. unilateral facial muscle movements.
    d. trauma-induced.
    e. the consequence of autosomal recessive disorders.

20. The tremor in Parkinson syndrome
    1. is produced by alternating agonist and
       antagonist joint muscles.
    2. is produced by decreased muscle tone in
       opposing muscle groups.
    3. is the result of inhibitory influences from the
       basal ganglia.
    4. is the result of increased output of pyramidal
       tract efferent impulses to skeletal muscles.

a. 1, 2, 3
b. 1, 3
c. 2, 4
d. 4
e. 1, 2, 3, 4

Match the disease to site of dysfunction.

21. Parkinson disease
22. myasthenia gravis
23. multiple sclerosis
24. Guillain-Barré syndrome
25. amyotrophic lateral sclerosis

a. cerebral cortex
b. basal ganglia
c. peripheral nerve myelin
d. neuromuscular junction
e. ventribular system of brain
f. corticospinal tracts and anterior roots
g. CNS myelin
h. muscles

Case Study

Mrs. B. is an overweight 71-year-old white female. Upon hospital admission, she had a severe right-sided headache, slurred speech, and some severe right-handed numbness with a weak hand grip on the left. Her smile was asymmetric with right-sided facial weakness that had persisted for 48 hours. Mrs. B. has a history of smoking moderately for 50 years and use of estrogen replacement for 20 years. Her mother had adult-onset diabetes and died of breast cancer at age 62; her father died of a gunshot accident at 29; one sister died of a subarachnoid hemorrhage at age 63, and another sister is hemiparietic because of a CVA. One brother is hypertensive, and three other younger siblings are apparently healthy.

Vital signs showed a normal temperature, elevated heart rate, normal respirations, but a severely elevated blood pressure. A lumbar puncture was negative for blood with normal protein and glucose levels. A normal electrocardiogram was found. EEG showed localized activity in the left hemisphere. A CT showed increased density on the left. Blood chemistry was normal except for elevated glucose.

How do you assess Mrs. B.'s history, her family history, and her symptoms and signs?

115

CHAPTER 16

Alterations of Neurologic Function in Children

Prerequisite Objectives

a. Identify the six embryologic stages of neurologic development.
   Review text page 588; refer to Figures 16-1 through 16-4.

Remember!

- Embryonic development of the nervous system occurs in six stages: (1) dorsal or posterior induction, (2) ventral or anterior induction, (3) proliferation, (4) migration, (5) organization, and (6) myelination.

---

b. Identify the normal immature infant neurologic reflexes.
   Refer to Table 16-1.

c. Identify the major differences between adult and infant neurological functioning.
   Review text pages 588-592.

Remember!

- Several differences between adults and children are notable. First, the head of a normal infant accounts for approximately one-fourth of the total height; whereas an adult's head is one-eighth of the total body height. Second, the bones of the infants skull are separated at the suture line to form anterior and posterior fontanelles or "soft spots." The posterior fontanelle may be open until two to three months of age; whereas the anterior fontanelle normally closes by 18 months. The adult's cranium is a closed cavity with sutures firmly holding the cranial bones together, while the infant's cranium has room for expansion through the fontanelles and increases in circumference during the first five years of life. An adult's head size cannot expand, regardless of trauma or increased production of cerebrospinal fluid. The infant's head circumference, on the other hand, increases in size as a result of normal growth up to age five years. The head is the fastest growing body part during infancy. In children, abnormal intracranial conditions characterized by increased intracranial pressure also may increase head circumference in excess of that expected with normal growth. Health care providers carefully monitor head growth during the first five years of life by measuring head circumference and comparing the results with a standardized growth chart.

Objectives

After successful study of this chapter, the learner will be able to:

1. Identify the major forms of central nervous system malformation and relate them to their clinical findings.

Study text pages 592-599; refer to Figures 16-5 through 16-11.

Neural tube defects are caused by an arrest in embryologic development and have an incidence of 0.7 to 1.0 per 1000 live births in the United States. A strong association with fetal death obscures the actual incidence somewhat. These can be subdivided into posterior defects or anencephaly, the myelodysplasias or defects of the vertebral column and spinal cord, and the less frequent anterior midline defects.

Anencephaly is the absence of skull and parts of the brain resulting from arrest in early closure of the anterior neural tube. It is a relatively common disorder that is fatal.

Encephalocele is herniation of the brain and meninges through a midline defect in the skull. An encephalocele may be located in the nasopharynx, in which case no obvious deformity is noted but may cause nasal congestion. Central nervous system (CNS) tissue may be seen on nasal examination. This form has a better prognosis for surgical repair. Size, location, and timing of the development of encephalocele determines the potential outcome for the child's development and cognition.

Meningocele is the protrusion of meninges through a vertebral defect. The spinal cord is not involved. The meningocele is present at birth as a protruding sac at the level of the defect. Abnormal neurological function may be present and hydrocephaly is a common complication. Damage and infection may result from manipulation of the sac. Surgical closure is optimal during the first 72 hours of life. The size and level of the defect determines the eventual outcome.

Myelomeningocele, or spina bifida, is a herniation of the meninges, spinal fluid, spinal cord, and nerves through a vertebral defect; 80 percent are located in the lumbosacral region. Myelomeningocele presents as a "sac on back." The covering membrane may leak cerebrospinal fluid (CSF). Function is dependent on the degree of spinal cord involvement. Deficits will be distal to the defect and include weakness, paralysis, spasticity, and either bowel or bladder dysfunction. These deficits may worsen with age because of tethering of the cord with development. Hydrocephalus occurs in 95 percent of cases. Myelomeningocele is detectable through prenatal ultrasound and alpha-fetoprotein sampling. Treatment includes early surgical correction of the defect and its complicating hydrocephaly and multidisciplinary therapy for related problems.

Spina bifida occulta is a less serious form of myelomeningocele, with the defect occurring in the lumbar or sacral area of the spine because of incomplete fusion of the vertebral laminae. Spina bifida occulta is more common than myelomeningocele and usually causes no neurologic deficits; it may occur in 10 to 15 percent of pregnancies. Physical findings may include abnormal hair growth along the spine, a midline sacral dimple with or without a sinus tract, angioma over the defect, or an overlying subcutaneous mass. Spina bifida occulta may cause tethering of the cord and result in dysfunctions during periods of rapid growth.

Craniosynostosis is the premature closure of cranial sutures during the first 20 months of life. Asymmetry of the skull or interference with brain growth may result if multiple sutures are involved. Diagnosis is made by physical examination, head circumference measurements, and radiologic studies. Surgical treatment is indicated for cases that restrict brain growth.

Microcephaly is a defect in brain growth as a whole. The brain may be 25 percent of normal with growth of the frontal lobes severely stunted. Primary microcephaly may be due to chromosomal abnormality, toxin exposure, radiation, or chemical exposure during periods of induction and major cell migration. Secondary microcephaly may be due to various insults during the third trimester. Manifestations range from decerebrate posturing and profound retardation to motor impairment and mild retardation.

Congenital hydrocephalus is characterized by an increase in the volume of CSF that may be due to overproduction, a defect in reabsorption, or blockage of the ventricular drainage system. The incidence rate is approximately two of every 1000 live births. The most frequent cause is congenital aqueduct stenosis, but other causes include brain tumors, cysts, trauma, arteriovenous malformations, infections, and blood clots. The resultant pathology is because of increased intracranial pressure, or pressure on the brain, that eventually causes tissue damage. At first, sutures and fontanelles of the skull are able to accommodate the increased fluid by separating, which allows the head to grow in diameter. This enlargement in utero may require cesarian delivery. After birth, the increasing pressure causes neurologic symptoms including irritability, high-pitched crying, vomiting, and lethargy; serious, irreversible brain damage; and eventually, death. Diagnosis is made by physical exam ination, radiologic imaging (CT or MRI), and head circumference measurement. Treatment includes surgical placement of a shunt from the affected ventricle to another cavity of the body, chiefly the peritoneal cavity. Though very effective, shunts are prone to blockage by infection or cellular debris. In the event of shunt malfunction, acute, life-threatening increases in intracranial pressure may result, which requires emergency surgery.

2. Compare and contrast the pathophysiology of three encephalopathic processes of childhood: cerebral palsy, phenylketonuria, and Reye syndrome.
Study text pages 599-603 and 605-606; refer to Figure 16-12 and Tables 16-4 and 16-5.

Cerebral palsy (CP) is a static encephalopathy meaning that the resulting damage does not change over time. Clinical manifestations, however, may change as the child continues to develop. CP affects nearly 400,000 children in the United States as a diverse group of syndromes classified according to the neurologic symptoms produced. These include spasticity, ataxia, dyskinesia, or a combination of all three. Many factors contribute to cerebral palsy, including birth asphyxia, low birth weight, vascular abnormalities, pre- or postnatal trauma, and a host of other insults that are not well understood. Treatment includes a multidisciplinary approach that encompasses the various neurologic and cognitive manifestations of the defect.

Phenylketonuria (PKU) is an encephalopathy caused by an inherited metabolic disorder and is progressive in nature. The disorder involves an inability to metabolize the amino acid phenylalanine and occurs once in every 10,000 births worldwide. A high level of phenylalanine causes insufficient amounts of other amino acids entering the brain that results in malformation, defective myelination, or cystic degeneration of the white and gray matter. Diagnosis is usually made by nonselective newborn screening. Treatment is to restrict phenylalanine in the diet, which generally results in normal growth and development.

Reye syndrome is an acute encephalopathy that is believed to be caused by an interaction of salicylate, viruses, and liver dysfunction. The pathophysiology includes induction of hypoglycemia, hyperammonemia, and an increase in short-chain fatty acids which lead to an encephalopathy frequently referred to as a hepatic encephalopathy. The brain eventually becomes severely edematous, which leads to tissue damage and transtentorial herniation. Clinical manifestations begin with vomiting and lethargy (stage 1) and progress to disorientation, delirium, central neurologic hyperventilation, and stupor (stage 2). Obtundation, coma, and decorticate rigidity ensue (stage 3), rapidly developing seizures, flaccidity, and respiratory arrest (stage 4). Avoiding aspirin administration during viral illnesses in children is the widely accepted preventive measure. Treatment ranges from rapid diagnosis and supportive therapy in the early stages to highly complicated neurointensive care in later stages.

3. Describe the seizure disorders of children and adults, noting their manifestations and etiology.
Study text pages 603-605; refer to Table 14-13.

Generalized seizures comprise 55 percent of all childhood seizure disorders; a greater incidence is seen in children than in adults. Seizure disorders change in pattern and frequency over time during childhood due to the maturation of neurons and their patterns of connection. The nervous system in children has decreased capability for generating well-organized seizures because the immature neuron is unable to generate long bursts of high-frequency signals and has relatively underdeveloped intracortical connections. Seizures during infancy and childhood may be the result of asphyxia, intracranial bleeding, CNS infection, electrolyte imbalance, or inborn errors of metabolism. Many seizure disorders are idiopathic, having no known cause. Frequently occurring seizure disorders in infancy and childhood include **infantile spasms**, **Lennox-Gastaut syndrome**, **juvenile myoclonic epilepsy**, and **febrile seizures**. Diagnosis includes the clinical features of the seizure, an electroencephalogram (EEG) to isolate seizure focus, and radiologic imaging for possible associated lesions. Treatment includes various standard drug therapies and, rarely, surgery for intractable or debilitating disorders which are amenable to surgical therapy.

4. Identify the most common pathogens responsible for bacterial meningitis in infancy and childhood; describe some common presentations at birth and their potential outcomes; characterize viral meningitis.
Study text pages 608-609.

Seventy percent of all cases of **meningitis** occurs in children less than 5 years of age. The most common bacterial pathogens are group B streptococci and gram-negative intestinal bacilli in infants from birth to two months of age; *H. influenzae* type B, *S. pneumoniae*, and *N. meningitidis* in children from two months to 12 years of age; and *N. meningitidis* in adolescents over 12 years of age. Headache, fever, irritability, photophobia, and nuchal and spinal rigidity often are presenting signs which follow an upper respiratory infection or otitis media. These symptoms, however, are more variable in the very young. Diagnosis is confirmed only by lumbar puncture and CSF culture. Meningitis may lead to death or profound brain damage, with 35 percent of survivors having sensory or motor dysfunction due to cranial nerve damage that occurs in the early phases of illness.

The hallmark of **viral meningitis** is a mononuclear response in the CSF instead of a neutrophilic response as in bacterial meningitis and normal sugar levels instead of decreased sugar levels as in bacterial meningitis. The symptoms are similar but milder than those in bacterial meningitis.

5. Identify the most common site of infection for human immunodeficiency virus (HIV) in children and identify the common effects of this infection.
Study text pages 609-610.

The site most commonly affected by **HIV** in infants and children is the CNS. Manifestations include progressive encephalopathy, deterioration of gross and fine motor skills, developmental and language delays, behavioral impairment, and onset of seizures.

6. Describe the types of brain tumors in children and characterize their presentation.
Study text pages 611-618; refer to Figures 16-14 through 16-17 and Tables 16-7 and 16-8.

Brain tumors are the most common solid tumor in childhood and the second most common neoplasm in children; leukemia is the most common neoplasm. Genetic, environmental, and immune factors are all implicated in causation. Parental employment and teratogen exposure also is a possible etiological factor. Most childhood brain tumors arise from glial tissue, with two-thirds of tumors found in the posterior fossa or infratentorial area. In contrast, two-thirds of adult tumors are found in the anterior fossa or supratentorial area. Brain tumors are unique in their presentation by virtue of their locations. **Infratentorial tumors** often present with signs of increased ICP because of a mass blockage of the 4th ventricle. Signs include early morning vomiting with neither nausea nor headache, lethargy, and somnolence. **Supratentorial tumors** frequently present with localized neurological findings such as truncal ataxia, impaired coordination, gait anomalies, and loss of balance. Diagnosis is confirmed by radiologic imaging. The most common brain tumors in childhood are **medulloblastoma, ependymoma, astrocytoma, brainstem glioma**, and **optic nerve glioma**. These tumors are generally amenable to a wide range of surgical, chemical, and radiation therapies. Prognosis is variable and specific to the individual process.

Practice Examination

True/False

____ 1. An infant of 11 months of age who displays a strong asymmetric tonic neck of fencer reflex is probably just "slow" in development and should be assumed to have normal neurological function.

____ 2. Ninety percent of neural tube defects are anencephaly.

____ 3. Anencephaly is the result of premature closure of the sutures of the skull.

____ 4. Environmental influences play an important role in neural tube defects.

____ 5. Encephalocele is the result of herniation of the brain and meninges through a defect of the lower vertebrae.

____ 6. Neurological function at birth is chiefly at the subcortical level.

____ 7. The prognosis for an individual with meningomyelocele is dependent on the level and extent of the defect.

____ 8. Hydrocephaly may be due to overproduction of CSF, blockage of CSF flow, or inhibition of reabsorption.

____ 9. Hydrocephaly is almost never a neural tube defect, because such defects usually permit leakage of the CSF out of the defect.

____ 10. Seizure disorders in children are usually static and resolve naturally due to the fact that the neurons and the neuronal pathways are constantly maturing.

____ 11. An obvious "sac" on the back of a newborn should be thoroughly probed and examined in order to determine where it is attached to underlying structures.

Fill-in-the-Blank

12. Aspirin administration during a viral illness has been associated with _____ syndrome, which is considered to be a _____ encephalopathy.

13. Early morning vomiting without associated nausea may be indicative of a _____ fossa brain tumor.

14. Focal neurological findings such as ataxia may be associated with an _____ fossa brain tumor.

15. A child becoming significantly more ill with symptoms of headache, lethargy, and stiff neck after several days of treatment for otitis media may be showing findings consistent with _____.

16. _____ is a disease associated with premature closure of the sutures of the skull.

Match the description with the alteration.

17. may restrict brain growth
18. may result from aqueductal stenosis
19. protrusion of the meninges through a vertebral defect
20. may require cesarian section for delivery
21. static disease that has changing findings over time
22. defect in metabolism of an amino acid with severe neurological involvement
23. associated with hypoglycemia, hyperammonemia, and short-chain fatty acids
24. very small head
25. infectious process that may cause profound damage to cranial nerves

a. meningitis
b. microcephaly
c. Reye Syndrome
d. PKU
e. cerebral palsy
f. hydrocephaly
g. meningocele
h. hydrocephaly
i. craniosynostosis

Case Study

Allen S. is an 11-year-old male caucasian who presents to the pediatric nurse practitioner's office for a school physical. His past medical history is unremarkable and the family history also is benign. After the examination has started, his mother requests that the practitioner pay particular attention to her son's lower back. He has an area "down there" that is extremely tender and has been tender as long as she can remember. The problem worsened this year when Allen was hit from behind while playing sandlot football and was paralyzed and "numb" from the hips down for approximately 15 minutes. When asked about the findings when he was taken to the emergency room for the injury, his mother states that she never sought care for him because his symptoms subsided within a few minutes and he "seemed fine!" The practitioner gently admonished and advised the mother that failure to seek care might have caused permanent damage in this case.

As the physical examination continues, it is noted that he has an exquisitely tender area over the lower lumbar spine and palpation causes pain in both legs. This area feels and appears perfectly normal. He is noted to have a very deep, dime-sized sacral dimple and highly fissured skin over the lower sacral spine. Deep tendon reflexes, strength, and sensation are all within normal limits. Bowel and bladder function are normal as well. Spine x-rays are ordered.

What do you expect the x-rays to reveal and what is the likely resolution of this alteration?

CHAPTER 17

Mechanisms of Hormonal Regulation

Objectives

After successful study of this chapter, the learner will be able to:

1. **Identify the functions of the endocrine system and describe the regulation of hormone secretion.**
   Review text pages 626-629; refer to Figures 17-2 and 17-3.

2. **Classify the types of hormones, their receptors, and proposed mechanisms of action.**
   Refer to Figure 17-4 and Tables 17-1 through 17-3.

3. **State the relationship between the hypothalamus and the pituitary; identify the hormones of the anterior pituitary and posterior pituitary, their target organs, and their functions.**
   Refer to Figures 17-5 through 17-8 and Tables 17-5 and 17-6.

4. **Distinguish between the thyroid hormones and identify their functions.**
   Refer to Figure 17-9 and Table 17-7.

5. **Cite the physiological effects of parathyroid hormone and the variables that affect its secretion.**
   Refer to Figures 17-10 and 17-11.

6. **Compare the sites of pancreatic somatostatin, insulin, and glucagon production and their roles in metabolism.**
   Review text pages 643-644; refer to Figures 17-12 and 17-13.

7. **Describe the effects of the adrenal cortical glucocorticoids, mineralocorticoids, and gonadotropins; note the adrenal medullary secretions and their roles.**
   Review text pages 644-649; refer to Figures 17-14 through 17-18.

8. **Describe endocrine gland changes that are associated with normal aging.**
   Review text pages 650-651.

Practice Examination

1. Organs that respond to a particular hormone are called the
   a. target organs.
   b. integrated organs.
   c. responder organs.
   d. hormone attack organs.
   e. None of the above is correct.

2. A major feature of the "plasma membrane receptor" mechanism of hormonal action is
   a. action of cyclic AMP.
   b. increased lysosomal activity.
   c. a "second messenger" is required.
   d. All of the above are correct.
   e. Both a and c are correct.

3. A major feature of the "activation of genes" mechanism of hormonal action is
   a. a "second messenger" is used.
   b. a hormone-golgi complex is used.
   c. the hormone enters the cell.
   d. lysosomal activity increases.
   e. All of the above are correct.

4. The only prominent example of positive feedback in the endocrine system involves
   a. insulin.
   b. oxytocin.
   c. hGH.
   d. aldosterone.
   e. ACTH.

5. The hypothalamus controls the adenohypophysis by direct involvement of
   a. nerve impulses.
   b. prostaglandins.
   c. cerebro-cortical controlling factors (CCCF).
   d. regulating hormones.
   e. None of the above is correct.

6. The target organ of prolactin is the
   a. melanocyte.
   b. mammary gland.
   c. ovum and sperm.
   d. adrenal medulla.
   e. uterine lining.

7. If calcium levels in the blood were too high, thyrocalcitonin (calcitonin) concentrations in the blood should
   a. increase, thereby inhibiting osteoclasts.
   b. increase, thereby stimulating osteoclasts.
   c. increase, but this would not affect osteoclasts.
   d. decrease, thereby inhibiting osteoclasts.
   e. decrease, thereby stimulating osteoclasts.

8. In the negative feedback mechanism controlling thyroid hormone secretion, which is the non-tropic hormone?
   a. TRH
   b. TSH
   c. thyroxine
   d. All of the above are tropic.

9. The control of parathyroid hormone is most accurately described as
   a. negative feedback controlled by the hypothalamus.
   b. positive feedback controlled by the pituitary.
   c. negative feedback involving the pituitary.
   d. negative feedback not involving the pituitary.
   e. Both a and c are correct.

Match the group of adrenocortical hormones with its function.

10. gonadocorticoids
11. glucocorticoids

a. blood cell formation
b. anti-inflammatory
c. aldosterone
d. usually no function
e. bone mineralization

12. The renin-angiotensin-aldosterone system begins to operate when renin is secreted by the
   a. adrenal cortex.
   b. adrenal medulla.
   c. pancreas.
   d. kidneys.
   e. None of the above is correct.

13. The effects of adrenal medullary hormones and the effects of sympathetic stimulation can be described as
   a. opposites in all respects.
   b. overlapping in some respects.
   c. opposites in some respects.
   d. variable depending on the sex involved.
   e. overlapping in most respects.

14. Which best describes the respective effects of insulin and glucagon on blood sugar?
   a. Insulin raises it, glucagon lowers it.
   b. Both raise blood sugar.
   c. Insulin lowers it, glucagon raises it.
   d. Both lower blood sugar.
   e. None of the above is correct.

15. The releasing hormones made in the hypothalamus travel to the anterior pituitary via the
   a. stem neurons.
   b. infundibular stem.
   c. hypophyseal stalk.
   d. hypophyseal arteries.

16. Which is a protein hormone?
   a. T_4
   b. aldosterone
   c. FSH
   d. insulin

17. Aldosterone maintains electrolyte balance by
   a. retention of potassium.
   b. elimination of sodium.
   c. retention of both Na and K.
   d. Both a and b are correct.
   e. None of the above is correct.

Match hormone to target organ.

18. ACTH
19. TSH
20. TRF
21. prolactin

a. mammary glands
b. adrenal cortex
c. adrenal medulla
d. thyroid gland
e. adenohypophysis

Match the hormone to its role.

22. epinephrine
23. glucocorticoids
24. mineralocorticoids
25. gonadocorticoids

a. immunity
b. growth inhibition
c. fight or flight
d. controls Na^+, H_2O, and K^+ excretion
e. normal metabolism and resistance to stress
f. minor sex hormones

Alterations of Hormonal Regulation

Prerequisite Objectives

a. Diagram the negative-feedback system of hormone secretion.
    Review text page 627.

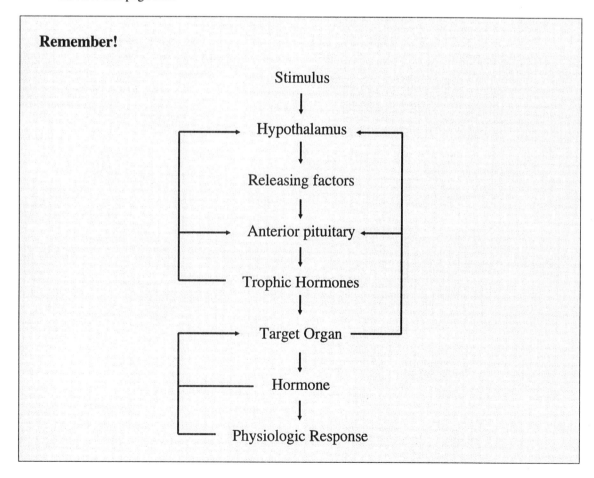

Remember!

Stimulus

↓

Hypothalamus

↓

Releasing factors

↓

Anterior pituitary

↓

Trophic Hormones

↓

Target Organ

↓

Hormone

↓

Physiologic Response

b. Describe hormone receptors as recognizing and signalling mechanisms for hormonal action.
   Review text pages 630-633; refer to Figure 17-4 and Table 17-4.

Remember!

- Hormone receptors are located on the plasma membrane or in the intracellular compartment of a target cell. Water-soluble hormones which include the protein hormones and epinephrine or norepinephrine cannot cross the cell membrane and interact or bind with receptors located in or on the cell membrane. Fat-soluble hormones, steroids, vitamin D, and thyroid hormones diffuse freely across the plasma and nuclear membranes to bind primarily with nuclear receptors.

- In the plasma membrane model, the hormones are called "first messengers." The receptors for the water-soluble hormones first recognize the hormone on the plasma membrane and then bind with the hormone. Once recognition and binding have occurred, the hormone-receptor complex initiates the transmission of an intracellular signal by a "second messenger"; the second messenger relays the message inside the cell where a response can occur. The best known second messenger is cyclic AMP (cAMP), although other substances are known as second messengers.

- For cells having cAMP as a second messenger, the purpose of these interactions is to activate the intracellular cyclic nucleotides such as adenylate cyclase. This enzyme converts adenosine triphosphate (ATP) to cAMP. Elevated levels of cAMP alter cell function in specific ways. An example of the function of cAMP as a second messenger can be seen in the action of epinephrine. The epinephrine-receptor complex interaction increases the synthesis of cAMP. Cyclic AMP, in turn, activates an elaborate enzyme cascade in which inactive enzymes are converted in sequence to active enzymes that lead to glycogen breakdown into glucose.

- In the lipid-soluble hormonal model, relatively small hydrophobic molecules cross the plasma membrane by simple diffusion. Once inside the cytosol, some hormones bind to receptor molecules in the cytoplasm and then diffuse into the nucleus. Hormones without cytoplasmic receptors diffuse directly into the nucleus and bind with an acceptor molecule. Once activated by hormones, the first messengers, the receptor likely binds to specific sites on the chromatin of the target cell. This causes RNA transcription and increased synthesis of specific proteins.

---

c. Identify the origins and functions of hormones.
   Review structure and function of endocrine glands in summary of Chapter 17 on pages 652-654.

Remember!

Site of Origin and Effects of Hormones

Site	Hormone	Effect
Hypothalamus	Releasing hormones	Act on anterior pituitary to release specific hormones
Posterior pituitary	Antidiuretic hormone (ADH)	Causes conservation of body water by promoting water resorption by renal tubules
	Oxytocin	Stimulates uterine contraction and lactation
Anterior pituitary	Adrenocorticotropic hormone (ACTH)	Stimulates production of glucocorticoids by adrenal cortex
	Melanocyte-stimulating hormone (MSH)	Stimulates pigment production in skin

(Continued)

Site	Hormone	Effect
	Growth hormone (GH)	Promotes growth of body tissues
	Thyroid-stimulating hormone (TSH)	Stimulates production and release of thyroid hormones
	Follicle-stimulating hormone (FSH)	Initiates maturation of ovarian follicles Stimulates spermatogenesis
	Prolactin	Stimulates secretion of breast milk
	Luteinizing hormone (LH)	Causes ovulation and stimulates ovary to produce estrogen and progesterone Stimulates androgen production by interstitial cells of testis
Thyroid	Thyroxine (T$_3$, *T$_4$*)	Increases rate of cellular metabolism
	Calcitonin	Osteoblastic, lowers serum calcium
Parathyroid	Parathyroid hormone (PTH)	Osteoclastic, raises serum calcium
Pancreatic Islets of Langerhans	Insulin	Promotes utilization of glucose, lowers serum glucose
	Glucagon	Promotes utilization of glycogen, raises serum glucose
Adrenal cortex	Glucocorticoids, mostly cortisol	Antagonizes effects of insulin, inhibits inflammatory response and fibroblastic activity
	Mineralocorticoid, mostly aldosterone	Promotes retention of sodium by renal tubules
	Androgens and estrogens	Secondary sex characteristics
Adrenal medulla	Catecholamines (epinephrine and norepinephrine)	Regulation of blood pressure by effects on vascular smooth muscle and heart

Objectives

After successful study of this chapter, the learner will be able to:

1. Identify the mechanisms causing hormonal alterations.

Study text pages 657-658; refer to Figure 18-1.

Any significantly elevated or depressed hormone levels have a variety of causes. Feedback systems may fail to function properly or may respond to inappropriate signals. Inadequate amounts of biologically free or active hormone occur when the secretory cells are unable to produce or obtain an adequate quantity of required hormone precursors or are unable to convert the percussors appropriately. A gland also may synthesize or release excessive amounts of hormone. Once in the circulation, hormones may be degraded too fast or too slow, or they may be inactivated by antibodies before reaching their target cell. Hormones produced by nonendocrine tissues may also result in abnormally elevated hormone levels.

The target cell may fail to respond to its hormone. The general types of abnormal target cell responses are receptor-associated disorders and intracellular disorders. **Receptor-associated disorders** may exhibit any of the following: decreased numbers of receptors, defective hormone-receptor binding, impaired receptor function with insensitivity to the hormone, presence of antibodies against specific receptors that either reduce available binding sites or mimic hormone action, or unusual expression by some tumor cells having abnormal receptor activity.

Intracellular disorders may involve inadequate synthesis of the second messenger, such as cAMP, needed to signal intracellular events. The target cell for water-soluble hormones such as insulin may not respond to hormone-receptor binding and thus fail to generate the required second messenger. The cell also may fail to respond to the second messenger if levels of intracellular enzymes or proteins are altered.

The target cell response for lipid-soluble hormones such as thyroid hormone are thought to occur less frequently than those affecting the water-soluble hormones. For lipid-soluble hormones, the number of intracellular receptors may be decreased or their receptors may have an altered affinity for hormones. Alterations of new messenger RNA or absence of substrates for new protein synthesis also may alter target cell response.

2. Distinguish between SIADH and diabetes insipidus.

Study text pages 659-661.

Diseases of the posterior pituitary are rare, but when occurring, they are usually related to abnormal antidiuretic hormone (ADH/vasopressin) secretion. **Syndrome of inappropriate ADH secretion** (SIADH) is characterized by high levels of ADH without normal physiologic stimuli for its release.

SIADH is associated with several forms of cancer because of the ectopic secretion of ADH by tumor cells. Tumors associated with SIADH include oat cell adenocarcinoma of the lung, carcinoma of the duodenum and pancreas, leukemia, lymphoma, and Hodgkin disease. SIADH may follow pituitary surgery as stored ADH is released in an unregulated fashion. SIADH may be seen in infectious pulmonary diseases because of the ectopic production of ADH by infected lung tissue or by increased posterior pituitary secretion of ADH in response to hypoxia. SIADH also may be associated with psychiatric disease and may occur after treatment with a variety of drugs that stimulate ADH release.

The main features of SIADH are water retention and solute loss, particularly sodium. This leads to hyponatremia and hypo-osmolality. As ADH is released continually, water retention results from the normal action of ADH on the renal tubules and collecting ducts. This action increases their permeability to water, thus increasing water reabsorption. Hyponatremia suppresses renin and aldosterone secretion, thus decreasing proximal tubule reabsorption of sodium.

Thirst, impaired taste, anorexia, dyspnea on exertion, fatigue, and dulled consciousness occur when the serum sodium falls from 140 to 130 mEq/L. Vomiting and abdominal cramps occur with a drop in sodium levels from 130 to 120 mEq/L. With a serum sodium level below 113 mEq/L, confusion, lethargy, muscle twitching, and convulsions may occur. Symptoms usually resolve with correction of hyponatremia. The treatment of SIADH involves the correction of any underlying casual problems, correction of severe hyponatremia by administration of hypertonic saline, and fluid restriction to 600 to 800 ml/ day.

Diabetes insipidus is related to an insufficiency of ADH leading to polyuria and polydipsia. There are three forms of diabetes insipidus: a neurogenic or central form, a nephrogenic form, and a psychogenic form. The **neurogenic form of diabetes** insipidus occurs when any organic lesion of the hypothalamus, infundibular stem, or posterior pituitary interferes with ADH synthesis, transport, or release. This results in too little ADH. **Nephrogenic diabetes insipidus** is an insensitivity of the renal tubule to ADH, particularly the collecting tubules. This diabetes is generally related to disorders and drugs that damage the renal tubules or inhibit the generation of cAMP in the tubules. The **psychogenic form** is caused by extremely large volume fluid intake. The clinical manifestations of diabetes insipidus are due to the absence of ADH. These signs and symptoms include polyuria, nocturia, continuous thirst, polydipsia, low urine, low urine osmolality, and high-normal plasma osmolality. Individuals with longstanding diabetes insipidus develop a large bladder capacity and distention of the kidney pelvis and calices with urine. Individuals who have excessive urine output and a low urine osmolality after a dehydration or water restriction test generally require ADH replacement with a synthetic vasopressin analogue. Drugs that potentiate the action of otherwise insufficient amounts of endogenous ADH may be used to stimulate ADH release from the hypothalamus in less severely affected individuals.

3. Describe the disorders of the anterior pituitary as either hypofunctions or hyperfunctions of the gland.

Study text pages 661-665; refer to Figures 18-3 through 18-6.

Anterior pituitary hypofunction may develop from infarction of the gland, removal or destruction of the gland, or space-occupying pituitary adenomas or aneurysms that compress secreting pituitary cells. **Hyperfunction of the anterior pituitary** generally involves an adenoma composed of secretory pituitary cells. An adenoma may lead to hypersecretion of the hormone produced by the adenoma and hyposecretion of another hormone due to the compressive effects of the tumor.

The pituitary gland is extremely vascular and is therefore extremely vulnerable to infarction. The pituitary gland may be susceptible to necrosis because its blood supply through the portal system is already partially deoxygenated. The likelihood of infarction is increased during pregnancy. The primary pathologic mechanism in postpartum pituitary infarction or **Sheehan syndrome** is vasospasm of the artery supplying the anterior pituitary. Following tissue necrosis, edema occurs which expands the pituitary within the fixed confines of the sella turcica. This further impedes blood supply to the pituitary and promotes hypofunction.

The signs and symptoms of hypofunction of the anterior pituitary are highly variable and depend on which hormones are affected. If all hormones are absent, a condition termed **panhypopituitarism** develops. The individual suffers from cortisol deficiency from lack of ACTH, thyroid deficiency from lack of thyroid-stimulating hormone (TSH), diabetes insipidus from lack of ADH, and gonadal failure and loss of secondary sex characteristics from absence of FSH and LH. Gonadotropic hyposecretion frequently results in menstrual irregularity in women. Decreased libido and diminished secondary sex characteristics in both men and women are present. Growth hormone and somatomedin levels are low and may affect children. Somatomedins directly promote bone growth, while GH causes the liver to produce somatomedins. These deficiencies do not generally develop in adults. When there is a growth hormone deficiency in children, hypopituitary **dwarfism** infrequently occurs. A dwarf has a normal face with normal proportions of head, trunk, and limbs; the dwarf also has normal intelligence.

In cases of hypopituitarism, the underlying disorder should be corrected as quickly as possible. Thyroid and cortisol replacement therapy may need to be initiated and maintained. Sex steroid replacement may be required depending on the needs and desires of the individual.

Pituitary adenomas that cause **hyperpituitarism** are usually benign, slow-growing tumors. Effects from an increase in tumor size include nonspecific complaints of headache, fatigue, neck pain or stiffness, and seizures. Visual changes produced by pressure on the optic chiasma include visual field impairments. If the tumor infiltrates other cranial nerves, various neuromuscular functions are affected. Hypersecretion of hormones secreted by the adenoma leads to symptoms associated with the particular hormone that is affected.

Acromegaly occurs in adults who are exposed to continuously excessive levels of growth hormone (GH). Acromegaly is uncommon. The most common cause of acromegaly is a primary autonomous GH-secreting pituitary adenoma. Acromegaly occurs more frequently in women than men and is a slowly progressive disease. If untreated, it is associated with a decreased life expectancy due to an increased occurrence of hypertension, congestive heart failure, and diabetes mellitus.

In the adult, after epiphyseal closure has occurred, increased amounts of GH and somatomedins cannot stimulate further long bone growth. Instead, these elevations cause connective tissue and cytoplasm increases.

Bony proliferation involves periosteal vertebral growth and enlargement of the facial bones and the bones of the hands and feet. The associated growth results in protrusion of the lower jaw and forehead. Because somatomedins stimulate cartilaginous growth, there is elongation of ribs at the bone-cartilage junction, causing a barrel-chested appearance and increased proliferation of cartilage in joints. Because of bony and soft-tissue overgrowth, nerves may be entrapped and damaged. This may be manifested by weakness, muscular atrophy, foot drop, and sensory changes in the hands. Because of a space-occupying lesion, central nervous system symptoms of headache, seizure activity, and visual disturbances may develop. The metabolic effects of GH hypersecretion include impaired carbohydrate tolerance and increased metabolic rate. Diabetes mellitus occurs when the pancreas is unable to secrete enough insulin to offset the effects of GH.

In children and adolescents whose epiphyseal plates have not yet closed, the effect of increased GH levels is **giantism**. Giantism is very rare because of early recognition and treatment of the adenoma. It occurs when the epiphyses are not fused and high levels of somatomedins stimulate excessive skeletal growth.

The goal of treatment is to protect the individual from the effects of tumor growth and to control hormone hypersecretion while minimizing damage to appropriately secreting portions of the pituitary. Surgery and radiation therapy are used, depending on the extent of tumor growth.

4. Characterize the manifestations of hypo-
   thyroidism and hyperthyroidism.
      Refer to Tables 18-1 and 18-2.

Manifestations of Hypothyroid and Hyperthyroid States

Characteristic	Hypothyroidism	Hyperthyroidism
Basal metabolic rate	Decreased	Increased
Sympathetic response	Decreased	Increased
Weight	Gain	Loss
Temperature tolerance	Cold intolerance Decreased sweating	Heat intolerance Increased sweating
Gastrointestinal function	Constipation Decreased appetite	Diarrhea Increased appetite
Cardiovascular function	Decreased cardiac output Bradycardia	Increased cardiac output Tachycardia and palpitations
Respiratory function	Hypoventilation	Dyspnea
Muscle tone and reflexes	Decreased	Increased
General appearance	Myxedematous Deep voice Impaired growth (child)	Exophthalmos Lid lag Decreased blinking Enlarged thyroid gland
General behavior	Mental retardation (infant) Mental and physical sluggishness Somnolence	Restlessness, irritability, anxiety Hyperkinesis Wakefulness

Note: Hypothyroidism is more common than hyperthyroidism.

5. Describe the disorders of hyperthyroidism;
   note the progressive states of severity.
      Study text pages 665-668; refer to Figure
      18-7.

Whenever thyroid hormones (TH) from any source exert greater-than-normal responses, **thyrotoxicosis** exists. **Hyperthyroidism** is a form of thyrotoxicosis in which excess thyroid hormones are secreted by the thyroid gland. Specific diseases that can cause hyperthyroidism include Graves disease and toxic multinodular goiter. Thyrotoxicosis other than hyperthyroidism in seen in subacute thyroiditis, increased TSH secretion, ectopic thyroid tissue, and ingestion of excessive TH. All forms of thyrotoxicosis share some common

characteristics because of increased circulating levels of thyroid hormones. The major types of therapy used to control the elevated levels of TH include drug therapy, radioactive iodine therapy, and surgery.

Graves disease is the most common form of hyperthyroidism and is likely associated with autoimmune abnormalities. Thyroid receptor antibody of the IgG class binds to the plasma membrane and initiates thyroid growth, vascularity, and hypersecretion of hormone. Ophthalmopathy appears in 50 to 70 percent of individuals with Graves disease. This disease is characterized by edema of the orbital contents, exophthalmos, and extraocular muscle weakness that sometimes leads to diplopia and pain, lacrimation, photophobia, and blurred vision.

Diffuse toxic goiter occurs when the thyroid gland enlarges in response to increased demand for TH. The demand for TH increases in puberty, pregnancy, iodine deficiency, and immunologic, viral, or genetic disorders. The increased number of follicles is compensatory in response to increased TSH levels. The thyroid gland returns to its original size when the stimulus for increased TH no longer exists. During the demand status, some follicular cells may be injured and produce less TH than the body requires. The remainder of the gland then functions to supply the body's need. Once thyrotoxicosis results, the condition is termed toxic multinodular goiter and the manifestations are similar to those of Graves disease, although infiltrative ophthalmopathy and myxedema do not occur.

Thyrotoxic crisis is rare but a dangerous worsening of the thyrotoxic state; death can occur within 48 hours without appropriate treatment. This condition occurs most frequently in individuals who have undiagnosed or partially treated severe hyperthyroidism and who are subjected to excessive stress from other causes. The systemic symptoms of thyrotoxic crisis include hyperthermia, tachycardia, high-output heart failure, agitation or delirium, and nausea, vomiting, or diarrhea contributing to fluid depletion. The symptoms may be attributed to increased beta-adrenergic receptors and catecholamines. The treatment is to reduce circulating TH levels by blocking thyroid hormone synthesis.

6. Describe the disorders of hypothyroidism.

Study text pages 668-671; refer to Figures 18-8 and 18-9.

Deficient production of TH by the thyroid gland results in hypothyroidism, which may be either primary or secondary. Primary causes include congenital defects or loss of thyroid tissue following treatment for hyperthyroidism and defective hormone synthesis resulting from antithyroid antibodies or endemic iodine deficiency. Causes of the less common secondary hypothyroidism are insufficient pituitary stimulation of the normal gland and peripheral resistance to TH.

Hypothyroidism can result from three distinct disorders. **Acute thyroiditis** is caused by bacterial infection of the thyroid gland and is rare. **Subacute thyroiditis** is a non-bacterial inflammation of the thyroid often preceded by a viral infection. Both conditions are accompanied by fever, tenderness, and enlargement of the thyroid. **Autoimmune thyroiditis** or **Hashimoto disease** results in destruction of thyroid tissue by circulating thyroid antibodies and infiltration of lymphocytes. Autoimmune thyroiditis may also be caused by an inherited immune defect.

The characteristic sign of severe or long-standing adult hypothyroidism is **myxedema.** In myxedema, the connective fibers are separated by an increased amount of protein and mucopolysaccharides. This protein-mucopolysaccharide complex binds water which develops nonpitting, boggy edema, especially around the eyes.

Myxedema coma is a medical emergency associated with severe hypothyroidism. Symptoms include hypothermia without shivering, hypoventilation, hypotension, hypoglycemia, and lactic acidosis. Older patients with severe vascular disease and with moderate or untreated hypothyroidism are particularly at risk for developing myxedema coma. It may also occur after overuse of narcotics or sedatives or after an acute illness in hypothyroid individuals.

Hypothyroidism in infants occurs because of absent thyroid tissue and hereditary defects in thyroid hormone synthesis. Signs may not be evident for at least four months after birth and include abdominal protrusion, umbilical hernia, subnormal temperature, lethargy, excessive sleeping, and slow pulse. Skeletal growth is stunted and the child will be dwarfed with short limbs if not treated. These signs constitute **cretinism**. Mental retardation in cretins is a function of the severity of hypothyroidism and the delay before initiation of thyroxine treatment.

Hypothyroidism is difficult to identify at birth, but high birth weight, hypothermia, delay in passing meconium, and neonatal jaundice are suggestive signs. There is a high probability of normal growth and intellectual function if treatment is started before the child is three or four months old.

Thyroid carcinoma is the most common endocrine malignancy but is still relatively rare. In approximately 10 percent of cases, any hyperplasia of the thyroid gland leads to thyroid carcinoma. The most consistent causal risk factor for the development of thyroid cancer is exposure to ionizing radiation during childhood. Changes in voice and swallowing and difficulty in breathing are related to tumor growth impinging on the esophagus or trachea. Treatment for this rare entity may include partial or total thyroidectomy, TSH suppressive therapy, radioactive iodine therapy, postoperative radiation therapy, and chemotherapy.

7. Distinguish between primary, secondary, and tertiary hyperparathyroidism and hypoparathyroidism.

Study text pages 671-674; refer to Table 18-3.

Approximately 80 percent of **primary hyperparathyroidism** disorders result from a chief cell adenoma with an increased secretion of parathyroid hormone (PTH). This causes hypercalcemia and decreased serum phosphate levels. **Secondary hyper-**

parathyroidism may be a compensatory response of the parathyroid glands to chronic hypocalcemia. Loss of calcium by failing kidneys leads to increased secretion of PTH. **Tertiary hyperparathyroidism** develops with hyperplasia of the parathyroid glands and a loss of sensitivity to normal circulating calcium levels. This hyperthyroidism frequently occurs in individuals with chronic renal failure. Tertiary hypersecretion of PTH causes excessive osteoclastic and osteolytic activity resulting in bone resorption. Pathologic fractures, kyphosis of the dorsal spine, and compression fractures of the vertebral bodies may occur.

Chronic hypercalcemia may be associated with insulin resistance, kidney stones, gastrointestinal disturbances, muscle weakness and lethargy, dehydration, and confusion. Long-term management of hypercalcemia uses drugs that decrease resorption of calcium from bone. Definitive treatment requires the surgical removal of the hyperplastic parathyroid glands.

Hypoparathyroidism is most commonly caused by damage to the parathyroid glands during thyroid surgery. In the absence of PTH, the ability to resorb calcium from bone and to regulate calcium reabsorption from the renal tubules are impaired. Hypocalcemia lowers the threshold for nerve and muscle excitation. Muscle spasms, hyperreflexia, clonic-tonic convulsions, laryngeal spasms, and, in severe cases, death from asphyxiation are seen with hypocalcemia. The treatment of hypoparathyroidism involves administration of calcium and vitamin D. Hypoplastic dentition, cataracts, bone deformities, and basal ganglia calcifications do not respond to the correction of hypocalcemia, but the other symptoms of hypocalcemia are reversible.

8. Describe the similarities and differences between insulin-dependent and non-insulin-dependent diabetes mellitus; note other types of diabetes mellitus.

Study text pages 674-681; refer to Tables 18-4 through 18-7.

Diabetes mellitus encompasses many etiologically unrelated diseases and includes many different causes of disturbed glucose tolerance. Diabetes mellitus is a syndrome characterized by chronic hyperglycemia and other disturbances of carbohydrate, fat, and protein metabolism. The four major classes of diabetes mellitus are insulin dependent diabetes mellitus (IDDM or type I diabetes mellitus), non-insulin-dependent diabetes mellitus (NIDDM or type II diabetes mellitus), malnutrition-related diabetes mellitus (MRDM), and other types of diabetes mellitus. Types I and II are the most common.

The diagnosis of diabetes is based on three observations: first, more than one fasting plasma glucose level greater than 140 mg/dL; second, elevated plasma glucose levels in response to an oral glucose tolerance test; and third, random plasma glucose levels above 200 mg/dL combined with classical symptoms or polydipsia, polyphagia, and polyuria. In individuals with poorly controlled diabetes, increases in the quantities of glycosylated hemoglobins are seen. Once a hemoglobin molecule is glycosylated, it remains that way.

Type I diabetes mellitus is characterized by a lack of insulin and a relative excess of glucagon and is most commonly diagnosed among whites under 30 years of age. In type I diabetes mellitus, beta cells are destroyed and islet cell antibodies appear. These antibodies tend to disappear with time. This disease seems to be caused by gradual process of autoimmune destruction in genetically susceptible individuals. Because of decreased use of glucose, glucose accumulates in the blood and is subsequently released in the urine. This in turn causes polyuria and polydipsia resulting from osmotic diuresis. Ketoacidosis, caused by increased levels of circulating ketones without the inhibiting effects of insulin; increased levels of circulating fatty acids; and weight loss are all manifestations of type I diabetes mellitus.

Type II diabetes mellitus is probably caused by genetic susceptibility that is triggered by environmental factors. The greatest risk factor for this diabetes is obesity. In the obese, insulin has a diminished ability to influence glucose uptake and metabolism. In type II diabetes, amyloid deposits in the islets, fatty atrophy of the pancreas and liver, and vascular sclerosis are generally present. Some insulin production continues in type II diabetes mellitus, but the mass and number of beta cells is decreased.

In the management of type I diabetes, insulin is most commonly given subcutaneously one to four times daily. The individual with type I diabetes mellitus must consume sufficient calories to achieve and maintain normal weight for height and age. Caloric intake should be regulated with consideration of age, activity, and severity of the diabetes. Approximately 55 to 60 percent of the total calories should be derived from carbohydrates, with less than 30 percent derived from fats, and 15 to 20 percent from proteins. Exercise by individuals with type I diabetes may result in hypoglycemia. Reducing the insulin dosage before exercising will reduce the possibility of hypoglycemia.

The treatment of the individual with type II diabetes requires appropriate meal planning as in type I diabetes; however, oral medication may be needed for optimal management. Oral hypoglycemic agents need a pancreas capable of synthesizing insulin. Thus, there must be some functioning beta cells. Insulin may also be used in the treatment of some individuals with type II diabetes. Exercise is as important aspect of treatment for the individual with type II diabetes. Exercise reduces after-meal blood glucose levels and diminishes insulin requirement. Increases in the level of good, high-density lipoprotein (HDL) cholesterol is achieved by exercise. Also, exercise adds to weight loss in the overweight individual.

Classifications of Diabetes and Glucose Intolerance States

Classification	Former Terminology	Characteristics
Diabetes mellitus(DM) Type I Insulin-dependent mellitus (IDDM)	Juvenile-onset diabetes	Few islet cells, acute onset at puberty, long preclinical record, insulin dependent, ketosis prone, autoimmune and genetic-environment etiology
Type II Non-insulin-dependent diabetes mellitus (NIDDM)	Adult-onset, maturity-onset diabetes (over age 40)	Usually not insulin dependent but they may use insulin, decreased islet cells because of age, not ketosis prone, frequently obese, likely an autosomal recessive disorder.
Malnutrition related diabetes (MRDM)	Pancreatic diabetes, topical diabetes	Severe protein malnutrition in tropical and developing countries, severe hyperglycemia without ketosis, etiology unknown
Other types Pancreatic disease Hormonal Drug or chemical-induced insulin receptor abnormalities	Secondary diabetes	Presence of diabetes and associated conditions
Impaired glucose tolerance (IGT)	Asymptomatic, chemical, subclinical, borderline, latent diabetes	Abnormal fasting glucose levels and glucose tolerance tests, 10-15% will convert to type II diabetes within 10 years
Gestational diabetes mellitus (GDM)	Same as above	Glucose intolerance develops during pregnancy (third trimester), increased risk of perinatal complications, increased risk of developing diabetes within 10-15 years after parturition

9. Identify the acute complications of diabetes mellitus; describe the features of each.

Study text pages 681-688; refer to Figures 18-10 and 18-11 and Tables 18-8 through 18-11.

Acute complications of diabetes mellitus include hypoglycemia or insulin shock, diabetic ketoacidosis (DKA), and hyperosmolar hyperglycemic nonketotic coma (HHNK).

Acute Complications of Diabetes Mellitus

Variable	Insulin Shock Hypoglycemia	DKA	HHNK
Onset	Rapid	Slow	Slowest
Symptoms	Weak, anxious, confused	Nausea, vomiting, polyuria, polyphagia, polydipsia, headache, irritable, comatose	Similar to DKA; stuporous, focal motor seizures
Skin	Cold, moist, pale	Hot, flushed, dry	Very dry
Mucous membranes	Normal	Dry	Extremely dry
Respiration	Normal	Hyperventilation, "fruity" or acetone odor to breath	Normal
Those at risk	Type I and II DM, fluctuating blood glucose levels, insufficient food intake, excessive exercise, oral medication, excessive insulin	Type I DM, stressful situations, omission of insulin	High carbohydrate diets, diuresis, hyperosmolar dialysis
Blood sugar/dL	30 mg or less in newborns, 60 mg or less in adults	300-800 + mg	600-4800 mg
Urine sugar	Low	High	High
Urine acetone	None	High	None, slight
Serum ketones	None	High	Moderate
Plasma pH	Normal	Acidic	Normal
Treatment	Fast-acting carbohydrate, intravenous glucose, subcutaneous glucagon	Low-dose insulin, electrolyte and fluid replacement	Fluid replacement with crystalloids and colloids

10. Describe the chronic complications of diabetes mellitus.

Study text pages 688-692; refer to Figures 18-12 and 18-13 and Tables 18-12 and 18-13.

Before the discovery of long-term insulin, the survival time of diabetics was short, especially for individuals with type I diabetes. Today, long-term survival is common. As a result, the problems of neuropathy, vascular disease, and infection have become important in clinical management of diabetic individuals.

Chronic Complications of Diabetes Mellitus

Insulin Deficiency

* Lipid mobilization

* Decreased glucose utilization

* Increased glucose production

Diabetic Neuropathies	Microvasular Disease	Macrovascular Disease	Infection
axonal and Schwann cell degenerations, altered motor nerve conduction, sensory alterations	* retinopathy * nephropathy capillary basement membrane thickening, decreased tissue perfusion or ischemia, hypertension	*coronary heart disease *CVA *peripheral vascular disease proliferation of fibrous plaques, atherosclerosis because of high serum lipids, ischemia	sensory impairment, atherosclerosis, ischemia, hypoxia, leukocytic impairment

11. Describe the etiology, pathogenesis, and manifestations of hyperfunction and hypofunction of the adrenal cortex.

Study text pages 692-700; refer to Figures 18-14 through 18-18 and Tables 18-14 and 18-15.

Cushing syndrome refers to excessive levels of circulating cortisol caused by hyperfunction of the adrenal cortex with or without pituitary involvement. **Cushing disease** refers specifically to pituitary-dependent hypercortisolism. Cushing-like syndrome may also develop as a result of the exogenous administration of cortisone. Elevated levels of pituitary ACTH account for approximately 75 to 80 percent of all cases of Cushing syndrome. Secretion of cortisol by an adrenal neoplasm accounts for approximately 10 percent of the cases of hypercorticoadrenalism.

Two observations consistently apply to individuals with Cushing syndrome: they lack diurnal or circadian secretion patterns of ACTH and cortisol, and they do not increase ACTH and cortisol secretion in response to a stressor. The elevated cortisol levels suppress hypothalamic CRH and pituitary ACTH secretion because normal feedback mechanisms still function. The low circulating levels of ACTH cause atrophy of the remaining normal portions of the adrenal cortex. This atrophy is considered reversible if the hypercortisolism is resolved, although recovery of cortisol-secreting activity of such cells may take several months.

Most of the clinical signs and symptoms of Cushing syndrome are caused by hypercortisolism. The most common feature is the accumulation of adipose tissue in the trunk, facial, and cervical areas. These have been described as "truncal obesity," "moon face," and "buffalo hump." Protein wasting is commonly observed in hypercortisolism and is caused by the catabolic effects of cortisol on peripheral tissues. Muscle wasting is especially obvious in the muscles of the extremities. Loss of the protein matrix in bone leads to osteoporosis and accompanying pathologic fractures, vertebral compression fractures, bone and back pain, kyphosis, and reduced height. Loss of collagen also leads to thin, weakened integumentary tissues through which capillaries are more visible. This accounts for the characteristic purple striae observed in the trunk area. Loss of collagenous support around small vessels makes them susceptible to rupture and easy bruising.

With elevated cortisol levels, vascular sensitivity to catecholamines is significantly increased, which leads to vasoconstriction and hypertension. Chronically elevated cortisol levels also cause suppression of the immune system and increased susceptibility to infections. Approximately 50 percent of individuals with Cushing syndrome experience irritability and depression. Without treatment, approximately 50 percent of individuals with Cushing syndrome die within five years of onset because of infection, suicide, complications from generalized arteriosclerosis, and hypertensive disease. Treatment is specific for the cause of hypercorticoadrenalism and includes medication, radiation, and surgery.

Hyperaldosteronism is characterized by excessive aldosterone secretion by the adrenal glands. An aldosterone secreting adenoma or excessive stimulation of the normal adrenal cortex by substances such as angiotensin, ACTH, or elevated potassium may cause hypersecretion. **Conn disease**, or **primary aldosteronism**, presents a clinical picture of hypertension, hypokalemia, renal potassium wasting, and neuromuscular manifestations. The most common cause of primary aldosteronism is the benign, single adrenal adenoma followed by multiple tumors or idiopathic hyperplasia of the adrenals. Because aldosterone secretion is normally stimulated by the renin-angiotensin system, **secondary hyperaldosteronism** can result from sustained elevated renin release and activation of angiotensin. Increased renin-angiotensin secretion occurs with decreased circulating blood volume and decreased delivery of blood to the kidneys.

Hypertension and hypokalemia are the essential manifestations of hyperaldosteronism. Hypertension usually results from increased intravascular volume and from altered serum sodium concentrations. If hypertension is sustained, left ventricular hypertrophy and progressive arteriosclerosis develops. Aldosterone-stimulated potassium loss can result in the typical manifestations of hypokalemia: hypokalemic alkalosis as potassium moves from the intracellular to extracellular space in exchange for hydrogen ions as well as renal loss of hydrogen ions to facilitate sodium reabsorption. Individuals with hypokalemic alkalosis may experience (1) tetany and paraesthesia, (2) skeletal muscle weakness, (3) cardiovascular alterations, and (4) loss of

urineconcentrating mechanisms leading to polyuria or nocturia. Treatment manages hypertension and hypokalemia with correction of any underlying causal abnormalities. If an aldosterone-secreting adenoma is present, it must be surgically removed.

Hypersecretion of adrenal androgens and estrogens may be caused by adrenal tumors, Cushing syndrome, or defects in steroid synthesis. The clinical manifestations depend on the hormone secreted, the sex of the individual, and the age at which the hypersecretion occurs. Hypersecretion of estrogens causes **feminization** or the development of female sex characteristics. Hypersecretion of androgens causes **virilization** or the development of male sex characteristics.

The effects of an estrogen-secreting tumor are most evident in males and cause gynecomastia, testicular atrophy, and decreased libido. In female children, such tumors may lead to early development of secondary sex characteristics. Androgen-secreting tumor changes are more easily observed in females and include excessive face and body hair growth or hirsutism, clitoral enlargement, deepening of the voice, amenorrhea, acne, and breast atrophy. In children, virilizing tumors promote precocious sexual development and bone aging. Treatment of androgen-secreting tumors usually involves surgical excision.

Hypocortisolism develops either because of inadequate stimulation of the adrenal glands by ACTH or because of an inability of the adrenals to produce and secrete the adrenal cortical hormones. Hypofunction of the adrenal cortex may affect glucocorticoid or mineralocorticoid secretion or a combination of both. Primary adrenal insufficiency is termed **Addison disease**, a relatively rare adult disease.

Addison disease is characterized by elevated serum ACTH levels with inadequate corticosteroid synthesis and output. The most common cause is idiopathic organ-specific autoimmune disease. A combination of cell membrane and cytoplasmic antibodies and cell-mediated immune mechanism contribute to the pathology of the disease. Apparently, a genetic defect in immune surveillance mechanisms causes a deficiency of immune suppressor cells. The symptoms of Addison disease are primarily a result of hypocortisolism and hypoaldosteronism. These manifestations include weakness, gastrointestinal disturbances, hypoglycemia, hyperpigmentation from increased ACTH secretion, and hypotension. The treatment of Addison disease involves glucocorticoid and possibly mineralocorticoid replacement therapy and dietary modifications to include adequate sodium. Hypocortisolism requires daily chronic glucocorticoid replacement therapy, and additional cortisol must be administered during acute stress.

12. Characterize adrenal medulla hyperfunction.
Study text pages 700-701; refer to Figure 18-18.

The most prominent cause of adrenal medulla hypersecretion is **pheochromocytoma**. Fewer than 10 percent of these tumors metastasize; if they do, they are usually found in the lungs, liver, bones, or para-aortic lymph glands. Most pheochromocytomas produce norepinephrine, although large tumors secrete both epinephrine and norepinephrine.

Pheochromocytomas cause excessive production of epinephrine and norepinephrine due to autonomous functioning of the tumor. The clinical manifestations of a pheochromocytoma include persistent hypertension associated with flushing, diaphoresis, tachycardia, palpitations, and constipation. Hypermetabolism may develop because of stimulation of the thyroid gland by the catecholamines. Glucose intolerance may occur because of catecholamine-induced inhibition of insulin release by the pancreas. The usual treatment of pheochromocytoma is surgical excision of the tumor. Medical therapy with adrenergic blocking agents is used to stabilize blood pressure prior to surgery.

Practice Examination

1. Which laboratory values would be expected in an individual with SIADH?
   a. serum sodium = 150 mEq/L and urine hypo-osmolality
   b. serum potassium = 5 mEq/L and serum hypo-osmolality
   c. serum sodium = 120 mEq/L and urine hypo-osmolality
   d. serum potassium = 3 mEq/L and serum hyper-osmolality

2. Hypopituitarism in an adult male likely includes all except
   a. dwarfism.
   b. impotence.
   c. muscular mass decrease.
   d. skin pallor.

3. Excessive secretion of hGH in an adult may cause
   a. acromegaly.
   b. giantism.
   c. hypoglycemia.
   d. decreased metabolic rate.

4. A characteristic shared by both diabetes mellitus and diabetes insipidus is
   a. elevated blood and urine glucose levels.
   b. inability to produce ADH.
   c. inability to produce insulin.
   d. polyuria.
   e. elevated blood urine and ketone body levels.

5. The manifestations of hyperthyroidism include all except
   a. diarrhea.
   b. constipation.
   c. heat intolerance.
   d. weight loss.
   e. wakefulness.

6. Hypothyroidism in adults is
   a. myxedema.
   b. Addison disease.
   c. Cushing disease.
   d. Graves disease.
   e. cretinism.

7. Treatment for Graves disease may include
   1. radioactive iodine.
   2. partial thyroidectomy
   3. antithyroid drugs
   4. TSH supplements

   a. 1, 2, 3
   b. 1, 3
   c. 2, 4
   d. 4
   e. 1, 2, 3, 4

8. Inadequate levels of thyroid hormones at birth may cause
   a. CNS abnormalities.
   b. immediate death.
   c. thyroid crisis.
   d. myxedema.
   e. dwarfism.

9. Hyperparathyroidism causes which of the following?
   1. increased osteoclastic activity
   2. decreased plasma calcium
   3. increased phosphorus absorption from GI tract
   4. hypocalcemia

   a. 1, 2
   b. 1
   c. 1, 2, 3
   d. 4

10. Manifestation of hypocalcemia include
    a. myopathy.
    b. lethargy.
    c. hypertension.
    d. tetany.
    e. bone cysts.

11. What is the most common cause of acromegaly?
    a. anterior pituitary adenoma
    b. overproduction of ACTH
    c. overproduction of TSH
    d. pituitary atrophy

12. If a 19-year-old woman were suffering from shortness of breath, weight loss, excessive sweating, exophthalmos, and irritability, what hormone would you expect to find elevated in her serum?
    a. cortisol
    b. thyroxine
    c. ACTH
    d. 17-ketosteroid

13. A 24-year-old female with a history of "juvenile-onset" diabetes is found in a stuporous state. She is hypotensive and has cold clammy skin. What is the likely etiology of her condition?
    a. hyperglycemia
    b. insulin reaction
    c. renal failure
    d. peripheral neuropathy

14. A 10-year-old male came into the ER comatose, suffering from metabolic acidosis, hyperkalemia, 4+ ketones, and blood glucose of 800 mg/dL. The most probable disease is
    a. cretinism.
    b. IDDM.
    c. NIDDM.
    d. IGT.
    e. GDM.

15. Your neighbor has not previously been diabetic but has gained 80 pounds the past year and is able to produce some insulin. Her fasting blood sugar is always elevated. She is being treated with oral insulin-stimulating drugs. This is likely
    a. diabetes insipidus.
    b. IDDM.
    c. NIDDM.
    d. IGT.
    e. GDM.

16. Common symptoms and signs of diabetes mellitus include all except
    a. hyperglycemia.
    b. blurred vision.
    c. increased muscle anabolism.
    d. persistent infection.
    e. polyuria.

17. Which laboratory finding is inconsistent with a diagnosis of insulin dependent diabetes mellitus (IDDM)?
    a. FBS (fasting blood sugar) of 90 mg%
    b. ketonuria
    c. blood glucose of 210 mg% after 1 hour following ingestion of 100 Gm glucose
    d. decreased serum insulin level
    e. All are consistent with IDDM.

18. Common complications to diabetes mellitus include all except
    a. retinopathy.
    b. peripheral neuropathy.
    c. nephropathy (kidney disease).
    d. None is common.
    e. All are common.

19. An individual with Type I diabetes mellitus while cross country running experiences hunger, lightheadedness, headache, confusion, and tachycardia. The likely cause of these manifestations is
    a. hyperglycemia.
    b. eating a snack before running.
    c. hypoglycemia because of running.
    d. Both a and b are correct.
    e. None of the above is correct.

20. Which is/are expected during hyperinsulinism?
    a. excess insulin
    b. high serum glucose
    c. epinephrine release
    d. All of the above are correct.
    e. Both a and c are correct.

21. Long-term corticosteroid therapy may cause
    1. delayed wound healing.   a. 1, 2, 3
    2. osteoporosis.   b. 4
    3. peptic ulcers.   c. 1, 3
    4. hyperkalemia.   d. 2, 4
                                        e. 1, 2, 3, 4

22. Which electrolyte changes occur in Addison disease?
    a. hypokalemia
    b. hypernatremia
    c. hyperkalemia
    d. hypocalcemia

23. A benign tumor of adrenal glands which causes hypersecretion of aldosterone is
    a. Addison disease.
    b. a pheochromocytoma.
    c. Cushing disease.
    d. Cushing syndrome.
    e. Conn disease.

Match the hypersecretion with the circumstance.

24. hypersecretion of aldosterone
25. hypersecretion of glucocorticoids

a. decreased cardiac output
b. hyperglycemia and/or osteoporosis
c. BMR (Basal Metabolic Rate) increases
d. hypernatremia
e. hyponatremia

Case Study

Scott, a 17-year-old high school football player, was brought to the hospital emergency room in a coma. According to his mother, he had lost weight during the last month in spite of eating large amounts of food. Besides losing weight, he was excessively thirsty and had frequently awakened his younger brother as he noisily voided several times during the night. The family history revealed others with diabetes mellitus. Physical examination was not significant except for tachycardia and hyperpnea.

Laboratory serum studies revealed:

Glucose on admission = 1000 mg/dl (high)
pH = 7.25 (low)
pCO_2 = 30 mm Hg (low)
HCO_3^- = 12 mEq/L (low)
ketones = 4+ (high)
glycosylated hemoglobin = 9% (high)

What to you think Scott's symptoms, signs, and diagnostic studies suggest regarding acute complications of diabetes mellitus?

Structure and Function of the Reproductive Systems

Objectives

After successful study of this chapter, the learner will be able to:

1. Describe the hormonal stimulation of the reproductive systems; note secondary sex characteristics.
Review text pages 714-715; refer to Figure 19-3.

2. Identify female external and internal genitalia.
Review text pages 715-721; refer to Figures 19-4 through 19-9.

3. Describe the time frame of the menstrual cycle, noting its differential hormonal effects, levels, and cellular events.
Review text pages 721-726; refer to Figure 19-11 and Tables 19-1 and 19-2.

4. Identify male external and internal genitalia.
Review text pages 726-731; refer to Figures 19-12 through 19-16.

5. Relate androgen production to spermatogenesis.
Review text pages 731-733; refer to Figures 19-17 and 19-18.

6. Describe the progressive and the cyclical hormonal changes associated with female breast tissue; note the lymphatic drainage.
Review text pages 733-735; refer to Figures 19-19 and 19-20.

7. List the tests to evaluate reproductive function.
Refer to Tables 19-4 and 19-5.

8. Identify normal changes in the female and male reproductive systems that occur with advancing age.
Review text pages 739-740.

Practice Examination

1. GnRH reaches the anterior pituitary gland through the hypothalamic hypophyseal-portal system and causes the release of
   1. growth hormone.
   2. FSH.
   3. ADH.
   4. LH.
   5. oxytocin.

   a. 1, 2, 3
   b. 3, 5
   c. 2
   d. 4
   e. 2, 4

2. Which is not a structure of the female external genitalia?
   a. vagina
   b. clitoris
   c. vestibule
   d. labia minor
   e. labia major

3. A new menstrual cycle has a rise in the levels of
   a. LH.
   b. GH.
   c. estrogen.
   d. progesterone.
   e. LSH.

4. Progesterone
   a. stimulates lactation.
   b. increases uterine tube motility.
   c. thins the endometrium.
   d. maintains the thickened endometrium.
   e. causes ovulation.

5. The ovaries produce
   a. ova, estrogen, and oxytocin.
   b. ova only.
   c. ova and estrogen.
   d. testosterone and semen.
   e. None of the above is correct.

6. During which days of the menstrual cycle does the endometrium achieve maximum development?
   a. 2-6
   b. 7-12
   c. 14
   d. 20-24
   e. 26-28

7. Hormones necessary for the growth and development of female breasts are
   a. estrogens and progesterone.
   b. oxytocin and ADH.
   c. androgens and steroids.
   d. gonadocorticoids.
   e. relaxin.

8. The structure that releases a mature ovum is the
   a. corpus albicans.
   b. graafian follicle.
   c. primary follicle.
   d. corpus luteum.
   e. infundibulum.

9. A major duct of the female reproductive system is the
   a. suspensory tube.
   b. uterosacral duct.
   c. broad duct.
   d. mesovarian duct.
   e. uterine tube.

10. Prostate is to the accessory gland as gonad is to the
    a. ejaculatory duct.
    b. ovary.
    c. bulbourethral gland.
    d. accessory gland.
    e. urethra.

11. Cells that produce testosterone are called
    a. interstitial endocrinocytes.
    b. testicular endocrine cells.
    c. sustentacular cells.
    d. spermatogonia.
    e. None of the above is correct.

12. The function of testosterone includes
    a. development of male gonads.
    b. bone and muscle growth.
    c. influencing sexual behavior.
    d. growth of testes.
    e. All of the above are correct.

13. Immediately after the sperm cells leave the ducts epididymis, they enter the
    a. ejaculatory duct.
    b. ductus deferens.
    c. urethra.
    d. exterior of the body.
    e. None of the above is correct.

14. A substance produced in the reproductive system mainly by the bulbourethral glands is
    a. fructose.
    b. HCl.
    c. mucus.
    d. an alkaline, viscous fluid.

15. Which of the following produce(s) a secretion that helps maintain the motility of spermatozoa?
    a. prostate
    b. penis
    c. greater vestibular glands
    d. interstitial tissues
    e. All of the above are correct.

16. Semen is
    a. vaginal secretions needed to activate sperm.
    b. the product of the testes.
    c. the sperm and secretions of the seminal vesicles, prostate, and bulbourethral gland.
    d. responsible for engorgement of the erectile tissue in the penis.
    e. the secretion that causes ovulation in the female.

17. The vulva consists of the
    a. labia majora and labia minora.
    b. clitoris.
    c. vaginal orifice.
    d. Both a and b are correct.
    e. a, b and c are correct.

18. The major difference between female and male hormone production is
    a. LH is without effect in the male.
    b. GnRH doesn't cause the release of FSH in the male.
    c. hormonal production is relatively constant in the male.
    d. Both a and b are correct.
    e. None of the above is correct.

19. The primary spermatocyte has
    a. 46 chromosomes.
    b. the same number of chromosomes as a sperm.
    c. 23 chromosomes.
    d. a diploid number of chromosomes.
    e. Both a and d are correct.

20. During the follicular/proliferative phase of the menstrual cycle,
    a. vascularity of breast tissue increases.
    b. vascularity of breast tissue decreases.
    c. progesterone constricts the ducts.
    d. Both b and c are correct.

21. Most of the lymphatic drainage of the female breast occurs through the
    a. axillary nodes.
    b. internal mammary nodes.
    c. subclavian nodes.
    d. brachial nodes.
    e. anterior pectoral nodes.

Match the aging reproductive changes with the term or response.

22. primary follicles resist gonadotropin stimulation
23. corpus luteum fails to develop
24. less effective erection
25. first menstruation

a. menarche
b. premenopause
c. menopause
d. vasomotor flush
e. vasocongestive response
f. luteal/secretory phase
g. follicular/proliferative phase

144

Alterations of the Reproductive Systems

Prerequisite Objectives

a. Describe the relationships of hormones to the normal menstrual cycle.
   Review text pages 723-725; refer to Figure 19-11.

Remember!

- The three phases of the menstrual cycle are the follicular/proliferative phase, the luteal/secretory phase, and menstruation. During menstruation, the functional layer of the endometrium disintegrates and is discharged through the vagina. Menstruation is followed by the follicular/proliferative phase. During this phase, the anterior pituitary gland secretes FSH, which causes an ovarian follicle to develop. While the follicle is developing, it secretes estrogen, which causes cells of the endometrium to proliferate. By the time the ovarian follicle is mature, the endometrial lining is restored. At this point, ovulation occurs.

- Ovulation marks the beginning of the luteal/secretory phase of the menstrual cycle. The ovarian follicle begins its transformation into a corpus luteum. LH from the anterior pituitary stimulates the corpus luteum to secrete progesterone which initiates the secretory phase of endometrial development. If conception occurs, the nutrient-laden endometrium is ready for implantation. If conception and implantation do not occur, the corpus luteum degenerates and ceases its production of progesterone and estrogen. Without progesterone or estrogen to maintain it, the endometrium enters the ischemic phase and disintegrates. Then, menstruation occurs, marking the beginning of another cycle.

b. Identify the circumstances required for normal reproductive function in the male and female.
   Review text page 738; refer to Tables 19-4 and 19-5.

Remember!

- The male must have normal numbers, amounts, structure, and motility of sperm with no obstruction along the reproductive tract. The female must have the cervix, uterus, and fallopian tubes adequately patent to allow passage of ovum and sperm. She must also have normal ovulation, an endometrium responding to hormones, and reproductive organs and tissues free of tumors or infections.

c. Characterize the structure and development of the female breast.
   Review text pages 733-735; refer to Figure 19-19.

Remember!

- The female breast is composed of 15 to 20 pyramid-shaped lobes which are separated and supported by Cooper ligaments. Each lobe contains 20 to 40 lobules which subdivide into many functional units called acini. Each acinus is lined with a layer of epithelial cells capable of secreting milk and a layer of subepithelial cells capable of contracting to squeeze milk from the acinus. The acini empty into a network of lobular collecting ducts that reach the skin through openings in the nipple. The lobes and lobules are surrounded and separated by muscle strands and fatty connective tissue. An extensive capillary network surrounds the acini. Lymphatic drainage of the breast occurs largely through the axillary nodes.

- The nipple is a pigmented, cylindrical structure that has multiple openings. The areola is the pigmented, circular area around the nipple. A number of sebaceous glands are located within the areola and aid in lubrication of the nipple during lactation. The nipple's smooth muscle is innervated by the sympathetic nervous system.

- During childhood, breast growth is latent and growth of the nipple and areola keeps pace with body surface. At the onset of puberty in the female, estrogen secretion stimulates mammary growth. Full differentiation and development of breast tissue are mediated by a variety of hormones including estrogen, progesterone, prolactin, growth hormone, thyroid hormone, insulin, and cortisol.

- During the reproductive years, the breast undergoes cyclic changes in response to changes in the levels of estrogen and progesterone associated with the menstrual cycle. Because the length of the menstrual cycle does not allow for complete regression of new cell growth, breast growth continues at a slow rate until approximately age 35. The number of acini increase with each cycle, so epithelial tissue proliferation is under the influence of hormones as long as secretion occurs.

Objectives

After successful study of this chapter, the learner will be able to:

1. **Distinguish between various menstrual disorders and their assorted hormonal alterations or causes; identify manifestations of premenstrual syndrome.**
   Study text pages 748-754; refer to Figure 20-1 and Tables 20-1 and 20-2.

Abnormal Menstrual Cycles

Disorder	*Alteration*
Primary dysmenorrhea	Excessive endometrial prostaglandin production
Painful menstruation	Increases myometrial contractions and constricts blood vessels
	(Continued)

Abnormal Menstrual Cycles *(cont'd)*

Disorder	*Alteration*
Amenorrhea	
Absence of menstruation	
Primary: menarche failure	Hypothalamus fails to synthesize Gn RH LH and FSH from pituitary are not secreted so no ovulation occurs, no menstruation nor secondary sex characteristics
Secondary: menstruation absence following menarche	Structural abnormalities, regulatory hormones inhibit ovulation
Dysfunctional Uterine Bleeding (DUB) Heavy or irregular bleeding caused by disturbance of menstrual cycle	Progesterone deficiency or estrogen excess Estrogen proliferates endometrium while progesterone limits it, large mass of tissue available for heavy, irregular bleeding
Polycystic Ovarian Syndrome (PCO) anovulation causes enlarged, polycystic ovaries	LH is elevated which increases androgen secretion by ovaries, androgen is converted to estrogen peripherally, excessive endometrial tissue and dysfunctional bleeding
Premenstrual Syndrome (PMS) cyclic physical, psychologic, or behavioral changes impair relationships	Abnormal nervous, immunologic, vascular, and gastrointestinal tissue response to menstrual cycle, fluctuating estrogen and progesterone levels, genetic

Premenstrual syndrome (PMS) is the cyclic recurrence in the luteal phase of the menstrual cycle of physical, psychologic, or behavioral changes distressing enough to impair interpersonal relationships or usual activities. It has been estimated that 5 to 10 percent of menstruating women have severe to disabling premenstrual symptoms and 50 percent or more have moderately distressing symptoms. Currently, it is believed that PMS is the end result of abnormal tissue response of nervous, immunologic, vascular, and gastrointestinal systems to the normal changes of the menstrual cycle. This biological response may or may not be triggered by fluctuating estrogen and progesterone levels.

A predisposition to PMS runs in families and is likely due to genetics and/or environment. There is some evidence that supports a relationship between the severity and frequency of premenstrual symptoms and perfectionism, increased stress, poor nutrition, lack of exercise, low self-esteem, and history of sexual abuse or family conflict. Depression, anger, irritability, and fatigue have been reported

as the most prominent and the most distressing symptoms; physical symptoms seem less prevalent and problematic.

Initial treatment requires education on PMS, self-help stress reduction techniques, elimination of contributing factors, or treatment of coexisting disorders and conflict resolution. Eating six meals a day; increasing intake of complex carbohydrates, fiber, and water; and decreasing caffeine, alcohol, sugar, and animal fat consumption may be beneficial. After a trial of nonpharmacologic therapies, medications may be added to the treatment plan even if their efficacy in the treatment of PMS is questionable.

2. Describe pelvic inflammatory disease.
Study text page 754; refer to Figures 20-2 and 20-3.

Pelvic inflammatory disease (PID) is an acute inflammatory process caused by infection. PID involves organs of the upper genital tract, the uterus, fallopian tubes or uterine tubes, or ovaries. In its most severe form, the entire peritoneal cavity may be involved. Infection of the fallopian tubes is salpingitis; infection of the ovaries is oophoritis. Most cases of PID are caused by sexually transmitted microorganisms that ascend from the vagina to the uterus, fallopian tubes, and ovaries. PID is considered a polymicrobial infection with the majority of cases being caused by gonorrheal or chlamydial microbes. These organisms may induce a response that causes tubo-necrosis with repeated infections, and may predispose a woman to PID. After one episode of pelvic infection, 15 to 25 percent of women develop long-term sequelae such as infertility, ectopic pregnancy, chronic pelvic pain, and pelvic adhesions. The incidence of complications increases markedly with repeated infections.

The clinical manifestations of PID are variable. Sixty-seven to 75 percent of women with salpingitis have subclinical infections. The first sign of the ascending infection may be the gradual onset of low bilateral abdominal pain often characterized as dull and steady. Symptoms are more likely to develop during or immediately after menstruation. The pain of PID may worsen with walking, jumping, or intercourse. Other manifestations of PID are difficult or painful urination and irregular bleeding. Other conditions causing pelvic pain must be excluded, such as ectopic pregnancy, threatened abortion, or appendicitis before treatment. Treatment involves bedrest, avoidance of intercourse, and combined antibiotic therapy. Twenty-five to 40 percent of women require hospitalization for intravenous administration of antibiotics and treatment of peritonitis or tubo-ovarian abscess.

3. Define and cite causes of vaginitis, cervicitis, vulvitis, and bartholinitis.

Study text pages 754-757; refer to Figure 20-4.

Vaginitis is an infection of the vagina mostly caused by sexually transmitted pathogens and *Candida albican*s. Since the acidic nature of vaginal secretions during the reproductive years provides protection against a variety of sexually transmitted pathogens, variables that alter the vaginal pH may predispose a woman to infection. The use of antibiotics may destroy *Lactobacillus acidophilus* which helps maintain an acidic vaginal pH. Thus, there may be an overgrowth of *C. albicans* which could cause a yeast vaginitis.

Cervicitis is an inflammation of the cervix usually caused by one or more sexually transmitted pathogens. A mucopurulent exudate drains from the external os.

Vulvitis is an inflammation of the skin of the vulva and often of the perianal area. Vulvitis can be caused by contact with soaps, detergents, lotions, hygienic sprays, menstrual pads, perfumed toilet paper, or nonabsorbent or tight-fitting clothes.

Bartholinitis is an inflammation of one or both of the ducts that lead from the vaginal opening to the Bartholin glands. The causes of bartholinitis are microorganisms that infect the lower female reproductive tract; this disorder is usually preceded by cervicitis, vaginitis, or urethritis. Infection or trauma causes inflammatory changes that narrow the distal portion of the duct, leading to obstruction and stasis of glandular secretions and causing further inflammation.

4. Characterize the benign growth and proliferative conditions of the female reproductive system.

Study text pages 758-762; refer to Figures 20-7 through 20-9.

Benign Lesions of the Female Reproductive System

	Cause	*Manifestations*
Ovarian Cyst		
follicular cyst	Ovarian follicle doesn't release ovum, fluid isn't reabsorbed from degenerating follicle	Pelvic and abdominal pain, menstrual irregularities
corpus luteum cyst	A persistent corpus luteum secretes progesterone	Pelvic pain, amenorrhea with subsequent heavy bleeding
Endometrial polyps	Estrogen stimulation	Premenstrual or intermenstrual bleeding
	(Continued)	

148

Benign Lesions of the Female Reproductive System *(cont'd)*

Lesion	Cause	Manifestations
Leiomyomas (smooth muscle tumor)	Unknown, hormonal fluctuations alter size	Abnormal or increased uterine bleeding, pain, pressure
Adenomyosis (endometrial tissue in the myometrium)	Repeated pregnancies	Dysmenorrhea, uterine enlargement and tenderness
Endometriosis (ectopic endometrial tissue)	Depressed T_c cells tolerate ectopic tissue, genetics	Ectopic tissues respond to hormonal stimulation, bleeding causes pelvic adhesions and pain

5. Characterize the malignant tumors of the female reproductive system.

Study text pages 762-769; refer to Figures 20-10 and 20-11 and Tables 20-5 through 20-7.

Malignant Tumors of the Female Reproductive System

	Cause	Manifestations
Cervical Cancer	STD, human papilloma virus, early sexual activity, multiple sex partners, smoking, diet, and vitamin deficiencies	Asymptomatic vaginal bleeding or discharge, grade of epithelial thickness enables precursor lesion diagnosis
Vaginal Cancer	Previous cervical cancer, nonsteroidal estrogens inhibit normal epithelial replacement	Asymptomatic, vaginal bleeding or discharge
Endometrial Cancer	Multiple risk factors: obesity, high fat diet, no pregnancies, late menopause, hypertension	Vaginal bleeding
Ovarian Cancer	Unknown, risk factors are similar to those for endometrial cancer	Diverse: pain and abdominal swelling, postmenopausal bleeding

6. Define terms used in female sexual dysfunction.

Study text pages 769-770; refer to Table 20-9.

Sexual anorexia or inhibited sexual desire may be a biological manifestation of depression, alcohol or other substance abuse, prolactin-secretin pituitary tumors, or testosterone deficiency. Beta-adrenergic blockers used for heart disease may also inhibit sexual desire.

Vaginismus is an involuntary muscle spasm in response to attempted penetration. Common causes include prior sexual trauma, fear of sex, or organic disorders.

Anorgasmia is the inability of the woman to reach or achieve orgasm. This inability ranges from difficulty in arousal to lack of orgasm. Any chronic illness may affect arousal. Orgasmic dysfunction is linked to organic causes in less than 5 percent of cases. Drugs such as narcotics, tranquilizers, antidepressants, and antihypertensive medications can inhibit orgasm.

Dyspareunia or painful intercourse is common. Inadequate lubrication may make penetration or intercourse unpleasant. Drugs with a drying effect, such as antihistamines, certain tranquilizers, and marijuana, and disorders such as diabetes, vaginal infections, and estrogen deficiency can decrease lubrication. Other causes of dyspareunia include infections and anatomical constraints around the introitus or the vulva.

Infertility is the inability to conceive after one year of unprotected intercourse and affects approximately 15 percent of all couples. Important causes of infertility in the female are malfunctions of the fallopian tubes, the ovaries, or the reproductive hormones. Endometriosis also may contribute to infertility.

7. By site, describe common disorders of the male reproductive system; distinguish between benign prostatic hypoplasia, prostatitis, and prostatic cancer.
Study text pages 770-782; refer to Figures 20-12 through 20-24.

Urethritis is an inflammatory process usually caused by sexually transmitted microorganisms. Nonsexual origins of urethritis are inflammation or infection as a result of urologic procedures, insertion of foreign bodies into the urethra, anatomic abnormalities, or trauma. Symptoms of urethritis include urtheral tingling or itching or a burning sensation when urinating. Frequency, urgency, and purulent or clear mucous-like discharge from the urethra may occur. Treatment is appropriate antibiotic therapy for infectious urethritis and avoidance of mechanical irritation.

Urethral stricture is a narrowing of the urethra because of scarring. The scars may be congenital but are more likely to result from trauma or untreated or severe urethral infections. Symptoms include urinary frequency and hesitancy, diminished force and size of the urinary stream, dribbling after voiding, and nocturia. Treatment is usually surgical and may involve urethral dilation, urethrotomy, or a variety of other surgical techniques.

Phimosis and **paraphimosis** are both disorders in which the penile foreskin, or prepuce, is "too tight" to be moved easily over the glans penis. In phimosis, the foreskin cannot be retracted back over the glans; whereas in paraphimosis the foreskin is retracted and cannot be moved forward to cover the glans. Phimosis can occur at any age and is most commonly caused by poor hygiene and chronic infection. Circumcision, if needed, is performed after infection has been eradicated. In paraphimosis, surgery must be performed to pre-

vent necrosis of the glans caused by constricted blood vessels.

Peyronie disease is a fibrotic condition that causes lateral curvature of the penis during erection. The problem usually affects middle-aged men and is associated with painful erection, painful intercourse for both partners, and poor erection distal to the involved area. There is no definitive treatment for Peyronie disease. Spontaneous remissions occur about 50 percent of the time. Pharmacologic therapies that increase oxygenation may hasten resolution. Surgical resection of the fibrous plaque followed by grafting have been successful.

Balanitis is an inflammation of the glans penis and usually occurs in conjunction with an inflammation of the prepuce. It is associated with poor hygiene and phimosis. The accumulation under the foreskin of glandular secretions, sloughed epithelial cells, and *Mycobacterium smegmatis* can irritate the glans directly or lead to infection. Balanitis is most commonly seen in men with poorly controlled diabetes mellitus and candidiasis. Antimicrobials are used to treat infection, and circumcision can prevent recurrences.

Penile cancer is rare in the United States. Although the exact etiology is unknown, cancer of the penis is likely a result of chronic irritation caused by smegma beneath a phimotic foreskin.

Varicocele, hydrocele, and spermatocele are common intrascrotal disorders. **Varicocele** is an abnormal dilation of a vein within the spermatic cord and most occur on the left side. They may be painful or tender. They occur in 10 to 15 percent of males, frequently after puberty. The cause of varicocele is incompetent or congenitally absent valves in the spermatic veins that normally prevent backflow of blood. Thus, blood pools in the veins rather than flowing into the venous system. Decreased blood flow through the testis interferes with spermatogenesis and can cause infertility. A **hydrocele** is a collection of fluid within the tunica vaginalis and is the most common cause of scrotal swelling. Hydroceles in infants are congenital malformations that frequently resolve spontaneously by one year of age. Hydroceles in adults may be caused by an imbalance between the secreting and absorptive capacities of scrotal tissues. The **spermatocele** is a cyst located between the head of the epididymis and the testis that usually is asymptomatic or produces mild discomfort that is relieved by scrotal support.

Cryptorchidism is a condition in which one or both testes fail to descend into the scrotum. It is the most common congenital condition involving the testes. In approximately 75 to 90 percent of infants with cryptorchidism, the testes descend into the scrotum by one year of age. The cause of cryptorchidism is not clear but may result from a developmental delay, a defect of the testis, deficient maternal gonadotropin stimulation, or some mechanical factor that prevents descent through the inguinal canal. Untreated cryptorchidism is associated with lowered sperm count and impaired fertility. Undescended testes are susceptible to neoplastic processes. Treatment often begins with administration of human chorionic gonadotropin. If hormonal therapy is not successful, the testis is located and moved into the scrotum surgically.

Torsion of the testis is a condition wherein the testis rotates on its vascular pedicle; this interrupts its blood supply. Onset may be spontaneous or follow physical exertion or trauma. If the torsion cannot be reduced manually, surgery must be performed within six hours after the onset of symptoms to preserve normal testicular function.

Orchitis is an acute inflammation of the testes and is uncommon except as a complication of systemic infection or as an extension of an associated epididymitis. Mumps is the most common infectious cause of orchitis and usually affects postpubertal males. The onset is sudden and occurs three to four days after the onset of parotitis. Irreversible damage to spermatogenesis results in about 30 percent of affected testes. Treatment is supportive and includes bed rest, scrotal support, elevation of the scrotum, hot or cold compresses, and analgesic agents for relief of pain. Appropriate antimicrobial drugs should be used for bacterial orchitis. Corticosteroids are indicated in proved cases of nonspecific granulomatous orchitis.

Testicular cancers are rare, accounting for approximately 1 percent of all male cancers; yet, they are the most common solid tumor of young adult men. The cure rate is greater than 95 percent. The etiology of testicular neoplasms is unknown. Because young men are affected most frequently, it is believed that high levels of androgens may contribute to carcinogenesis. A genetic predisposition exists. Cryptorchidism also is statistically associated with the development of testicular cancer. Apparently, the undescended testis has a developmental defect or undergoes gradual involution and degeneration over time which may contribute to neoplastic changes.

Painless testicular enlargement usually is the first sign of testicular cancer. Enlargement is gradual and may be accompanied by a sensation of testicular heaviness or dull ache in the lower abdomen. Occasionally, acute pain occurs because of rapid growth; then, there may be hemorrhage and necrosis. Besides surgery, treatment involves radiation and chemotherapy singly or in combination. Orchiectomy does not affect sexual function.

Epididymitis, inflammation of the epididymis, generally occurs in sexually active young males. In young men, the usual cause is a sexually transmitted microorganism. In men over 35 years of age, intestinal bacteria and *Psuedomonas aeruginosa*

found in urinary tract infections and prostatitis may also cause epididymitis. The pathogenic microorganism reaches the epididymis by ascending the vas deferens from an infected urethra or bladder. Acute and severe scrotal or inguinal pain is caused by inflammation of the epididymis and surrounding tissues. The individual may have pyuria and bacteriuria and a history of urinary symptoms including urethral discharge. Complications of epididymitis include abscess formation, infarction of the testis, recurrent infection, scarring of epididymal endothelium, and infertility. Treatment includes antibiotic therapy for the infection and various measures to provide symptomatic relief. The individual's sexual partner should be treated with antibiotics if the causative microorganism is a sexually transmitted pathogen.

Benign prostatic hyperplasia (BPH) is also called benign prostatic hypertrophy and causes problems as enlarged prostatic tissue compresses the prostatic urethra. More than half of all men between 60 and 69 years of age have prostatic enlargement. During the third decade of life, the prostate reaches adult size. Between 40 and 45 years of age, benign hyperplasia begins and continues slowly until death. Current etiologic theories of BPH implicate estrogen/androgen synergism or undefined prostatic growth factors with possible additional hormonal involvement.

BPH begins in the periurethral glands, which are the inner glands or layers of the prostate. As nodular hyperplasia and cellular hypertrophy progress, the compressed prostatic urethra usually, but not always, causes bladder outflow obstruction. During the early stages of urethral obstruction, the detrusor muscle hypertrophies to expel urine against increasing urethral resistance. The urge to urinate frequently, some delay in starting urination, and decreased force of the urinary stream develop. Over a period of several years, the bladder is unable to empty all of the urine and urine retention becomes chronic.

Progressive bladder distention causes sacculations or diverticular outpouchings of the bladder wall. The ureters may be obstructed as they pass through the hypertrophied detrusor muscle. Bladder or kidney infection then develops. Hyperplastic tissue may be removed surgically, drugs can be used to relax the smooth muscle of the bladder, and a specific drug may shrink the prostate gland by interrupting the action of hormones.

Prostatitis is an inflammation of the prostate usually limited to a few of the gland's excretory ducts. Prostatitis is categorized as acute bacterial prostatitis, chronic bacterial prostatitis, or nonbacterial prostatitis.

Acute bacterial prostatitis is an ascending infection of the urinary tract that tends to occur in men between the ages of 30 and 50 but also is associated with BPH in older men. Coliform bacteria are common causes of acute bacterial prostatitis. Symptoms include dysuria and urinary frequency and lower abdominal and suprapubic discomfort. The individual may also have a slow, small urinary stream, inability to empty the bladder, and the need to urinate frequently during the night. Systemic signs of infection include sudden onset of a high fever, fatigue, joint pain, and muscle pain. Long-term, broad-spectrum antibiotics may be required to resolve the infection and control its spread. Pain relievers, antipyretics, bed rest, and adequate hydration are also used therapeutically.

Chronic bacterial prostatitis is characterized by recurrent urinary tract infections and the persistence of pathogenic bacteria. This prostatitis is the most common recurrent urinary tract infection in men. Symptoms are variable and may be similar to those of acute bacterial prostatitis. The prostate may be only slightly enlarged, but fibrosis causes it to be firm and irregular in shape. Treatment of chronic bacterial prostatitis is difficult mainly because fibrosis blocks passage of antibiotics into prostatic tissues. Therefore, therapeutic levels are hard to achieve. The usual treatment is a 12-week course of antibiotics. If chronic bacterial prostatitis is not cured medically, a radical transurethral prostatectomy may be required.

Nonbacterial prostatitis is the most common prostatitis syndrome and consists of prostatic inflammation without evidence of bacterial infection. Its etiology is unclear. Men with nonbacterial prostatitis may complain of continuous or spasmodic pain in the suprapubic, infrapubic, scrotal, penile, or inguinal area. The prostate gland generally feels normal upon palpation. Nonbacterial prostatitis is diagnosis by exclusion. There is no generally accepted treatment for nonbacterial prostatitis. A course of antibiotics for both affected individuals and sexual partners may minimize symptoms.

Prostatic cancer accounts for more than 13 percent of all cancer deaths and more than 28 percent of all cancers in men in the United States; only lung cancer accounts for more male deaths. Prostatic cancer rarely occurs in men under the age of 40. Incidence increases with advancing age; over 80 percent of all prostate cancers are diagnosed in men over age 65. It is believed that both genetic and environmental influences play a role in the etiology of prostate cancer. Male hormones play an additional role as a tumor-promoter. There is no clear evidence of a causal link between BPH and prostate cancer even though they frequently occur together. More than 95 percent of prostatic neoplasms are adenocarcinomas and most occur in the periphery of the prostate. The aggressiveness of the neoplasm appears to be related to the degree of differentiation rather than the size of the tumor. Local extension is usually posterior, although late in the disease the tumor may invade the rectum or encroach on the prostatic urethra and cause bladder outlet obstruction. Sites of distant metastasis occur via lymph and blood vessels and include the lymph nodes, bones, lungs, liver, and adrenals. The pelvis, lumbar spine, femur, thoracic spine, and ribs are the most common sites of bone metastasis.

Prostatic cancer often causes no symptoms until it is far advanced. The first manifestations of disease are slow urinary stream, hesitancy, incomplete emptying, frequency, nocturia, and dysuria. Unlike the symptoms of obstruction caused by BPH, the symptoms of obstruction caused by prostatic cancer are progressive and do not temporarily remit. Symptoms of late disease include bone pain at sites of bone metastasis, edema of the lower extremities, enlarged lymph nodes, liver enlargement, pathologic bone fractures, and mental confusion associated with brain metastases. Transrectal ultrasound (TRUS), prostatic-specific antigen (PSA) blood tests, and digital examination can validate the symptoms of prostatic cancer. Treatment options include hormonal therapy, chemotherapy, radiation therapy, surgery, or any combination of these. Symptomatic relief of urinary obstruction, bladder outlet obstruction, colon obstruction, and spinal cord compression may be required.

8. Describe sexual dysfunction in the male.
Study text pages 782-783.

Male **sexual dysfunction** is the impairment of erection, emission, and ejaculation. In men over 40 years of age, organic factors are involved in more than 50 percent of dysfunctional cases. Some arterial diseases diminish or interrupt circulation to the penis thus preventing engorgement of erectile tissues in the corpora cavernosa and corpus spongiosum; erection is not possible. Inadequate secretion of the pituitary gonadotropins, feminizing tumors, estrogen therapy, and testicular atrophy from any cause decrease testosterone levels and contribute to sexual dysfunction. Neurologic disorders can interfere with the important sympathetic, parasympathetic, and central nervous system mechanisms of erection, emission, and ejaculation. Upper motor neuron lesions prevent emission and ejaculation. Lesions affecting the lower motor neurons usually prevent erection and often prevent emission and ejaculation. Diabetes mellitus causes both peripheral vascular and neurologic pathology which leads to erectile dysfunction. Pelvic surgery can create erectile dysfunction by severing small nerve branches that are essential for erection. Men who are taking antihypertensives, antidepressants, antihistamines, antispasmodics, sedatives or tranquilizers, barbiturates, diuretics, sex hormone preparations, narcotics, or psychoactive drugs or who consume ethyl alcohol experience sexual dysfunction.

9. Differentiate between benign and malignant female breast disease.

Study text pages 783-793; refer to Figures 20-25 through 20-27 and Tables 20-12 through 20-18.

Many terms have been used to describe benign breast lesions of epithelial origin. **Fibrocystic disease** or physiologic nodularity is one description, and it is manifested by palpable lumps in the breast. These lumps fluctuate with the menstrual cycle and may become progressively worse until menopause. This terminology is unfortunate since physiologic nodularity is present in approximately 50 percent of menstruating women. Also, some of the lesions called fibrocystic disease are associated with an increased risk of breast cancer. Having these epithelial processes grouped together under one term generates significant confusion regarding prognosis.

Breast cancer is the most common cancer in American women and the second biggest killer after lung cancer. Breast cancer afflicts approximately one in every eight women. The risk of breast cancer increases as age advances and is the greatest in women aged 45 to 64. The risk factor and possible etiologies of breast cancer can be classified as reproductive, hormonal, environmental, and familial.

Benign/Malignant Female Breast Disorders

Disorder	Risks	Pathophysiology	Manifestations	Treatment
Fibrocystic disease *microcysts *macrocysts *adenosis *apocrine change *fibrosis *fibroadenomas *ductal hyperplasia	Puberty to lifetime, nonproliferative lesions demonstrate no added risk for cancer, proliferative lesions without atypia have slightly increased risk, proliferation with atypia have a high risk for cancer development	Increased estrogen levels, alterations in estrogen-to-progetesterone ratio	Fluctuating pain, pain increases as menstruation approaches, fluctuating lesion size, multiple lesions	Cyst drainage, surgical excision, pain relief by synthetic androgen
Breast Cancer	Increasing age: Lifetime, 1 in 8 at age 30, 1 in 2500 at age 40, 1 in 200 at age 50, 1 in 50 at age 60, 1 in 25 at age 70, 1 in 15 at age 80, 1 in 10 No full term pregnancies, long reproductive life, ionizing radiation, high fat diet, alcohol ingestion, first-degree relatives	Estrogens have a proliferative effect on mammary gland epithelium, estrogens may increase susceptibility to environmental carcinogens, transforming growth factor (TgF), autosomal dominant inheritance on chromosome 17	Painless lumps, skin retraction over lesion, nipple puckering and discharge After metastasis: palpable axillary lymph nodes, bone pain, pleural effusion, jaundice, hypercalcemia leading to nausea, vomiting, and renal stones	Surgery to remove lesion, radiation to prevent metastasis, chemotherapy, hormones for hormone-dependent tumors

Practice Examination

1. The cause of dysmenorrhea usually involves
   a. excessive endometrial prostaglandin production.
   b. failure of ovarian follicle maturation.
   c. decreased myometrial contractions.
   d. purulent material draining from the uterine tube.

2. Secondary amenorrhea is
   a. failure to begin menstruation by age 20.
   b. menarche failure.
   c. increased myometrial vasculature constriction.
   d. the absence of menstruation following menarche.

3. What is the likely pathophysiology of PMS?
   a. Elevated prolactin levels cause salt and water retention.
   b. Elevated aldosterone levels cause salt and water retention.
   c. An abnormal nervous, immunologic, vascular, and gastrointestinal response to the menstrual cycle likely occurs.
   d. Both a and b are correct.

4. Acute pelvic inflammatory disease (PID)
   1. primarily affects males.
   2. is usually caused by viruses.
   3. never causes peritonitis.
   4. involves the epididymis.
   5. may cause infertility or tubular pregnancy.

   a. 1, 3
   b. 2, 4
   c. 2, 3, 4
   d. 4, 5
   e. 5

5. A yeast vaginitis may be caused by
   a. an overgrowth of *C. albicans.*
   b. a declining number of lactobacilli.
   c. chronic use of antibiotics.
   d. a, b, and c are correct.
   e. None of the above is correct.

6. Vulvitis is
   a. inflammation of the cervix.
   b. can be caused by contact with perfumed toilet paper or menstrual pads.
   c. inflammation of the Bartholin glands.
   d. vaginal infection spread to the labia.
   e. Both b and c are correct.

7. Anovulatory cycles having prolonged estrogen levels and absent progesterone production are found in
   a. cervical cancer.
   b. corpus luteum cysts.
   c. adenomyosis.
   d. endometrial hyperplasia.
   e. Both b and c are correct.

8. Depressed T-cell function is associated with
   a. follicular cysts.
   b. endometrial polyps.
   c. leiomyomas.
   d. adenomyosis.
   e. endometriosis.

9. It is possible that repeated pregnancies cause
    a. ovarian cysts.
    b. endometriosis.
    c. leiomyomas.
    d. adenomyosis.
    e. polyps.

10. A 42-year-old retired prostitute who became sexually active at age 14 is at risk to develop
    a. endometriosis.
    b. cervical carcinoma.
    c. breast cancer.
    d. uterine carcinoma.

11. Your neighbor's obese grandmother has hypertension and breast cancer. Her risk factors are greatest for
    _____ cancer.
    a. cervical
    b. vaginal
    c. endometrial
    d. ovarian

12. Painful intercourse is
    a. inability to achieve orgasm.
    b. inhibited sexual desire.
    c. muscle spasm in response to attempted penetration.
    d. dyspareunia.

13. Elevated serum gonadotropins suggest
    a. testicular disease.
    b. genital organ inflammation.
    c. prostatic carcinoma.
    d. gynecomastia.

14. Phimosis is
    a. thickening of the fascia in the erectile tissue of the corpora cavernosa.
    b. the condition of a retracted foreskin that cannot be moved forward.
    c. a condition in which the foreskin cannot be retracted.
    d. caused by poor hygiene and chronic infection.
    e. Both c and d are correct.

15. A varicocele is an intrascrotal disorder
    a. that results in a collection of fluid within the tunica vaginalis.
    b. occurring because of independent or congenitally absent values in the spermatic veins.
    c. located between the head of the epididymis and the testis.
    d. that does not interfere with spermatogenesis.

16. Cryptorchidism is
    a. underdevelopment of the testes.
    b. the absence of scrotal tissue.
    c. relieved by scrotal support.
    d. failure of testes to descend into the scrotum.
    e. an imbalance between secreting and absorptive capacities of scrotal tissues.

17. The infectious cause of orchitis is
    a. streptococci.
    b. gonococci.
    c. chlamydial organisms.
    d. mumps virus.

18. Which organisms can cause epididymitis?
    a. enterobacteriaceae
    b. *Neisseria gonorrhoeae*
    c. *Chlamydia trachomatis*
    d. a, b, and c are correct.
    e. None of the above is correct.

19. In benign prostatic hyperplasia, enlargement of periurethral tissue of the prostate causes
    a. obstruction of the urethra.
    b. inflammation of the testis.
    c. decreased urinary outflow from the bladder.
    d. abnormal dilation of a vein within the spermatic cord.
    e. tension of the spermatic cord and testis.

20. A major cause of recurrent urinary tract infections in the male is
    a. orchitis.
    b. balanitis.
    c. epididymitis.
    d. chronic bacterial protastitis.
    e. nonbacterial prostatitis.

21. A symptom or sign of late stage prostatic cancer is
    a. a slow urinary stream.
    b. frequency of urination.
    c. incomplete emptying.
    d. mental confusion.
    e. a, b, and c are correct.

22. Male sexual dysfunction may be caused by
    a. infection around the introitus.
    b. diabetes mellitus.
    c. infected hymenal remnants.
    d. None of the above is correct.

Match the characteristic with the benign or malignant female breast disorder.

23. fluctuating lesion size   a. fibrocystic disease
24. palpable axillary lymph nodes   b. breast cancer
25. gene on chromosome 17

Case Study

Mrs. B. is a 46-year-old female who consults her physician about the nature of a lump in her left breast. About three months ago, her spouse noticed a small lump in her left breast; however, she was unconcerned since she experienced small lumps in her breast around the times of her menses. However, this lump seemed to be growing and did not seem to fluctuate in size as in the past. Three small lumps that fluctuated in size were noticed by Mrs. B in her right breast. She states she is in excellent health, exercises daily, and neither smokes nor drinks alcohol.

Mrs. B. is the mother of two preteen children. After the birth of her last child, she took birth control pills for eight years and then selected an alternative method of birth control. Her onset of menses occurred at age 10. Her family history reveals that her mother and one of three aunts died of breast cancer; otherwise, the history is noncontributing.

On examination, a two- to three-centimeter mass was palpated in the upper quadrant of her left breast. This mass was firm, fixed to the chest wall, and slightly tender to touch. The skin and nipple appeared normal. Under the left axilla, a node about the size of a pea was palpable. Three one- to two-centimeter soft, movable masses were palpated in Mrs. B.'s right breast.

Mammography confirmed the presence of a three-centimeter mass in the left breast and four 1.5-centimeter masses in the right breast. All other diagnostic procedures were negative.

What do you think about Mrs. B.'s history and examination?

Sexually Transmitted Diseases

Prerequisite Objectives

a. Identify the female reproductive structures.
   Review text pages 715-721.

Remember!

- The external genitalia collectively are called the vulva and comprise the structures visible externally: the mons pubis, the labia majora, the labia minora, the clitoris, and the vestibule. The urethral meatus, the vaginal opening and two sets of glands — Skene glands and Bartholin glands — open onto the vestibule. The internal organs of the female reproductive system are two ovaries, two fallopian tubes or uterine tubes, the uterus, and the vagina. The ovaries are the primary female reproductive organs. They are located on both sides of the uterus and are suspended and supported by ligaments.

- The fallopian tubes extend from the ovaries to the uterus and open into the uterine cavity thus providing a direct communication from the peritoneal cavity to the uterine cavity. The uterus lies centrally in the pelvis and is divided structurally into the body, or corpus, and the cervix. The inner layer, the endometrium, consists of surface epithelium, glands, and connective tissue. The endometrium is shed during menstruation. At the lowest portion of the corpus is the internal os of the cervix. The external os is at the lower end of the cervix. The canal of the cervix provides a direct communication from the cavity of the uterine body through the internal os and the external os to the vagina.

- The vagina extends from the cervix of the uterus to the vaginal opening. Thus, there is continuous communication from outside the body to the peritoneal cavity through the reproductive system structures.

---

b. Identify the male reproductive structures.
   Review text pages 726-731.

Remember!

- The male reproductive structures are the penis, the testes in the scrotal sac, the duct system which includes the epididymis, the vas deferens, the ejaculatory ducts, and the urethra, and the accessory glands which include the seminal vesicles, the prostate, and the bulbourethral glands.

- The testes are divided internally into lobules that contain the seminiferous tubules and Leydig cells. Sperm production takes place in the seminiferous tubules; Leydig cells secrete testosterone. On the posterior portion of each testis is a coiled duct, the epididymis. The head of the epididymis is connected with the seminiferous tubule of the testis and its tail is continuous with the vas deferens. The vas deferens is the excretory duct of the testis. It extends to the duct of the seminal vesicle and joins with it to form the ejaculatory duct. The ejaculatory duct joins the urethra, which is the common passageway to outside the body for both sperm and urine. The accessory glands communicate with the duct system. The prostate surrounds the neck of the bladder and the upper urethra. Its glandular ducts open into the urethra. The bulbourethral glands, or Cowper's glands, are located near the urethral meatus. The penis is composed of three elongated cylindrical masses of erectile tissue which comprise the shaft of the penis. The inner, ventral mass is the corpus spongiosum, which contains the urethra. The two outer, dorsal, parallel masses are the corpus cavernosa. The distal end of the penis or the glans is covered by the prepuce, or foreskin.

---

c. Identify tests used to diagnose STDs.
   Refer to Table 19-3.

Remember!

Diagnostic Tests for Common STDs

Tests for gonorrhea	
Culture	Isolation and detection of *Neisseria gonorrhoeae* in urethral, anal, and/or pharyngeal secretions
Gram stain	Direct smear and staining of cervical or urethral discharge to identify gram-negative intracellular diplococci within polymorphonuclear (PMN) leukocytes
Tests for syphilis	Detection of antibodies to *Treponema pallidum*
RPR	Rapid plasma reagin
FTA	Fluorescent treponemal antibody absorption test
Darkfield Exam	Direct smear of serous exudate from moist lesions to detect *Treponema pallidum* with corkscrew appearance
Tests for *Chlamydia*	
Antigen detection	Direct immunofluorescence staining of cervical and/or urethral specimens to detect monoclonal antibodies
Tissue culture	Isolation and detection of *Chlamydia trachomatis* from epithelial cells of endocervix and urethra

(Continued)

Diagnostic Tests for Common STDs

Tests for HIV infection

ELISA (enzyme-linked immunoabsorbent assay)	Detects the presence of antibodies to human immunodeficiency virus (HIV)
IFA (indirect fluorescent antibody)	A more specific, definitive test for HIV
WB (Western blot)	An even more specific, definitive test for HIV

Tests for other viral infections

TORCH test	Detects elevations of IgA or IgM caused by toxoplasma, rubella, cytomegalovirus, syphilis, and herpes simplex in mother and newborn infant; herpes requires more specific, follow-up testing if positive
Cytomegalovirus	Cell culture with samples from urine, cervix, semen, saliva, and blood can reveal cytopathic effects of virus

Objectives

After successful study of this chapter, the learner will be able to:

1. State the current status of sexually transmitted diseases.

Study text pages 800-801; refer to Table 21-1.

Within the past decade, the study and categorization of **STD**s has broadened to include bacterial, viral, and other agents as causes of STDs. The viral induced STDs are generally considered incurable. It is estimated by the World Health Organization that 250 million cases of STD occur each year in the world. In many countries STDs have reached epidemic proportions. The magnitude of the occurrence of STDs has a significant impact on the mortality and morbidity of adults and exposed infants. The incidence and increase in STDs is due to increased premarital sex, an increase in the divorce rate, nonmonogamy among married people, and bisexuality. These factors contribute to the increase in numbers of sexual partners and an increased exposure to STDs. The number of individuals who fail to take protective measures when engaging in sexual activities also contributes to the problem. STDs are prevalent among all individuals in all socioeconomic groups.

2. Characterize the bacterial, bacterial-like STDs, focusing on infectious agents, manifestations, and complications.

Study text pages 801-814.

Bacterial, Bacterial-like STDs

Disease/Infectious Agent	Manifestations	Major Complications
Gonorrhea		
Neisseria gonorrhoeae (gm-negative diplococcus)	Possibly asymptomatic, urethritis, cervicitis, mucopurulent discharge, anorectal infection, pharyngitis conjunctivitis, ophthalmia, neonatatoun	Epididymitis and lymphangitis, salpingitis, infertility, disseminated blood stream infection, neonatal blindness
Syphilis		
Treponema pallidum (anaerobic spirochete)	Primary: nonpainful chancre at site of invasion. Secondary: systemic involvement with skin rash and lymphadenopathy. Tertiary: gummas. Congenital: dental deformations, destructive bone lesions	Destructive lesions in cardiovascular and nervous system
Chancroid		
Haemophilus ducreyi (gm-negative bacillus)	Papule erodes into painful ulcer, superficial exudate, painful lymphadenopathy	
Granuloma inguinale		
Calymmatobacterium granulomatis (Predominant in tropical climates) (gm-negative bacillus)	Painless, indurated, subcutaneous nodule of distal penis and introitus	Possible spread to bones, joints, and liver
Bacterial vaginosis		
Gardnerella vaginitis and other anaerobes (gm-negative bacilli)	Thin and scant malodorous vaginal discharge	
Urogenital infections		
Lymphogranuloma venereum (endemic in southern hemisphere) *Chlamydia trachomatis* (gm-negative intracellular microbe)	Commonly associated with other STDs thus not common STD, purulent discharge, cervicitis, urethritis, proctitis, newborn conjunctivitis and pneumonia, tender lymph node and inguinal buboes	Epididymitis, Reiter syndrome, arthritis; in secondary LGV there may be disrupted lymph node function, meningitis, or pneumonitis
Mycoplasmosis		
Mycoplasma hominis (no cell walls)	Urethritis, salpingitis, postpartum fever	

Note: Treatment of bacterial, bacterial-like STDs is with appropriate antibiotics.

3. Characterize the viral STDs focusing on infectious agents, manifestations, and complications.

Study text pages 814-818.

Viral STDs

Disease/Infectious Agent	Manifestations	Major Complications
Genital herpes Herpes simplex virus (HSV-1 or HSV-2) (latent virus in trigeminal ganglion or dorsal sacral nerve roots)	Painful blister-like lesions on external genitalia and genital tract, pharyngitis, aseptic meningitis, hepatitis	Predisposition to cervical cancer, spontaneous abortion, neonatal morbidity and mortality from CNS involvement
Condylomata acuminata (warts) Human papillomavirus (HPV)	Soft, skin-colored single or clustered growths	Cervical and vulva cancer, anorectal and penile cancer
Molluscum contagiosum molluscum contagiosum virus (STD and fomites)	Flesh-colored papules with a thick, creamy core	

Note: Treatment for HSV is not curative but oral and topical antiviral agents (acyclovir) are used to lower recurrence; HPV lesions are treated with topical agents and surgery; and molluscum contagiosum can be treated by curettage or cryotherapy.

4. Characterize the parasitic STDs by infectious agents and manifestations.

Study text pages 819-821.

Parasitic STDs

Disease/Infectious Agent	Manifestations
Trichomoniasis *Trichomonas vaginalis* (protozoa)	Damages squamous epithelial cells so vaginal walls are erythematous, vaginal discharge, pruritus
Scabies *Sarcoptes scabiei* (female itch mite)	Intense pruritus, papules near the burrow sites
Pediculosis pubis (crabs) *Phthirus pubis* (crab louse, STD and fomites)	Pruritus, lice and nits are visible to naked eye

Note: Treatment is by antitrichosomal agents, scabicides, prescription creams, and effective hygiene practices.

5. Identify systemic infections that may be transmitted sexually.

Study text pages 821-824.

Other Systems Affected by STDs

Disease/Infectious Agent	Transmission Mode	Manifestations
Shigellosis Shigella (gm-negative bacillus) and Campylobacteria enteritis Campylobacter (gm-negative bacillus)	Contact with infected feces by anal-oral or genital-anal contact	Fever, abdominal distension, diarrhea, dysentery with bloody discharge
Giardiasis *Giardia lamblia* (protozoa)	Anal-oral or genital-anal contact	Sudden and explosive diarrhea, distension, flatulence, epigastric pain, nausea and vomiting
Amebiasis *Entamoeba histolytica* (protozoa)	Anal-oral or genital-anal contact	Mild diarrhea to severe dysentery, may spread to liver
Hepatitis B Hepatitis B virus	Needle puncture, blood transfusion, cuts in mucous membranes and skin, perinatal transmission	Rash, urticaria, polyarthralgias, arthritis, jaundice, liver enlargement with infected body fluids, neonatal death
AIDS Human immunodeficiency virus (HIV)	Inoculation with contaminated blood, perinatal transmission	Depressed immune system, opportunistic infections, malignancies
Cytomegalic inclusion disease Cytomegalovirus (CMV)	Interpersonal contact or direct transfer of cells or body fluids, perinatal transmission	Mild subclinical illness, life-threatening in the immunocompromised, congenitally infected may have hepatosplenomegaly and neurological deficits

Note: Treatment is as earlier indicated for bacterial, protozoan, and viral diseases.

Practice Examination

Match the STD with its causative agent.

1. gonorrhea
2. syphilis
3. condylomata acuminata
4. pediculosis pubis
5. amebiasis

a. *Hemophilus ducreyi*
b. *Mycoplasma hominis*
c. *Neisseria gonorrhoreae*
d. *Gardnerella vaginalis*
e. *Treponema pallidum*
f. human papillomavirus
g. *Sarcoptes scabiei*
h. *Phthirus pubis*
i. *Entamoeba histolytica*
j. *Trichomonas vaginalis*

True/False

____ 6. Gonococcal infection of the newborn is manifested as mental retardation.

____ 7. The organism that causes syphilis can be identified by a gram-stained slide.

____ 8. The organism that causes trichomoniasis is a protozoa.

____ 9. A clinical manifestation associated with HVS-2 infection is painful blister-like lesions.

____ 10. *Treponema pallidum* spirochetes cross the placental barrier.

____ 11. Chlamydial infections in the newborn may result in blindness and deafness.

____ 12. Transmission of AIDS in children most often occurs because of contact with an affected individual.

____ 13. A gram-negative bacillus causes gonorrhea.

____ 14. Women who have gonorrhea are frequently asymptomatic.

____ 15. The secondary stage of syphilis is characterized by a chancre.

____ 16. *Treponema pallidum* is a protozoa.

____ 17. Acyclovir is a treatment for genital herpes.

____ 18. *Condylomata acuminata* are warts.

____ 19. Pruritus is not a manifestation of scabies.

____ 20. Genital herpes predisposes to cervical cancer.

____ 21. Human papillomaviruses may lead to penile cancer.

____ 22. Mycoplasmosis results in a malodorous vaginal discharge.

____ 23. Reiter syndrome is gonorrhea.

____ 24. Giardiasis may exhibit epigastric pain.

____ 25. Neonatal infection with hepatis B virus may result in neonatal death.

Case Study

Ms. C.T., a 23-year-old recently divorced female, presented to her physician for her annual gynecologic examination. She states that she is experiencing a gray-white, creamy vaginal discharge that has a heavy, fishy order. She admits to having more than one current sex partner and a history of multiple sex partners and to using nonbarrier contraception.

C.T.'s physical examination reveals lower abdominal and pelvic pain; all other physical signs are normal except she has a slightly elevated temperature. There are no blisters on the vulva. Her pelvic examination shows cervical edematous congestion and a mucopurulent discharge. A gram stain of the mucopurulent discharge revealed no intracellular gram-negative diplococci within the polymorphonuclear leukocytes.

What do you consider the most likely cause of Ms.C.T.'s signs and symptoms? What tests might be ordered to validate a presumptive diagnosis?

CHAPTER 22

Structure and Function of the Hematologic System

Objectives

After successful study of this chapter, the learner will be able to:

1. **Identify the constituents of blood plasma.**
   Review text page 831; refer to Table 22-1.

2. **Identify the structural characteristics, normal values, and functions of the cellular elements of blood.**
   Review text pages 831-836; refer to Table 22-2.

3. **Diagram the differentiation of the cellular elements of blood; note the effects of colony stimulating factors.**
   Refer to Figures 22-5 through 22-7 and Table 22-4.

4. **Define erythropoiesis and identify the nutritional requirements necessary for erythropoiesis to occur.**
   Review text pages 840-845; refer to Figures 22-8 through 22-10 and Table 22-6.

5. **Describe the sequence of events in hemostasis.**
   Review text pages 847-853; refer to Figures 22-12 through 22-14 and Table 22-7.

6. **Diagram the fibrinolytic system.**
   Refer to Figure 22-15.

7. **Describe the types of information that can be obtained from bone marrow biopsy and various blood tests.**
   Refer to Tables 22-8 and 22-9.

8. **Describe changes occurring within the hemologic system with aging.**
   Review text page 857.

Practice Examination

1. Which does not constitute a plasma component?
   a. colloids
   b. electrolytes
   c. gases
   d. glucose
   e. platelets

2. Which is the most abundant protein in blood plasma?
   a. fibrinogen
   b. albumins
   c. globulins
   d. immunoglobulins
   e. hormones

3. A fragment of megakaryocyte cytoplasm is the
   a. reticulocyte.
   b. normoblast.
   c. promyelocyte.
   d. proerythroblast.
   e. platelet.

4. The progenitor of granulocytes is a
   a. pronormoblast.
   b. promegakaryocyte.
   c. prolymphoblast.
   d. premyeloblast.

5. Which is the correct sequence in the development of erythrocytes?
   a. polychromatophilic erythroblast - normoblast - reticulocyte
   b. normoblast - reticulocyte - basophilic erythroblast
   c. normoblast - committed proerythroblast - reticulocyte
   d. normoblast - basophilic erythroblast - reticulocyte

6. A differential count of WBCs includes all except
   a. granulocytes.
   b. a granulocytes.
   c. reticulocytes.
   d. monocytes.
   e. lymphocytes.

7. The purpose of the mean corpuscular volume (MCV) is to measure the
   a. amount of hemoglobin.
   b. hematocrit.
   c. size of the RBC.
   d. size of platelets.

8. The normal platelet count/mm^3 of blood is about
   a. $4\text{-}10 \times 10^3$.
   b. $50\text{-}100 \times 10^3$.
   c. $150\text{-}300 \times 10^3$.
   d. 5×10^6.
   e. $150\text{-}300 \times 10^6$.

9. The hematocrit is the
   a. number of RBCs in plasma.
   b. aqueous portion of blood.
   c. criterium of blood flow.
   d. percentage of RBCs in a given volume of blood.
   e. amount of hemoglobin by weight in blood.

10. If the total leukocytic count of an individual was 7000/mm^3, about how many neutrophils would normally be present in a mm^3 of blood?
    a. 400
    b. 700
    c. 2100
    d. 3000
    e. 4200

11. Which granulocyte functions in antibody-mediated defense against parasites?
    a. lymphocytes
    b. monocytes
    c. neutrophils
    d. esophils
    e. basophils

12. Erythropoietin
    a. causes a rise in circulatory RBCs.
    b. is a glycoprotein.
    c. causes recycling of iron for production of RBCs.
    d. is released by the kidney to stimulate erythrocyte and platelet formation.
    e. Both a and b are correct.

13. Which of the following is not an agranulocyte?
    a. basophil
    b. lymphocyte
    c. monocyte
    d. reticulocyte
    e. Both a and d are correct.

14. In tissue, which are the most effective phagocytes?
    a. neutrophils and basophils
    b. lymphocytes and eosinophils
    c. basophils and monocytes
    d. neutrophils and monocytes
    e. None of the above is correct.

15. Which vitamins are needed for erythropoiesis?
    a. C and E
    b. B$_2$ and B$_{12}$
    c. A and D
    d. Both a and b are correct.
    e. a, b, and c are correct.

Match colony-stimulating factor with the cell that is stimulated.

16. IL-3
17. G-CSP

a. erythrocytes
b. macrophage, neutrophil
c. neutrophil, eosinophil, and basophil
d. normoblast
e. erythroblast

18. Which is not used to measure RBC indices?
    a. differential count
    b. reticulocyte count
    c. erythrocyte count
    d. hemoglobin determination
    e. MCHC

19. Which test reflects bone marrow activity?
    a. reticulocyte count
    b. MCH
    c. MCV
    d. HCT

20. As an individual ages,
    a. the erythrocyte life span is shortened.
    b. lymphocytic function decreases.
    c. platelet numbers decrease.
    d. All of the above are correct.

21. Hemostasis involves all except
    a. vasoconstriction.
    b. platelet plug formation.
    c. intrinsic pathway activities.
    d. clot formation.
    e. erythropoiesis.

22. When a blood vessel is damaged,
    a. subendothelial collagen is exposed.
    b. platelets are attracted to collagen.
    c. platelets degranulate.
    d. Both a and b are correct.
    e. a, b and c are correct.

23. The biochemical mediators released by adhering platelets cause
    a. vasodilation of the injured vessel.
    b. vasoconstriction of the injured vessel.
    c. the inflammatory process to proceed.
    d. All of the above are correct.

24. Which is a correct sequence in coagulation?
    a. X - tissue thromboplastin - XA
    b. prothrombin activator complex - X - XA
    c. fibrinogen - thrombin - stabilizer fibrin
    d. damaged tissue - tissue thromboplastin - X

25. Which is a correct sequence in fibrinolysis?
    a. fibrin - plasminogen
    b. FDP - fibrinogen
    c. plasminogen - XIIa
    d. plasmin - fibrin

Alterations of Erythrocyte Function

Prerequisite Objective

a. Identify the differentiation sequence, function, and normal values for erythrocytes.
   Review text pages 831-834 and 838-845; refer to Figures 22-7 through 22-10.

Remember!

Differentiation of Erythrocytes

Uncommitted Pluripotential Stem Cell

⬇ ⟵ Erythropoietin

Proerythroblast (Very large nucleus)

⬇

Basophilic Erythroblast (Hemoglobin synthesis begins)

⬇

Intermediate Polychromatic Erythroblast
(Last stage of DNA synthesis and cell division, hemoglobin synthesis continues)

⬇

Orthochromatic Normoblast
(The nucleus shrinks and undergoes autolysis and resorption, additional hemoglobin is synthesized)

⬇

Reticulocyte
(Larger than mature RBC, no nucleus, enters vascular circulation of the bone marrow by diapedesis)

⬇

Erythrocyte
(Reticulum of the nucleus resorbed, disk shape achieved)

- The function of erythrocytes is to transport gas to and from the tissue cells and lungs. The normal adult range of values for erythrocytes is:

    Number = 4.2 - 6.2 million/mm^3

    Hematocrit = 42 - 48%

    Hemoglobin = 12-16.5 gm/100 ml

Note: Reticulocytes normally comprise less than one percent of the RBCs found in blood.

(Continued)

Objectives

After successful study of this chapter, the learner will be able to:

1. Define anemia.

Study text page 861.

Anemia is a reduction in the total number of circulating erythrocytes or a decrease in the quality or quantity of hemoglobin. Anemic conditions are usually a result of impaired erythrocyte production, blood loss, increased erythrocyte destruction, or a combination of the three.

2. Classify the anemias.

Study text page 861; refer to Tables 23-1 and 23-2.

Whether there is decreased/defective production or destruction of erythrocytes, anemias are classified according to their **etiologic basis** or **morphologic appearance**. Descriptions of anemias based on erythrocyte morphologic appearance refer to the cell's size and hemoglobin content. The morphologic classification is widely used. Terms that refer to cellular size end with "cytic." Terms that describe hemoglobin content end with "chromic." An erythrocyte can be **macrocytic**, meaning abnormally large, or **microcytic**, meaning abnormally small, and **hyperchromic**, containing an unusually high concentration of hemoglobin within its cytoplasm, or **hypochromic**, containing an abnormally low concentration of hemoglobin. For comparison, cells of normal size are termed **normocytic** and cells with normal amounts of hemoglobin are termed **normochromic**. In some anemias, the erythrocytes take on various sizes or they have various shapes; this is **anisocytosis** or **poikilocytosis**, respectively.

3. Describe the pathophysiology of the clinical manifestations of anemias.

Study text pages 861-864; refer to Table 23-2.

Compensation for reduced oxygen-carrying capacity of the blood requires the cardiovascular, respiratory, and hematologic systems to respond. A reduction in the number of circulating erythrocytes after hemorrhage affects the consistency and volume of the blood. To compensate for reduced blood volume, fluids from the interstitium move into the blood vessels and plasma volume expands. The thinner, less viscous blood flows faster and more turbulently than normal blood. Increased blood flow within the heart can cause ventricular dysfunction, cardiac dilation, and heart valve insufficiency. Hypoxia of anemia causes arterioles, capillaries, and venules to dilate, which speeds blood flow even more. As venous return to the heart increases, the heart must pump harder and faster to meet normal oxygen demand and to prevent cardiopulmonary congestion. Congestive heart failure can develop. Tissue hypoxia also causes the rate and depth of breathing to increase in an attempt to make more oxygen available to the remaining erythrocytes. When anemia is severe or sudden in onset, peripheral blood vessels constrict to direct available blood flow to the vital organs. A number of systemic symptoms occur subsequent to this shunting of blood. Decreased blood flow is sensed by the kidneys, and in an effort to improve kidney perfusion, the renal renin-angiotensin response is activated. This results in salt and water retention, causing increased workload for the heart. The individual will experience shortness of breath or dyspnea, a rapid pounding heartbeat, dizziness, and fatigue even when at rest.

The skin, mucous membranes, lips, nailbeds, and conjunctivae become pale due to reduced hemoglobin concentration or yellowish due to accumulation in the skin of products of red blood cell breakdown or hemolysis. Decreased oxygen delivery to the skin results in impaired healing and loss of elasticity. Thinning and early graying of the hair can occur.

If the anemia is due to vitamin B_{12} deficiency, the nervous system is affected. Myelin degeneration may occur with loss of nerve fibers in the spinal cord. Paresthesias, gait disturbances, extreme weakness, spasticity, and reflex abnormalities may then result.

Decreased oxygen supply to the gastrointestinal tract often produces abdominal pain, nausea, vomiting, and anorexia. Low-grade fever, less than

101° F, occurs in some anemic individuals and may be the result of leukocytic pyrogens being released from ischemic tissues. Therapeutic intervention for any anemic condition requires treatment of the underlying disorder and palliation of symptoms. Therapies for anemia include transfusions, dietary corrections, and administration of supplemental vitamins or iron.

4. Develop a comparative chart of the macrocytic-normochromic, microcytic-hypochromic, and normocytic-normochromic anemias.
Study text pages 864-875.

Anemias

Anemia	Etiology	High Risk Groups	Symptoms
Macrocytic-normochromic			
Pernicious	Insufficient influence of vitamin B$_{12}$ on developing cells because of deficient IF, antibodies develop against parietal cells, gastrectomy or ilectomy therapies, chronic gastritis	Anglo-Saxon and Scandinavian populations	*Typical, digestive symptoms from lack of HC1 and enzymes, glossitis, peripheral neuropathy: tingling numbness, loss of vibratory sense
Folate (Folic Acid)	Dietary deficiency inhibits DNA synthesis	Alcoholics, pregnant women, chronically malnourished	*Typical, similar to pernicious except no neurologic disorders
Microcytic-hypochromic			
Iron Deficiency	Excessive bleeding which depletes iron, poor diet, no meat	Premenopausal, adolescents, children, infants on milk, minor blood loss, elderly	*Typical
Sideroblastic	Dysfunctional iron uptake by erythroblasts, decreased heme synthesis, enzymes, etc. genetic	Acquired from drugs: ethanol, lead, chloramphenicol,	*Typical, mild hepatomegaly and splenomegaly
Thalassemia	Genetics, persistence of fetal hemoglobin (HbF) after birth, phagocytosis of cell	Italians, Greeks	*Typical
			(Continued)

171

Anemias *(cont'd)*

Anemia	Etiology	High Risk Groups	Symptoms
Normocytic-normochromic			
Aplastic	Radiation, drugs, lesions within red bone marrow, immune response that halts erythropoiesis	Anyone	*Typical, infection, bleeding
Post-hemorrhagic	Sudden blood loss	Surgery, trauma	Shock, acidosis
Hemolytic	Premature dysfunction of mature erythrocytes in circulation, genetics result in fragile cells, acquired from infections, drugs, IgG of warm or cold, IgM, antibodies	Anyone	Splenomegaly, jaundice
Chronic Inflammation	Bacterial toxins, cytokines from activated macrophages and lymphocytes, reduced iron in blood	AIDS, autoimmunity, neoplasms	Mild because of disability caused by chronic condition
Sickle Cell	Genetic trait causes abnormal hemoglobin and increased lysis of sickled cells	8% of African-Americans	*Typical, develop during heavy exercise

*Typical symptoms: fatigue, weakness, dyspnea, pallor
Treatment: Remove cause if possible and replace the deficient element.

5. Describe the types, causes, manifestations, and treatment of polycythemia vera.
Study text pages 875-876; refer to Table 23-5.

Polycythemia vera is an unusual disease that causes excessively large numbers of erythrocytes in the blood. It is typically accompanied by increased circulating platelets and granulocytes. There are essentially two types of polycythemia vera: primary or absolute and secondary or relative. The primary form of polycythemia vera is relatively rare and tends to occur in men between the ages of 40 and 60 of Jewish or European ancestry. Rarely is polycythemia vera found in children or multiple members of a single family. The cause of secondary polycythemia, the more common form, is essentially a physiologic response to hypoxia. It is not uncommon to find an increased red cell count in individuals living at high altitudes, in smokers, and in individuals with congestive heart failure or chronic obstructive pulmonary disease.

Erythrocytosis causes blood volume and blood viscosity to increase simply because of increased erythrocytes. The liver and spleen become increasingly congested with erythrocytes as increased viscosity causes blood flow to slow. Eventually, the thick, sticky, slow-flowing blood becomes an ideal environment for clotting and acidosis. If thrombi obstruct vessels, tissue or organ infarction develops.

The clinical signs of polycythemia vera include ruddy, red color of the face, hands, feet, ears, and mucous membranes, engorgement of retinal and sublingual veins, elevated blood pressure, splenomegaly, and hepatomegaly. Symptoms include headache, a feeling of fullness in the head, dizziness, weakness, itching, sweating, epigastric distress, fatigue on exertion, backache, and visual disturbances. The clinical manifestations of vascu-

172

lar disease likely predominate. Angina pectoris, calf pain associated with vasospasms during walking, thrombosis, and cerebral insufficiency can occur.

Treatment for polycythemia vera consists of reducing erythrocytosis and blood volume, controlling symptoms, and preventing thrombosis. Erythrocytosis and blood volume are reduced by phlebotomy, wherein a vein is opened and blood is removed according to need. Smokers should be urged to quit, and patients with congestive heart failure and chronic obstructive pulmonary disease require appropriate pharmaceutical intervention. Radioactive phosphorus is sometimes given orally or intravenously to suppress erythropoiesis, with 18 months usually elapsing between treatments. Although polycythemia vera is a chronic disorder, appropriate therapy can prevent significant morbidity and mortality.

Practice Examination

1. Anemia refers to a deficiency of
   a. blood plasma.
   b. erythrocytes.
   c. platelets.
   d. hemoglobin.
   e. Both b and d are correct.

2. Morphological classification of anemia is based on all except
   a. size.
   b. color.
   c. shape.
   d. cause.

3. Tissue hypoxia causes
   a. arterioles, capillaries, and venules to constrict.
   b. the heart to contract less forcefully.
   c. the rate and depth of breathing to increase.
   d. Both a and b are correct.
   e. a, b, and c are correct.

Match the etiology of the anemia with its morphologic appearance.

4. vitamin B_{12} deficiency
5. iron deficiency
6. folic acid deficiency
7. bone marrow depression
8. chronic infection
9. hemolysis
10. posthemorrhagic
11. decreased heme synthesis
12. impaired synthesis of beta chain of hemoglobin
13. malignancy

  a. macrocytic-normochromic
  b. microcytic-hypochromic
  c. normocytic-normochromic

14. Which symptoms are consistent with aplastic anemia but not with pernicious anemia?
   a. petechia and purpura
   b. pallor
   c. fatigue
   d. hypoxia
   e. neuropathy

15. If a reticulocyte count were done on a patient with iron deficiency anemia because of chronic bleeding, it would be
    a. high.
    b. low.
    c. normal.

16. A 40-year-old white pregnant female with four children experienced weakness, loss of appetite, and pallor. Her CBC revealed the following:
    macrocytic RBCs 2.5 x 10^6/mm3
    hemocrit of 32%
    hemoglobin of 8.7gm%
    She most likely has
    a. sickle cell anemia.
    b. folic acid anemia.
    c. iron deficiency anemia.
    d. pernicious anemia.
    e. None of the above is correct.

17. The cause of macrocytic-normochromic anemia is
    a. iron deficiency.
    b. deficiency of vitamin B_{12} and folic acid.
    c. an enzyme deficiency.
    d. inheritance of abnormal hemoglobin structure.
    e. None of the above is correct.

18. Sickle-cell crisis is due to
    a. occlusion of small capillaries.
    b. autoimmune attack on RBCs.
    c. hemolysis of platelets.
    d. internal bleeding.
    e. All of the above are correct.

19. Chronic diseases associated with anemia include all but
    a. systemic lupus erythematosus.
    b. polycythemia vera.
    c. Hodgkin disease.
    d. rheumatoid arthritis.
    e. All of the above are associated with anemia.

20. An individual having chronic gastritis and tingling in his/her fingers requires which of the following for treatment?
    a. oral B_{12}
    b. B_{12} by intramuscular injection
    c. ferrous fumarate by intramuscular injection
    d. oral folate
    e. transfusions

21. Individuals at risk for iron deficiency anemia include
    a. those having undergone a gastrectomy.
    b. Italians.
    c. those with neoplastic disease.
    d. warm antibodies.
    e. those with minor, chronic blood loss.

22. The symptoms of sickle cell anemia
    a. include glossitis.
    b. develop during heavy exercise.
    c. include bleeding and recurrent infections.
    d. include neuropathy.
    e. include jaundice.

23. Primary (absolute) polycythemia occurs when there is
    a. an increase in circulating red blood cells.
    b. a decrease of circulating plasma.
    c. a physiologic response to hypoxia.
    d. obstructive pulmonary disease in an individual.

24. Secondary (relative) polycythemia may be caused by
    a. dehydration.
    b. chronic obstructive pulmonary disease.
    c. living at high altitudes.
    d. Both b and c are correct.
    e. a, b, and c are correct.

25. The symptoms of polycythemia vera are essentially caused by
    a. fewer erythrocytes than normal.
    b. decreased blood volume.
    c. increased blood viscosity.
    d. increased rate of blood flow.

Case Study

Ann is a healthy 26-year-old white female of Italian descent. Since the beginning of this current golf season, Ann has noted increased shortness of breath and low levels of energy and enthusiasm. These symptoms seem worse during her menses. Today, while playing poorly in a golf tournament at a high, mountainous course, she became light-headed and was taken by her golfing partner to the emergency clinic of a multi-specialty medical group.

The attending physician's notes indicated a temperature of 98° F, an elevated heart rate and respiratory rate, and low blood pressure. She states that menorrhagia and dysmenorrhea have been a problem for 10-12 years and she takes 1000 mg of aspirin every 3-4 hours for six days during menstruation. During the summer months while playing golf, she also takes aspirin to avoid "stiffness in my joints."

Laboratory values:

Hemoglobin = 8g/dl
Hematocrit = 32%
Erythrocyte count = $3.1 \times 10^6/mm^3$
RBC smear showed microcytic and hypochromic cells.
Reticulocyte count = 1.5%
Other laboratory values were within normal limits.

Considering the circumstances and the preliminary work-up, what type of anemia is most likely for Ann? Which clinical sign shows her body is attempting to compensate for anemia?

CHAPTER 24

Alterations of Leukocyte, Lymphoid, and Hemostatic Function

Prerequisite Objectives

a. Identify the differentiation sequence for granulocytes, agranulocytes, and platelets.
    Refer to Figure 22-5.

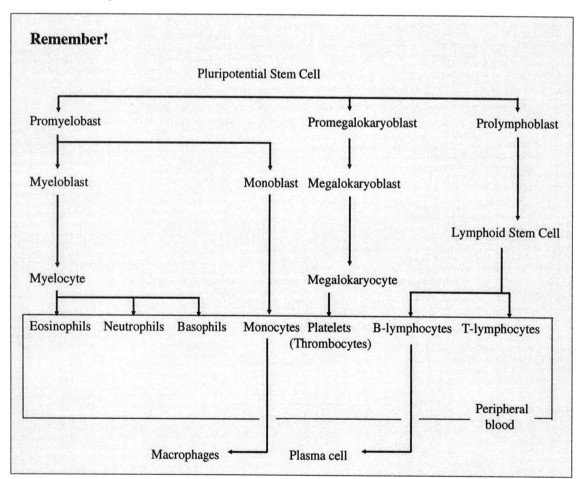

Remember!

Pluripotential Stem Cell

Promyelobast   Promegalokaryoblast   Prolymphoblast

Myeloblast   Monoblast Megalokaryoblast

Lymphoid Stem Cell

Myelocyte   Megalokaryocyte

Eosinophils Neutrophils Basophils Monocytes Platelets B-lymphocytes T-lymphocytes
(Thrombocytes)

Peripheral
blood

Macrophages   Plasma cell

b. Identify the normal numbers in circulating blood, the function, and life span of leukocytes and platelets.
Refer to Table 22-2.

Remember!

Cellular Components of the Blood

Cell	Normal amounts in	Function	Life span
Leukocyte	5000-10,000/mm^3	Bodily defense mechanisms	
Lymphocyte	25% to 33% of leukocytes	Immunity	Days or years
Monocyte and macrophage	3% to 7% of leukocytes	Phagocytosis, mononuclear phagocyte system	Months or years
Eosinophil	1% to 4% of leukocytes	Phagocytosis, antibody-mediated defense against parasites, allergic reactions, recovery phase of infection	Unknown
Neutrophil	57% to 67% of leukocytes	Phagocytosis, particularly during early phase of inflammation/infection	4 days
Basophil	0% to 0.75% of leukocytes	Unknown, but associated with allergic reactions and mechanical irritation	Unknown
Platelet	140,000 to 340,000/mm3	Hemostasis following vascular injury, normal coagulation and clot formation/reactions	8 to 11 days

c. Summarize briefly the coagulation cascade and the fibrinolytic system.
Refer to Figures 22-14 and 22-15.

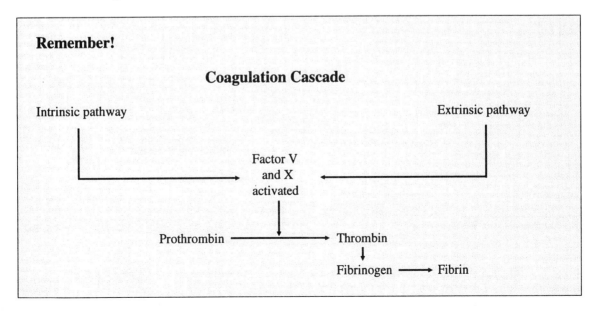

Remember!

Coagulation Cascade

Intrinsic pathway   Extrinsic pathway

Factor V and X activated

Prothrombin ⟶ Thrombin

Fibrinogen ⟶ Fibrin

Objectives

After successful study of this chapter, the learner will be able to:

1. Describe terms associated with high or low leukocyte counts and the causes of the alterations.
> Study text pages 879-882; refer to Tables 24-1 and 24-2.

Leukocytosis exists when the leukocyte count is higher than normal; **leukopenia** is a condition in which the leukocyte count is lower than normal. Leukocytosis is a normal, protective response to invading microorganisms, strenuous exercise, emotional changes, temperature changes, anesthesia, surgery, pregnancy, some drugs, hormones, and toxins. Malignancies and hematologic disorders also cause leukocytosis. Increased levels of circulating neutrophils, eosinophils, basophils, and monocytes are chiefly a physiologic response to infection. Elevations can also occur as a result of polycythemia vera and chronic myelocytic leukoma that increase stem cell proliferation in the bone marrow. Leukopenia is never beneficial. As the leukocyte count falls below 1000 per cubic millimeter, the individual is at risk for infection. The risk for very serious life-threatening infections develops with counts below 500/mm^3. Leukopenia can be caused by radiation, anaphylactic shock, systemic lupus erythematosus, and certain chemotherapeutic agents. Decreased leukocytic counts occur when infectious processes delete the circulating granulocytes and monocytes. Infectious agents draw them out of the circulation and into infected tissues faster than they can be replaced. Decreases can also be caused by disorders that suppress marrow function.

Granulocytosis or **neutrophilia** is prevalent in the early stages of infection or inflammation when stored neutrophils from the venous sinuses are released into the circulating blood. Emptying of the venous sinuses stimulates granulopoiesis to replenish normal stores of granulocytes in the marrow. **Neutropenia** or low neutrophilic count may be caused by decreased or ineffective neutrophil production because the marrow is producing other formed elements. Also, autoimmunity, reduced neutrophil survival, and abnormal neutrophil distribution and sequestration in tissues lead to neutropenia. When the demand for neutrophils exceeds the circulatory supply, the marrow releases immature neutrophils and other leukocytes into the blood; this is called a **shift to the left.** The shift to the left is sometimes called a leukemoid reaction because the morphologic findings in blood smears are similar to those of individuals with leukemia. As infection or inflammation diminishes and granulopoiesis replenishes the circulating granulocytes, a **shift to the right** or back to normal occurs. Neutropenia exists when the neutrophil count is less than 2,000 per ml. If neutrophils are reduced below 500/ml and the entire granulocyte count is extremely low, a very serious condition called **agranulocytosis** results. The usual cause of agranulocytosis is interference with hematopoiesis in the bone marrow or increased cell destruction in the circulation. Chemotherapeutic agents used in the treatment of hematologic and other malignancies and some drugs cause bone marrow suppression. Clinical manifestations of agranulocytosis include respiratory infection, general malaise, septicemia, fever, tachycardia, and ulcers in the mouth and colon. If untreated, sepsis caused by agranulocytosis can result in death within three to six days.

Eosinophilia is an absolute increase in the total numbers of circulating eosinophils. Allergic disorders associated with asthma, hay fever, parasitic invasion, and drug reactions are frequently the cause of eosinophilia. Chemiotaxic factor of anaphylaxis (CTF-A) and histamine released from mast cells attract eosinophils to the area. **Eosinopenia** is a decrease in circulating eosinophils generally due to migration of eosinophils into inflammatory sites. It may also be seen in Cushing syndrome as a result of stress due to surgery, shock, trauma, burns, or mental distress.

Basophilia is quite rare and is generally seen as a response to inflammation and hypersensitivity reactions of the immediate type. An increase in basophils is also seen in chronic myeloid leukemia and myeloid metaplasia. **Basopenia** is seen in hyperthyroidism, acute infection, and long-term therapy with steroids, as well as during ovulation and pregnancy.

Monocytosis, an increase in monocytes, is often transient and correlates poorly with disease states. When present, it is most commonly associated with bacterial infections during the late stages of recovery when needed to phagocytize any surviving microorganisms and debris. Monocytosis is seen in chronic infections such as tuberculosis and subacute bacterial endocarditis. **Monocytopenia**, a decrease in monocytes, is rare but has been identified with hairy cell leukemia and prednisone therapy.

A **lymphocytosis** is rare in acute bacterial infections and occurs most often in acute viral infections, especially those caused by the Epstein-Barr virus (EBV). **Lymphocytopenia** may be associated with neoplasias, immune deficiencies, and destruction by drugs. It may be that the lymphocytopenia associated with heart failure and other acute illnesses is caused by elevated levels of cortisol. Lymphocytopenia is a major problem in AIDS. The lymphocytopenia seen with this condition is caused by the HIV virus, which is cytopathic for T-helper lymphocytes.

2. Describe the pathogenesis of infectious mononucleosis.

Study text page 882.

Infectious mononucleosis is an acute infection of B-lymphocytes. The most common etiologic virus is the Epstein-Barr virus (EBV); however, cytomegalovirus (CMV) and other viruses as well as *Toxoplasma gondii* have been identified as causative agents for this disease. Infectious mononucleosis usually affects young adults between the ages of 15 and 30. Splenomegaly occurs in about one half of affected individuals. The proliferation of clones of B- and T-cells and removal of dead and damaged leukocytes are largely responsible for the swelling of cervical lymphoid tissues. The incubation period for infectious mononucleosis is approximately 30 to 50 days. The accompanying sore throat is caused by inflammation at the site of viral entry. Laboratory findings include an increase in relative and absolute lymphocyte and monocyte counts and 10 to 20 percent atypical forms. The atypical lymphocytes are large with oval, horseshoe-shaped or indented nuclei and vacuolated, spongy cytoplasm. During the first week of infec-

tion, the leukocyte count may be normal or slightly low. After the first week, the leukocyte count, which is predominantly lymphocytes and monocytes, rises to 10,000 to 20,000 per microliter and persists at this level from four to eight weeks. Platelet counts are low. An agglutination test shows the presence of heterophilic antibodies, which are agglutins against sheep red blood cells.

Infectious mononucleosis is usually self-limiting with recovery occurring in few weeks. Treatment consists of rest and alleviation of symptoms with analgesics.

3. Classify, contrast, and describe the manifestations of leukemia.

Study text pages 882-888; refer to Figures 24-1 and 24-2 and Table 24-3.

Leukemia is a malignant disorder of the blood and blood-forming organs, exhibiting an uncontrolled proliferation of dysfunctional leukocytes. The excessive proliferation of leukemic cells crowds the bone marrow and causes decreased production and function of normal hematopoietic cells.

The two major forms of leukemia are acute and chronic. They are classified by predominant cell type and the rate at which the affected individual develops clinical symptoms. Acute leukemia is characterized by undifferentiated immature or blastic cells. The onset of disease is abrupt and rapid, and the affected individual has a short survival time. In chronic leukemia, the predominant cell appears mature but does not function normally. The onset of disease is gradual and the prolonged clinical course results in a relatively longer survival time. Leukemia occurs with varying frequencies at different ages and is about 10 times more frequent in adults than in children in the United States.

Causal risk factors acting together with a genetic predisposition can alter nuclear DNA of a single cell, and then the leukemic cell profilerates. The leukemic cell is unable to mature and respond to normal regulatory mechanisms. Abnormal chromosomes are reported in 40 to 50 percent of patients with acute leukemia. Studies indicate a significant tendency for leukemia to recur in families. Hereditary abnormalities are also associated with an increased incidence of leukemia.

Acquired disorders that progress to acute leukemia include chronic myelocytic leukemia (CML), polycythemia vera, Hodgkin disease, multiple myeloma, ovarian cancer, chronic lymphocytic leukemia (CLL), and sideroblastic anemia. Large doses of ionizing radiation also are associated with an increased incidence in myelogenous leukemia. Drugs such as chloramphenicol and certain alkylating agents cause bone marrow depression and also can predispose an individual to leukemia. Acute myelogenous leukemia (AML) is the most frequently reported secondary cancer following high doses of chemotherapy used for some other cancers.

Leukemias

| | Myelogenous | | Lymphocytic | |
	AML or ANLL	CML	ALL	CLL
Age	Adults or children	Adults, < 50 years of age	Children	Adults, > 50 years of age
Onset	Acute	Gradual	Acute	Gradual
Sign/symptoms	Pallor petechial hemorrhage, lymphadenopathy	Splenomegaly, hepatomegaly, Philadelphia chromosome	Same as AML or ANLL	Splenomegaly, hepatomegaly, lymphadenopathy
Presence of Blasts	High	Low	High	Rare
Treatment	Chemotherapy, marrow transplants	No cure: chemotherapy, marrow transplants	Chemotherapy, marrow transplants	No cure: chemotherapy, marrow transplants
Survival	Days to months	Months to years	Months (untreated) Years (treated)	Years

4. Differentiate multiple myeloma from the leukemias.
Study text pages 888-890.

Multiple myeloma is a B-cell cancer arising from a hematopoietic stem cell that is associated with mature plasma-cell structure and function. Data suggest that this disorder originates in the bone marrow and probably moves through the circulation to and from lymph nodes. The nodes are required for their cellular development. Subsequently, the neoplastic cells return to the bone marrow or soft-tissue sites. These cells use adhesion molecules for return and attachment to sites that provide appropriate environment for expansion and maturation. Development of myeloma is governed by cytokines; IL-6 is likely the major myeloma growth factor. Chemotherapy, radiation therapy, plasmapheresis, and marrow transplant have been used for treatment. With chemotherapy and aggressive management of complications, a median survival of 24 to 30 months and a 10-year survival rate of three percent can be achieved.

Multiple Myeloma/Common Leukemias

Characteristic	Multiple Myeloma	Common Leukemias
Malignant proliferation of WBC in the bone marrow	Yes	Yes
Anemia	Yes	Yes
Bleeding	Yes	Yes
Recurrent infections	Yes	Yes
Plasma cells	Yes	No
Ineffective immunoglobins	Yes	No
Bence-Jones protein in urine	Yes	No
Pathologic bone fractures	Yes	No
WBC blood elevation	No	Yes
Osteocytic lesions	Yes	Possible
Elevated calcium serum	Yes	Possible
Bone pain	Yes	Possible
Renal disease	Yes	Possible

5. Compare Hodgkin disease and non-Hodgkin lymphomas.

Study text pages 891-896; refer to Figures 24-5 through 24-9 and Tables 24-4 and 24-5.

Lymphomas are tumors of (1) primary lymphoid tissue or the thymus and bone marrow and (2) secondary lymphoid tissue or lymph nodes, the spleen, tonsils, and intestinal lymphoid tissue. Most lymphomas are neoplasms of secondary lymphoid tissue involving mostly lymph nodes and/or spleen. The major types of malignant lymphomas are **Hodgkin disease** and **non-Hodgkin lymphoma.** Bone marrow involvement occurs more often in non-Hodgkin lymphoma than in Hodgkin disease. Hodgkin disease uses one of four histologic types for classification. Non-Hodgkin lymphoma has several classifications that eventually may become standardized into three types having histologic subdivisions within each type.

Malignant Lymphomas

	Hodgkin	*Non-Hodgkin*
Cause	Unknown: herpes virus, immunosuppression Epstein-Barr virus	Unknown:
Cellular deviation	*Monocyte-macrophage, T-cells	B-cells
Age of onset	2 peaks 20s and 30s, 60s and 70s	> 50
Nodes involved	Cervical, inguinal, axillary, retroperitoneal	Cervical, axillary, inguinal, femoral
Extranodal involvement	Uncommon	More common
Symptoms	Painless mass, fever, night sweats, weakness, weight loss	Similar to Hodgkin plus pleural effusion, abdominal pain, splenomegaly
Curability	> 75%	< 25%
Treatment	Radiotherapy or surgery for localized, chemotherapy for generalized for both leukemias	

Note: Reed-Sternberg cell is a malignant tissue macrophage that is scattered among normal cells.

6. Describe thrombocytopenia and thrombocytosis.

Study text pages 897-898.

Thrombocytopenia exists when the platelet count is below 100,000 platelets per cubic millimeter of blood. Hemorrhage from minor trauma can occur with counts of 50,000 or less. Spontaneous bleeding can occur with counts between 20,000 and 10, 000. Severe bleeding results if the count is below 10,000. Such bleeding can be fatal if it occurs in the gastrointestinal tract, respiratory system, or central nervous system.

Primary idiopathic thrombocytopenia purpura (ITP) may be either acute or chronic. It is thought to be an autoimmune disorder in which an IgG autoantibody is formed that binds to and destroys the platelets. The acute form is most common in children and young adults and is usually preceded by a viral infection. Chronic ITP is more common in females between the ages of 10 and 50. The individual most commonly presents with mucosal or skin bleeding, which often is manifested as menor-rhagia, purpura, and petechiae.

Secondary thrombocytopenia is caused by conditions associated with drug hypersensitivities that produce antibodies, viral and bacterial infections, and some autoimmune conditions. Viruses inhibit platelet production, destroy circulating platelets, or form viral antigen-antibody complexes.

Thrombocytosis has a platelet count greater than 400,000 per cubic millimeter of blood. Transient thrombocytosis is a normal, physiologic response to stress, infection, trauma, exercise, and ovulation. It is usually asymptomatic until the count exceeds 1 million/mm^3. Then, intravascular clot formation or thrombosis, hemorrhage, or other abnormalities can occur.

Primary thrombocytosis is a myeloproliferative disorder in which megakaryocytes in the marrow are produced in excess. Clinical manifestations of primary thrombocytosis include thrombosis of peripheral blood vessels or, in severe cases, thrombosis of hepatic, mesenteric, or pulmonary vessels. Splenomegaly and easy bruising also occur. In individuals with thrombotic and hemorrhagic complications, the platelet count is lowered by use of chemotherapy agents or phlebotomy.

Secondary thrombocytosis occurs following splenectomy because platelets that normally would be stored in the spleen remain in circulating blood. Secondary thrombocytosis may be seen in conjunction with hemolytic anemias and some polycythemias or as a compensation following thrombocytopenia.

7. Identify the causes of coagulation disorders; characterize disseminated intravascular coagulation.

Study text pages 898-904; refer to Figure 24-10 and Table 24-6.

Disorders of coagulation are usually caused by defects or deficiencies of one or more of the clotting factors. Abnormalities of clotting factors prevent the enzymatic reactions by which these factors are normally transformed from circulating plasma proteins to a stable fibrin clot. Two common inherited disorders are the hemophilias and Von Willebrand disease. These are caused by deficiencies of clotting factors. The hemophilias lack the clotting factors VIII and IX while Von Willebrand has low levels of factor VIII and impaired platelet function. The partial thromboplastin time (PTT), which measures the intrinsic pathway, would likely be prolonged.

Other coagulation defects are acquired and usually result from deficient synthesis of clotting factors by an impaired liver. A deficiency of vitamin K, which is necessary for normal synthesis of the clotting factors by the liver, is an acquired coagulation defect. Deficiencies of vitamin K occur because of insufficient dietary intake, the absence of bile salts necessary for vitamin K absorption, intestinal malabsorption syndromes, and oral antibiotics that kill resident intestinal bacteria that normally provide a source of vitamin K.

Any cardiovascular abnormality that speeds, slows, or obstructs blood flow can create conditions for coagulation within the vessels. Coagulation is also stimulated by tissue thromboplastin that is released by damaged or dead tissue; any condition of tissue decay or damage releases tissue thromboplastin and can cause coagulation. Damage to inflamed vessels causes platelet activation, which in turn activates the coagulation cascade. In these acquired conditions, normal hemostatic function proves detrimental to the body by excessively consuming coagulation factors or by overwhelming normal control of clot formation and breakdown.

Hypercoagulability may be hereditary or be acquired. Hereditary hypercoagulability may result from a deficiency of protein C, protein S, or antithrombin III. These are vitamin K-dependent inhibitors of coagulation and are synthesized by the liver. Inheritance of protein C deficiency and antithrombin III are autosomal dominant. Protein S deficiency is inherited as a codominant autosomal recessive disorder. Other inherited conditions that may predispose to hypercoagulability include decreased fibrinolysis and the presence of antiphospholipid antibodies. The acquired hypercoagulable states are mostly because of conditional venous stasis. The most common clinical states that predispose to thromboembolic conditions are major surgery, acute myocardial infarction, congestive heart failure, limb paralysis, spinal injury, malignancy, advanced age, the postpartum period, and extended bedrest. Factors that promote thrombus formation are referred to as the triad of Virchow and include (1) loss of vessel wall integrity, (2) abnormalities of blood flow, and (3) alterations in the blood factors and platelets.

Disseminated intravascular coagulation (DIC) is an acquired coagulation disorder having a variety of predisposing conditions. DIC is a paradoxical condition in which clotting and hemorrhage occur within the vascular system simultaneously. The development of DIC is generally associated with three pathologic processes, including endothelial damage, release of tissue thromboplastin (TTP), and direct activation of factor X. Gram-negative sepsis, septic shock, hypoxia, and low flow states associated with cardiopulmonary arrest can damage the endothelium and precipitate DIC by activating the intrinsic clotting pathway. Endotoxins of gram-negatives activate both intrinsic and extrinsic clotting pathways. Release of tissue thromboplastin is associated with burns, brain injury, myocardial infarctions, surgeries, obstetric accidents, and malignancies. Excessive amounts of TTP in the circulation activate the extrinsic clotting pathway.

Activation of factor X is stimulated by various substances that enter the bloodstream. Pancreatic and hepatic enzymes and venom from snakebites act in this manner. DIC also can be precipitated by blood transfusion. Transfused blood dilutes the clotting factors and circulating, naturally occurring antithrombins. Antigen-antibody reactions are responsible for the development of DIC following anaphylaxis as procoagulant material is released from disrupted platelets. In DIC, the extrinsic system is most often involved. When either system is activated, widespread, unrestricted coagulation occurs throughout the body, leading to thrombic events within the vasculature. The clotting factors are consumed as widespread clotting develops. Thrombosis in the presence of hemorrhage comprises this paradoxical alteration. The amount of thrombin that enters the systemic circulation during DIC greatly exceeds the ability of the body's naturally occurring antithrombins. The obstruction that results from circulatory deposition of thrombin interferes with blood flow and causes widespread organ hypoperfusion that can lead to ischemia, infarction, and necrosis with manifestations of multisystem organ dysfunction. Plasmin, which is present because of overstimulation of the clotting cascade, begins to degrade fibrin before a stable clot can develop. As fibrin is broken down by plasmin, fibrin degradation products (FDPs) are released into the circulation; these are potent anticoagulants. The macrophage system likely is unable to clear the blood of FDPs because of lack of fibronectin. The clearance of particulate matter or fibrin clumps is mediated by the adhesive properties of fibronectin.

Treatment of DIC attempts to remove the underlying pathology, restore an appropriate balance between coagulation and fibrinolysis, and maintain organ viability. Once the underlying pathology has been removed, coagulation factors can be restored by a normally functioning liver within 24 to 48 hours. Heparin therapy as an anticoagulant may be a way of restoring balance between coagulation and fibrinolysis; however, its use may be beneficial or harmful. Heparin is indicated when organ function is compromised by microthrombi. In DIC precipitated by septic shock or during bleeding, heparin is contraindicated. Organ viability is treated primarily by adequate fluid replacement to assure adequate circulating blood volume so optimal tissue perfusion can be maintained.

Practice Examination

Match the leukocytic alteration with its cause.

1. eosinophilia
2. leukopenia
3. granulocytosis
4. eosinopenia
5. lymphocytosis

a. immune deficiencies
b. allergic disorders
c. radiation
d. early stage of infection
e. AIDS
f. surgical stress
g. acute viral infections

6. Leukocytosis is found in all except
   a. inflammatory responses.
   b. allergic responses.
   c. bacterial infections.
   d. bone marrow depression.

7. What is the most notable characteristic of infectious mononucleosis?
   a. A short incubation period of less than one week.
   b. It usually affects preteens.
   c. Atypical lymphocytes account for some of the lymphocytosis.
   d. Lymphocytosis persists for less than one week.

8. Which likely does not play a role in leukemia?
   a. radiation
   b. Down syndrome
   c. polycythemia vera
   d. chloramphenicol
   e. diet

9. The group most likely to be affected by ALL is
   a. young adults.
   b. middle age adults.
   c. older adults.
   d. children.

10. Signs and symptoms of acute leukemia include all except
   a. splenomegaly.
   b. petechiae.
   c. lymphadenopathy.
   d. polycythemia.
   e. pallor.

11. CML is characterized by its
   a. acute onset.
   b. high incidence in children.
   c. presence of the Philadelphia chromosome.
   d. survival time of days to months.

12. A bone marrow analysis in a 3-year-old female reveals an abnormally high number of lymphoblasts. The likely diagnosis is
   a. AML.
   b. ALL.
   c. CML.
   d. CLL.

13. Clinical manifestations of multiple myeloma include all but
   a. bone pain.
   b. decreased serum calcium.
   c. m-protein.
   d. renal damage.
   e. pathological fractures.

Match the characteristic with the malignant lymphoma.

14. high curability
15. Epstein-Barr virus
16. Reed-Sternberg cell
17. more frequent extranodal involvement
18. B-cells

a. Hodgkin
b. non-Hodgkin

19. Thrombocytopenia may be caused by all except
   a. an IgG autoantibody.
   b. drug hypersensitivities.
   c. viruses stimulating platelet production.
   d. bacterial infections consuming platelets.
   e. viruses destroying circulating platelets.

20. A thrombocytopenia with a platelet count between 50,000/mm^3 and 40,000/mm^3 likely will cause
   a. hemorrhage from minor trauma.
   b. spontaneous bleeding.
   c. death.
   d. polycythemia.

21. Bleeding time may be prolonged in
   1. thrombocytopia.
   2. thrombocytopathy.
   3. hypoprothrombinemia.
   4. hemophilias.
   5. Von Willebrand disease.

   a. 1
   b. 3
   c. 1, 2, 3
   d. 4, 5
   e. 1, 2, 3, 4, 5

22. Thromboembolic disease can be caused by all except
    a. injured vessel walls.
    b. tissue damage that releases excessive tissue thromboplastin.
    c. obstructed blood flow.
    d. deficient dietary intake of vitamin K.
    e. polycythemia.

23. Hypercoagulability may result because
    a. of a genetic deficiency of protein C, protein S, or antithrombin III.
    b. venous states.
    c. loss of vessel wall integrity.
    d. Both b and c are correct.
    e. a, b, and c are correct.

24. DIC is associated with
    a. endothelial damage.
    b. activation of factor X.
    c. release of tissue thromboplastin.
    d. Both a and c are correct.
    e. a, b, and c are correct.

25. Heparin may sometimes be used to treat DIC because it
    a. stimulates platelet aggregation.
    b. stimulates conversion of fibrinogen to fibrin.
    c. stimulates fibrinolysis.
    d. All of the above are correct.
    e. prevents thromboplastin from activating the coagulation mechanisms.

Case Study

L.L., a nine-year-old male, was brought to his dentist for a regular pre-school check-up. Past dental visits were routine, except that two years ago, L.L. missed one appointment because of chicken pox. The dentist and mother were having a chatty conversation when L.L.'s mother stated that her son recently had stopped showing interest in sports and complained of fatigue. During the dental examination, the dentist noted gingival bleeding whenever the tissue was lightly probed. Three nontender lymph nodes were palpable in the submandibular nodes. No other abnormalities were noted. The dentist advised the mother to take L.L. to the medical clinic next door.

The physical examination by the physician showed LL's skin to be pale with ecchymoses and petechiae of the trunk. The spleen and liver were not palpable and the remaining examination was unremarkable. A sample of blood was withdrawn.

The CBC revealed:

Hemoglobin = 9.2 gm/dl
Hemocrit = 30%
RBCs = 3×10^6/mm^3
WBC = 16×10^3/mm^3
Neutrophils = 8×10^3/mm^3
Basophils = 250/mm^3

Eosinophils = 445/mm^3
Monocytes = 1,900/mm^3
Lymphocytes = 4,500/mm^3
Blasts = much higher than normal
Platelets = 30×10^3/mm^3

Considering the examinations and CBC, what would the physician likely conclude and do?

Alterations in Hematologic Function in Children

Prerequisite Objectives

a. Describe fetal and neonatal hematopoiesis.
   Review text pages 909-911; refer to Figures 22-7 and 25-1 and Table 25-1.

Remember!

- When the developing embryo becomes too large for oxygenation of tissues by simple diffusion, the production of erythrocytes begins within the vessels of the yolk sac. At approximately the eighth week of gestation, erythrocyte production shifts from the vessels to the liver sinusoids, the spleen, and lymph nodes. Erythropoiesis in these sites reaches a peak at approximately four months. Hepatic blood cellular formation declines steadily thereafter but does not disappear entirely during the remainder of gestation. By the fifth month of gestation, hematopoiesis begins to occur in the marrow and increases rapidly until marrow fills the entire bone marrow space. By the time of delivery, the marrow is the only significant site of hematopoiesis. During childhood, hematopoietic tissue retreats to the vertebrae, ribs, sternum, pelvis, scapulae, skull, and proximal ends of the femur and humerus. A biochemically distinct type of hemoglobin is synthesized during fetal life and is composed of two alpha and two gamma chains of polypeptides; whereas the adult hemoglobins are composed of two alpha and two beta chains.

---

b. Identify the postnatal changes occurring in the blood throughout childhood.
   Review text pages 911-912; refer to Table 25-1.

Remember!

- Blood cell counts tend to rise above adult levels at birth and then decline gradually throughout childhood. The immediate rise in values is the result of accelerated hematopoiesis during fetal life, the trauma of birth, and cutting of the umbilical cord. These events surrounding the birth also are accompanied by a "shift to the left," or the presence of large numbers of immature erythrocytes and leukocytes in peripheral blood. The shift to the left usually disappears within the first two to three months of life.

Objectives

After successful study of this chapter, the learner will be able to:

1. Describe the etiology of childhood iron deficiency anemia and identify appropriate preventive, diagnostic, and treatment measures.

Study text pages 912-914; refer to Table 25-2.

Iron deficiency anemia is the most common childhood anemia and is caused by poor dietary iron intake, occult blood, or both. Iron stores in the form of hemosiderin are at their lowest level in the term infant at 16 to 20 weeks of age. Thereafter, dietary intake must supply iron requirements. Early exposure to cow's milk protein often causes hemorrhagic bowel inflammation and occult blood loss in the infant. The highest incidence of iron deficiency anemia occurs at six months to two years of age and peaks again in adolescence during rapid growth periods. The onset of menstruation in females also is a contributor. Poor socioeconomic status also can be a significant factor. Iron stores are best measured by serum ferritin and total iron-binding capacity. There are few symptoms in infants and young children until moderate anemia develops. Anemia in infants can be avoided by ingestion of iron-fortified formulas instead of cow's milk in early infancy and iron-rich solid foods at appropriate ages. Treatment for iron deficiency anemia is oral or parenteral iron supplements; oral supplements are preferred.

2. Compare and contrast the two major causes of hemolytic disease of the newborn.

Study text pages 914-916; refer to Figure 25-2 and Table 25-2.

The two major causes of **hemolytic disease of the newborn (HDN)** are **blood type incompatibility** and **Rh factor incompatibility**. Blood type incompatibility is a mild form of hemolytic disease. Rh incompatibility is potentially much more severe. Blood type incompatibility in the mother occurs when maternal antibodies to fetal erythrocytes are formed because of a prior incompatible pregnancy, other antigenetic factors, or exposure of the mother to fetal erythrocytes during pregnancy. Incompatibility in the infant occurs when sufficient antibody, usually IgG, crosses the placenta from the mother to the infant or when maternal antibodies attach to and damage fetal erythrocytes. ABO incompatibility occurs in 20 to 25 percent of pregnancies with only one in 10 cases producing HDN. Usual causes are a type O mother with a type A or B infant, a type A mother with a type B infant, or a type B mother with a type A infant. Hemolysis in the newborn is usually limited and requires no treatment; however, mild hemolysis may contribute to hyperbilirubinemia. Rh incompatibility occurs in less than 10 percent of pregnancies and rarely is a problem during the first pregnancy; the first pregnancy initiates sensitization. Rh incompatibility becomes a greater problem with subsequent pregnancies. It should be noted that HDN caused by Rh incompatibility occurs in only 5 percent of pregnancies after five or more pregnancies. In the most severe form, Rh incompatibility will lead to **hydrops fetalis** with severe anemia, edema, central nervous system damage, and fetal death. It may also contribute to severe hyperbilirubinemia. Blood typing in mothers and infants reveals those at risk. Indirect Coombs' test reveals antibodies in mothers and direct Coombs' test reveals antibodies bound to fetal erythrocytes. Inutero testing through the umbilical vein is now available. Immunoprophylaxis with Rh immunoglobulin (RhoGAM) for at-risk mothers has been very successful.

3. Identify the etiology, pathophysiology, and ethnic groups at risk for glucose-6-phosphate dehydrogenase deficiency.

Study text page 917.

Glucose-6-phosphate dehydrogenase deficiency (G-6-PD) is an X-linked recessive disorder fully expressed in homozygous males. G-6-PD is primarily a problem in African Americans where the incidence may be 10 percent; a frequency range of 5 to 40 percent exists in Sephardic Jews, Greeks, Iranians, Chinese, Filipinos, and Indonesians. G-6-PD is caused by a defect of an enzyme that enables erythrocytes to maintain normal function in the presence of certain substances such as sulfa drugs, salicylates, quinolones, antimalarials, and fava beans, which are a dietary staple in the Mediterranean area. Exposure to these substances causes hemolysis, often of a very severe nature, that resolves when the offending substance is removed. Episodes may result in shock or death. Males at risk for G-6-PD should be tested prior to being exposed to certain oxidant drugs.

4. Describe childhood sickle cell disease and identify its most common forms of presentation.

Study text pages 919-923; refer to Figures 24-4 through 24-7 and Table 25-3.

Intravascular sickling may be present in infants six to eight weeks of age, but clinical manifestations usually do not become apparent until six months of age because of the persistence of fetal hemoglobin. The parent's medical history and clinical findings may generate an index of suspicion about the child. The sickle solubility test and hemoglobin electrophoresis are used to assist diagnosis. Prenatal chorionic villus sampling is now available. Acute complications or crises occur in **sickle cell disease** and may be provoked by infection, exposure to cold, low PO_2, acidosis, or localized hypoxemia. Infections are frequent in childhood and may generate various degrees of other triggers. **Vasoocclusive crises** result from a "log-jam" effect produced by stiff, sickled erythrocytes in the microcirculation. Symptoms include symmetric swelling of the hands and feet, which may be the first clinical manifestation in infancy. In older children, swollen painful joints, priapism, severe abdominal pain from infarctions of abdominal organs, and strokes may occur. Other complications include sickle cell retinopathy, renal necrosis, and necrosis of the femoral head. **Sequestration crises** occur only in the young child. Large amounts of blood may pool in the liver and spleen which can contain as much as one-fifth of the blood volume and, thus, precipitate shock. Up to a 50 percent mortality rate has been reported with these crises. **Aplastic crises** may occur because of the decreased survival of sickled erythrocytes, which is 10 to 20 days, and may lead to aplastic anemia if compensatory mechanisms are not intact. Most sickle cell deaths are due to overwhelming sepsis.

5. Describe the usual manifestations of childhood hemophilias and their complications.
Study text pages 925-928; refer to Tables 25-4 and 25-5.

Hemophilia or spontaneous bleeding is rare in the first year of life, although significant bleeding may occur during circumcision. However, this is an unusual complication, as hemostasis in these infants is achieved through the extrinsic pathway that does not require factors VIII, IX, or XI. **Hematoma** formation is a more common problem during the first year of life and may be due to injections, firm holding, or the many accidents that occur in the development of movement in children. These accidents may also precipitate hemarthrosis. By three to four years of age, 90 percent of children have had persistent bleeding due to minor trauma. Hemarthrosis also causes joint pain, limits movement, and promotes degenerative joint changes. Spontaneous hematuria and epistaxis are bothersome but rarely serious. Life-threatening intracranial and cervical bleeding may result from normal childhood injury.

6. Describe the pathophysiology of idiopathic thrombocytopenic purpura and identify its most likely etiology.
Study text pages 928-929.

Idiopathic thrombocytopenic purpura (ITP) is the most common thrombocytopenic purpura of childhood. Antiplatelet antibodies attach to platelets that are then sequestered in the spleen where they are destroyed by mononuclear phagocytes. Destruction far exceeds production and thrombocytosis occurs. Classic symptoms of bruising and petechiae are usually preceded from one to four weeks by a viral illness that may cause sensitization of the platelets that triggers an antibody response; high levels of IgG have been found on the platelets of affected children. The prognosis is excellent. The acute phase lasts one to two weeks, although thrombocytopenia may persist longer. Complete recovery is approximately 75 percent at three months after onset with 90 percent recovering by nine to 12 months. Although serious complications are few, severe intracranial bleeding does occur in less than 1 percent of cases and can be devastating. Corticosteroids are indicated in some cases to suppress the body's immune response system to platelets. Splenectomy is reserved for severe, chronic cases.

7. Describe proposed causative factors and common manifestations for childhood leukemias.
Study text pages 929-934; refer to Table 25-6.

Leukemia, in its various forms, is the most common childhood cancer; it comprises 35 percent of the neoplasms of children. Acute lymphoblastic leukemia (ALL) represents 80 to 85 percent of all childhood leukemias. Peak incidence of ALL occurs between two and six years of age and is twice as common in white children as in nonwhite children. The etiology of leukemia is probably multifactorial, with genetic predisposition, environment, and viruses playing a role. Exposure to high levels of radiation also has become an established etiological factor. The appearance of symptoms may be rapid or slow but generally reflects the effects of bone marrow failure. Findings include decreased red blood cells and platelets and changes in white blood cells. Pallor, fatigue, petechiae, purpura, and fever are generally present. Fever may be due to a hypermetabolic state brought on by the rapid production and destruction of leukemic cells or because of a secondary infection due to neutropenia. Although white blood cell counts are generally less than $50,000/mm^3$ in most forms of leukemia, they may exceed $100,000/mm^3$. Renal failure may ensue because of high uric acid levels that produce precipitates of urates in the renal tubules. This phenomenon is the result of rapid cellular breakdown which liberates high levels of purines that are then metabolized into uric acid. Other symptoms, such as bone and joint pain, may be due to infiltration of leukemic cells into other organs. The central nervous system is a common site of extramedullary infiltration, although few children have this problem at diagnosis. Prognosis for the childhood leukemias is variable; however, 60 to 70 percent of children with ALL can be cured.

Practice Examination

True/False

_____ 1. Early initiation of iron-rich cow's milk in an infant's diet is an excellent preventive measure against iron deficiency anemia.

_____ 2. Although a frequent problem, ABO incompatibility seldom results in significant disease.

_____ 3. Sequestration crisis is a serious complication of sickle cell disease unique to childhood.

_____ 4. Rh incompatibility is a problem only of Rh positive women bearing an Rh negative fetus during a second pregnancy.

_____ 5. Since hemostasis in the newborn is chiefly attained through the extrinsic pathway, serious bleeding in the newborn period is usually not a problem in hemophiliacs.

_____ 6. Idiopathic thrombocytopenic purpura is a genetically transmitted disease.

_____ 7. Leukemias are multifactorial diseases with genetic disposition, environment, and bacterial infections playing a role in their etiology.

8. Which of the following is the most frequent blood disorder of infancy and childhood?
   a. iron deficiency anemia
   b. pernicious anemia
   c. folate deficiency anemia
   d. sideroblastic anemia

9. Maternal-fetal blood incompatibility may exist in which of the following conditions?
   a. mother Rh-positive, fetus Rh-negative
   b. mother Rh-negative, fetus Rh-positive
   c. Rh-negative father, Rh-positive mother
   d. Rh-negative father, Rh-negative mother

10. G-6-PD may be classified as
    a. an inherited disorder.
    b. an X-linked, recessive disorder.
    c. an autosomal, recessive disorder.
    d. Both a and b are correct.
    e. Both a and c are correct.

11. Which of the following is a correct statement?
    a. Sickle cell disease is an autosomal dominant disorder.
    b. Sickle cell disease is an X-linked recessive disorder.
    c. Sickle cell disease is an X-linked dominant disorder.
    d. Sickle cell disease is an autosomal recessive disorder.

12. Idiopathic thrombocytopenic purpura (ITP) involves antibodies against
    a. neutrophils.
    b. eosinophils.
    c. platelets.
    d. basophils.

13. Which of the following are factors associated with iron deficiency anemia?
    a. rapid growth
    b. low socioeconomic status
    c. cow's milk for infants
    d. Both a and c are correct.
    e. a, b, and c are correct.

14. What is the most likely cause of idiopathic thrombocytopenic purpura?
    a. stress and fatigue
    b. genetic predisposition
    c. prolonged occult bleeding
    d. viral sensitization
    e. Both b and c are correct.

15. Acute exacerbations of G-6-PD may be triggered by all except
    a. sulfa drugs.
    b. quinolones.
    c. fava beans.
    d. viral infections.

16. In sickle cell disease, vasoocclusive crisis is the result of
    a. damage to platelets due to IgG.
    b. "plugging" of peripheral blood vessels by "stiff" sickled erythrocytes.
    c. ingestion of sulfa drugs.
    d. sequestration of large numbers of erythrocytes in the spleen.

17. Which factors may play a part in the development of childhood leukemia?
    a. genetic predisposition
    b. environmental factors
    c. viral infections
    d. radiation
    e. All of the above are correct.

18. Which statement is true about acute lymphocytic leukemia?
    a. It is the most common childhood leukemia.
    b. It usually occurs between two and six years of age.
    c. It is uniformly fatal.
    d. It is easily predicted through genetic testing.
    e. Both a and b are correct.

Match the circumstance with the alteration.

19. leukocyte counts approaching 100,000/mm^3
20. low platelet counts
21. lack of coagulation factors VIII, IX, XI
22. may present early as symmetric, painful swelling of hands and feet
23. may cause severe hemolysis in the newborn period
24. may result in aplastic crises
25. may result in hydrops fetalis or fetal death

a. the leukemias
b. ITP
c. sickle cell disease
d. Rh incompatibility
e. the hemophilias

191

Case Study

   Steven D. is a 10-year-old caucasian boy seeking physician attention because of possible physical abuse observed by his gym teacher. The teacher noticed severe bruising over much of his upper body when his shirt "rode up" during an exercise. Steven emphatically states that he has never been abused by anyone and has had the bruising for two to three days. He denies any accidents and didn't tell anyone about his bruises because he thought they might "get me into trouble." He also denies any systemic symptoms but acknowledges he had a "bad cold" nearly a month ago. His mother is very confused and concerned. She cannot explain the bruises either and did not see them before today as her son does all of his own hygiene and is quite modest about revealing his body even to family members. Steven's physical examination is benign except for multiple, irregular dark purple bruises over most of his torso and lower extremities. He also has a "shower" of light petechiae over his shoulders and neck. His complete blood count is well within normal limits except for a low platelet count of 18,000/mm^3.

   What is Steven's diagnosis? What are the diagnostic clinical manifestations and what is the treatment?

C H A P T E R 26

Structure and Function of the Cardiovascular and Lymphatic Systems

---

Objectives

After successful study of this chapter, the learner will be able to:

1. **Describe the function of the circulatory system; distinguish between pulmonary and systemic circulation.**
   Review text page 944; refer to Figure 26-1.

2. **Describe the heart wall and the chambers, fibrous skeleton, valves, and great vessels of the heart; trace the blood flow through the heart and indicate factors that regulate blood flow.**
   Review text pages 944-951; refer to Figures 26-2 through 26-7.

3. **Describe the coronary arteries, veins, and lymphatic vessels.**
   Review text pages 951-953; refer to Figure 26-8.

4. **Describe the initiation of and conduction sequence of electrical impulses through the heart; identify the autonomic innervation and its effects on the heart.**
   Review text pages 953-959; refer to Figures 26-9 through 26-12 and Table 26-2.

5. **Identify the structure and characteristics of myocardial cells.**
   Review text pages 959-963; refer to Figures 26-13 through 26-17.

6. **Use the Frank-Starling law and Laplace law to demonstrate interrelationships that affect cardiac function.**
   Review text pages 963-968; refer to Figures 26-18 through 26-20.

7. **Contrast the structure and function of arteries, capillaries, and veins.**
   Review text pages 969-974; refer to Figures 26-22 through 26-27.

8. **Describe the determinants of blood flow.**
   Review text pages 975-980; refer to Figures 26-28 through 26-31.

9. **Identify the factors that regulate arterial and venous blood pressure.**
   Review text pages 980-983; refer to Figures 26-32 and 26-33.

10. **Describe the normal structure and function of the lymphatic system.**
    Review text pages 983-986; refer to Figures 26-34 and 26-35.

11. **Note the changes that aging causes in the cardiovascular system.**
    Review text pages 993-994; refer to Table 26-7.

Practice Examination

1. Oxygenated blood flows through the
   a. superior vena cava.
   b. pulmonary veins.
   c. pulmonary arteries.
   d. coronary veins.
   e. None of the above is correct.

2. The hepatic vein
   a. carries blood from the vena cava to the liver.
   b. carries blood from the liver to the vena cava.
   c. carries blood from the aorta to the liver.
   d. carries blood from the liver to the aorta.

3. The position of the heart in the mediastinum is
   a. inferior to the diaphragm and between the lungs.
   b. medial to the lungs, superior to the diaphragm.
   c. posterior to the trachea, anterior to the esophagus.
   d. posterior to the lungs and anterior to the diaphragm.

4. The pericardial space is found between the
   a. myocardium and parietal pericardium.
   b. endocardium and visceral pericardium.
   c. visceral and parietal pericardium.
   d. visceral and epicardial pericardium.

5. In the normal cardiac cycle,
   1. the right atrium and right ventricles contract simultaneously.
   2. the two atria contract simultaneously while the two ventricles relax.
   3. the two ventricles contract simultaneously while the two atria relax.
   4. both the ventricles and atria contract simultaneously to increase cardiac output.

   a. 1, 4
   b. 2, 3
   c. 1, 2
   d. 2, 4

6. The QRS complex of the EKG represents
   a. atrial depolarization.
   b. ventricular depolarization.
   c. atrial contraction.
   d. ventricular repolarization.
   e. atrial repolarization.

7. A person having a heart rate of 100, a systolic blood pressure of 200, and a stroke volume of 40 would have an average cardiac output of
   a. 0.5 milliliters.
   b. 5 liters.
   c. 4 milliliters.
   d. 8000 milliliters.
   e. None of the above is correct.

8. During atrial systole,
   a. the AV valves are open.
   b. the atria are filling.
   c. the ventricles are emptying.
   d. the semilunar valves are open.

9. Which does not significantly affect heart rate?
   a. temperature
   b. age
   c. presence of heart murmur
   d. Na and K ions

10. One cardiac cycle
    a. has a duration which changes if the heart rate changes.
    b. usually requires less than one second to complete.
    c. is equal to stroke volume times heart rate.
    d. pumps approximately five liters of blood.
    e. Both a and b are correct.

11. A patient who is hemorrhaging severely will be pale because
    a. peripheral vasoconstriction is a homeostatic response to low BP.
    b. peripheral vasodilation is a homeostatic response to low BP.
    c. constriction of the cranial arteries is a homeostatic response to low BP.
    d. None of the above is correct.

12. When the intraventricular pressure becomes greater than the pressure in the pulmonary arteries,
    a. the semilunars will open.
    b. the semilunars will close.
    c. the AV valves will open.
    d. the AV valves will close.

13. The two distinct heart sounds, lubb and dupp, are most directly related to
    a. pulse pressure in the aorta.
    b. the contraction of the ventricles.
    c. turbulence from closing of valves.
    d. contraction of the atria.

14. Another name for the mitral valve is the
    a. aortic semilunar valve.
    b. pulmonary semilunar valve.
    c. tricuspid valve.
    d. bicuspid valve.

15. Starling "law of the heart" concerns the
    a. relationship between the length of the cardiac muscle fiber and the strength of contraction.
    b. relationship between stroke volume and arterial resistance.
    c. relationship between rapidity of nerve conduction and stroke volume.
    d. relationship between systolic rate and cardiac output.

16. What three factors assist the return of venous blood to the heart?
    1. peripheral pooling   a. 1, 2, 4
    2. venous valves   b. 2, 4, 5
    3. increased intra-abdominal pressure   c. 2, 3, 4
    4. respiratory movements   d. 2, 3, 5
    5. contraction of skeletal muscles

17. Blood pressure is measured by the
    a. pressure exerted on the ventricular walls during systole.
    b. pressure exerted by the blood on the wall of any blood vessel.
    c. pressure exerted on arteries by the blood.
    d. product of the stroke volume times heart rate.

18. Place the portions of the pulmonary circulation in correct sequence.
    1. pulmonary veins
    2. pulmonary arteries
    3. lungs
    4. right ventricle
    5. left atrium

    a. 1, 5, 3, 2, 4
    b. 4, 2, 3, 1, 5
    c. 4, 1, 3, 2, 5
    d. 5, 2, 3, 1, 4
    e. 5, 1, 3, 2, 4

19. The heart beat is initiated by the
    a. coronary sinus.
    b. atrioventricular bundle.
    c. right ventricle.
    d. SA node.
    e. AV node.

20. If the sympathetic nervous system stimulation of the heart predominates over parasympathetic nervous stimulation, the heart will
    a. increase its rate.
    b. contract with greater force and at a slower rate.
    c. decrease its rate and force of contraction.
    d. contract with less force and at a higher rate.

21. When fluids have a turbulent flow,
    a. more energy is lost than with laminar flow.
    b. it is a sign of greater blood viscosity.
    c. the fluids have greater velocity than with laminar flow.
    d. there is greater hydrostatic pressure than if the fluids had laminar flow.

22. Identify the normal sequence of an electrical impulse through the heart's conduction system.
    1. atrioventricular bundle
    2. AV node
    3. Purkinje fibers
    4. SA node
    5. right and left bundle branches

    a. 4, 1, 2, 5, 3
    b. 4, 2, 5, 1, 3
    c. 2, 4, 1, 5, 3
    d. 4, 2, 1, 5, 3

23. Which factors might increase resistance to the flow of blood through the blood vessels?
    a. an increased inner radius or diameter of blood vessels
    b. decreased numbers of capillaries
    c. decreased blood viscosity
    d. decreased numbers of red blood cells

24. Depolarization of cardiac muscle cells occurs because of
    a. decreased permeability of the cell membrane to potassium.
    b. rapid extracellular movement of sodium into the cardiac cell.
    c. rapid intracellular movement of sodium out of the cardiac cell.
    d. rapid extracellular movement of calcium into the cardiac cell.
    e. rapid intracellular movement of calcium out of the cardiac cell.

25. Which is true?
    a. Lymphatic walls consist of multiple layers of flattened endothelial cells.
    b. Lymph from the entire body, except the upper right quadrant, eventually drains into the thoracic duct.
    c. The thoracic duct has approximately the same diameter as the great veins.
    d. Lymph contains more proteins than does blood plasma.
    e. The lymphatic system, like the circulatory system, is a closed circuit.

CHAPTER 27

Alterations of Cardiovascular Function

Prerequisite Objectives

a. Describe the flow of blood through the heart and identify the coronary vessels.
   Review text pages 948-951; refer to Figures 26-5 and 26-8.

Remember!

- The pumping action of the heart consists of contraction and relaxation of the myocardial layer of the heart wall. During relaxation, termed diastole, blood fills the chambers. The contraction that follows, termed systole, forces the blood from the chamber into the pulmonary or systemic circulation. During diastole, blood from the veins of the systemic circulation enters the thin-walled right atrium from the superior vena cava and the inferior vena cava. Venous blood from the coronary circulation enters the right atrium through the coronary sinus. The right atrium fills and its fluid pressure pushes open the right atrioventricular or tricuspid valve. Blood fills the right ventricle. The same sequence of events occurs a fraction of a second earlier in the left heart. The four pulmonary veins, two from the right lung and two from the left lung, carry oxygenated blood from the pulmonary circulation to the left atrium. As the left atrium fills, its fluid pressure pushes the cusps of the mitral valve open and blood flows into the left ventricle. Left atrial contraction, or "atrial kick," provides a significant increase of blood to the left ventricle. Blood circulates from the left ventricle and returns to the right atrium because of a progressive fall in pressure from the left ventricle to the right atrium of approximately 120 mm Hg. Blood always flows from a higher pressure area toward a lower pressure area.

- The blood within the heart chambers does not supply oxygen and other nutrients to the cells of the heart. Like all other organs, heart structures are nourished by vessels of the systemic circulation. The coronary circulation consists of coronary arteries and the cardiac veins. The right and left coronary arteries traverse the epicardium and branch several times. The left coronary artery arises from a single opening behind the left cusp of the aortic semilunar valve. It divides into two branches, the left anterior descending artery and the circumflex artery. The left anterior descending artery delivers blood to portions of the left and right ventricles and much of the interventricular septum. The circumflex artery supplies blood to the left atrium and the lateral wall of the left ventricle. The circumflex artery often branches to the posterior surfaces of the left atrium and left ventricle. The right coronary artery originates from an opening behind the right aortic cusp. Three major branches of the right coronary artery supply blood to the right atrium, upper right ventricle, and both ventricles.

(Continued)

Remember! *(cont'd)*

- Collateral arteries are connections or anastomoses between two branches of the same coronary artery or connections of branches of the right coronary artery with branches of the left. They are particularly common within the interventricular and interatrial septa, at the apex of the heart, over the anterior surface of the right ventricle, and around the sinus node. The heart has an extensive capillary network with about one capillary per muscle cell. Blood travels from the arteries to the arterioles, then into the capillaries, where exchange of oxygen and other nutrients takes place.

- Blood from the coronary arteries drains into the cardiac veins which travel alongside the arteries. The cardiac veins feed into the great cardiac vein and then into the coronary sinus located between the atria and ventricles. The coronary sinus empties into the right atrium.

b. Describe the conduction system of the heart.
   Review text pages 953-959; refer to Figures 26-9 through 26-12.

Remember!

- Continuous, rhythmic repetition of the cardiac cycle or systole and diastole depends on the continuous, rhythmic transmission of electrical impulses. As an electrical impulse passes from cell to cell in the myocardium, it stimulates the fibers to shorten. Shortening causes muscular contraction or systole. After the action potential passes, the fibers relax and return to their resting length; this relaxation is diastole.

- The myocardium differs from other muscle tissues; it contains its own intrinsic conduction system. It can generate and transmit action potentials without stimulation from the nervous system. These cells are concentrated at certain sites in the myocardium called nodes. Although the heart is innervated by both sympathetic and parasympathetic fibers, neural impulses are not needed to maintain the cardiac cycle.

- Normally, electrical impulses arise in the sinoatrial node or SA node, often called the pacemaker of the heart. The SA node lies only a millimeter or less beneath the visceral pericardium, making it vulnerable to injury and disease, especially pericardial inflammation. There are numerous autonomic nerve endings within the node which enable the node to respond to the nervous system. In the resting adult, the SA node generates about 75 action potentials per minute. Each action potential travels rapidly from cell to cell and through special pathways in the atrial myocardium which causes both atria to contract. Atrial contraction initiates systole. Transmission of the action potential from the atrial to the ventricular myocardium occurs through muscle fibers of the conduction system. The action potential travels first to the atrioventricular node or AV node, then to the atrioventricular bundle, then to the common bundle, and finally through the bundle branches of the interventricular septum to Purkinje fibers in the heart wall.

- The extensive network of Purkinje fibers enables the rapid spread of the impulse to the ventricular apices.

- Electrical activation of the muscle cells, or depolarization, is caused by the movement of electrically charged solutes, primarily sodium and potassium, across cardiac cell membranes. Deactivation, or repolarization, occurs by ion movement in the opposite direction. Movement of ions into and out of the cell creates an electrical or voltage difference across the cell membrane. This difference or potential of charged ions causes the impulse to flow within cells and from cell to cell.

(Continued)

- Sympathetic neural stimulation of the myocardium and coronary vessels depends on the presence of adrenergic receptors that are able to bind specifically with neurotransmitters of the sympathetic nervous system. The effects of sympathetic stimulation depend on which adrenergic receptors are most plentiful on the cells of the effector tissue and whether the neurotransmitter is norepinephrine or epinephrine. Beta1 receptors are found mostly in the AV and SA nodes, Purkinje fibers, and the atrial and ventricular myocardium. Norepinephrine binding with B_1 receptors increases the rate of impulse generation and conduction and also the strength of myocardial contraction during systole. These effects enable the heart to pump more blood. At the same time, epinephrine binds with B_2 receptors which are most plentiful in the coronary arterioles. This causes the coronary arterioles to dilate and supplies the hard-working myocardium with more oxygen and nutrients.

c. Describe the interrelationships between myocardial stretch and chamber wall dimensions and the contractible force of the heart.
    Review text pages 963-966; refer to Figures 26-18 and 26-19.

Remember!

- Cardiac muscle, like other muscle, increases its strength of contraction within certain limits when it is stretched. The Frank-Starling law of the heart states that there is a direct relationship between the volume of blood in the heart and stretch or length of cardiac fibers at the end of diastole and the force of contraction during the next systole. The greater the stretch from preload blood volume, the stronger the contraction. The failing or dilated heart may not be able to respond to increased filling because its fibers are already lengthened maximally.

- Laplace's law states the relationships between wall thickness, pressure, and wall tension. Wall tension is related directly to the product of intraventricular pressure and internal radius and inversely to the wall thickness. Stated another way, wall tension equals intraventricular pressure times radius of space divided by wall thickness. If solved for pressure, the pressure or contractible force is directly related to wall thickness and wall tension and indirectly related to the radius. The thicker the wall and greater the wall tension and smaller the radius, the greater the force of contraction. With a dilated chamber or vessel, the myocardial fibers in the wall must develop greater tension to produce a given pressure within the chamber or vessel.

d. Establish the determinants of blood flow.
    Review text pages 975-980; refer to Figures 26-28 and 26-29.

Remember!

- Blood flow is determined primarily by two factors: pressure and resistance. Pressure in a liquid system is the force exerted on the liquid per unit area. Fluid moves from the arterial "side" of the capillaries, which is a region of greater pressure, to the venous side, which is a region of lesser pressure. Resistance opposes force. In the cardiovascular system, most opposition to blood flow is because of the diameter and length of the blood vessels themselves.

- The relationship between blood flow, pressure, and resistance can be stated as Q equals P divided by R, where Q is blood flow, P is the pressure difference, and R is resistance.

(Continued)

Remember! (cont'd)

- Resistance to fluid flow considers the length of the tube or vessel, the viscosity of the fluid, and the radius of the lumen. According to Poiseuille's formula, the resistance equals viscosity of blood times length of vessel divided by the fourth power of the lumen's radius.

- Because this equation was derived using straight, rigid tubes with steady, streamlined flow, it cannot be applied exactly to the vascular system. Nevertheless, it is a useful model for vascular resistance assessment. Small changes in the lumen's radius lead to large changes in vascular resistance. Because vessel length is relatively constant, length is not as important as lumen size in determining flow through a single vessel. However, blood flowing through the distributing arteries encounters more resistance than blood flowing through the capillary bed. In the capillary bed, flow is distributed among many short, tiny branches.

- If R equals viscosity times length divided by the fourth power of radius is substituted into the formula Q equals P divided by R, a helpful summary of likely factors affecting blood flow rate can be expressed. Now, blood flow equals pressure times radius to the fourth power divided by the viscosity times the length. The higher the pressure and greater the vessel radius and the less the viscosity of blood and length of vessel, the greater the flow of blood.

e. Establish the determinants of blood pressure.
Review text pages 980-982; refer to Figures 26-32 and 26-33.

Remember!

- The mean arterial pressure, which is the average pressure in the arteries throughout the cardiac cycle, depends on the elastic properties of the arterial walls and the mean volume of blood in the arterial system. The main determinants of venous blood pressure are the volume of fluid within the veins and the compliance or distensibility of their vessel walls. Veins have much thinner walls than arteries and are more distensible than arteries. The venous system accommodates approximately 60 percent of the total blood volume at any given moment with a venous pressure averaging less than 10 mm Hg. Conversely, the arteries accommodate about 15 percent of the total blood volume with a pressure of about 100 mm Hg. Some important relationships are:

- Mean blood pressure equals cardiac output times peripheral resistance.

- Cardiac output equals heart rate times stroke volume.

- Peripheral resistance equals blood viscosity times vessel length divided by vessel radius raised to the fourth power.

- Blood pressure equals heart rate times stroke volume times viscosity times length divided by the radius to the fourth power. The higher the heart rate, stroke volume, blood viscosity, and vessel length and the less the vessel radius to the fourth power, the greater the blood pressure.

Objectives

After successful study of this chapter, the learner will be able to:

1. Distinguish between arteriosclerosis and atherosclerosis; describe the development of atheromatous plaque and its manifestations.
> Study text pages 1001-1004; refer to Figures 27-1 and 27-2 and Table 27-1.

Arteriosclerosis is a chronic disease of the arterial system characterized by abnormal thickening and hardening of the vessel walls. Smooth muscle cells and collagen fibers migrate into the tunica intima causing it to stiffen and thicken; this decreases the artery's ability to change lumen size.

Atherosclerosis is a form of arteriosclerosis in which the thickening of vessel walls is caused by hardening of soft deposits of intraarterial fat and fibrin that reduce lumen size. Atherosclerosis can take several forms depending on the anatomic vessel location, the individual's age, genetic and physiologic status, and the risk factors to which each individual may have been exposed. It is the leading contributor to coronary artery and cerebrovascular disease.

Lipid deposition is an early event in atherogenesis and occurs with excessive influx and deposition of cholesterol into the arterial wall. The lesions of atherosclerosis occur primarily within the tunica intima or the innermost layer. These lesions include the fatty streak, fibrous plaque, and the complicated lesion. The early **fatty streak** is a flat, yellow, lipid-filled smooth muscle cell that causes no obstruction of the affected vessel.

Fibrous plaque is the characteristic lesion of advancing atherosclerosis and consists of lipid-laden smooth muscle cells surrounded by collagen, elastic fibers, and a mucoprotein matrix. The lesion is elevated and protrudes into the lumen of the artery. The growing mass fixes to the inner wall of the tunica intima and may invade the muscular tunica media. Fibrous plaques likely develop from fatty streaks. The core of the fibrous plaque consists of lipids and debris from cellular necrosis caused by insufficient blood supply. If the lesion progresses sufficiently, it occludes the arterial lumen at arterial bifurcations, curves, or regions where the arteries taper.

Complicated lesions occur as the fibrous plaques are altered by hemorrhage, calcification, cellular necrosis, and blood clots throughout the intimal layer. As the altered complex structure becomes rigid, it causes extensive vascular occlusion.

Atherosclerotic lesions generally cause no symptoms until 60 percent or more of the tissue's arterial blood supply is occluded. If plaque formation occurs slowly, collateral arteries may develop to provide tissues with adequate blood supply. Atherosclerosis may have many different manifestations. High blood pressure develops if atherosclerosis elevates systemic vascular resistance. Cerebral or myocardial ischemia is a life-threatening manifestation of atherosclerosis that occurrs in the vessels of the brain or heart.

Dietary modifications are always the first treatment for atherosclerosis. Daily cholesterol intake must be reduced to 250 to 300 mg. Total blood cholesterol levels of less than 200 mg/dl, with low density lipoproteins (LDL) less than 130 mg/dl, are desirable. Drugs that decrease lipidemia are prescribed if serum lipoproteins are not reduced by dietary modification or if lipid levels are dangerously elevated in an individual requiring a lengthy time for significant dietary change and weight reduction.

2. Distinguish between primary, secondary, complicated, and malignant hypertension.
> Study text pages 1004-1011; refer to Figures 27-3 through 27-5 and Tables 27-2 through 27-4.

Individuals are diagnosed as having hypertension when the average of two or more diastolic blood pressure measurements made on two or more consecutive clinical visits is 90 mm Hg or higher or when the average of systolic blood pressure measurements made on two or more consecutive visits is greater than 140 mm Hg.

Hypertension is caused by increases in cardiac output, total peripheral resistance, or both. Cardiac output is increased by any condition that increases heart rate or stroke volume; whereas peripheral resistance is increased by any factor that increases blood viscosity or reduces vessel diameter.

A specific cause for **primary hypertension**, which is also called essential or idiopathic hypertension, has not been identified; a combination of genetic and environmental factors likely is responsible for its development. Primary hypertension affects 92 to 95 percent of hypertensive individuals. Factors associated with primary hypertension include (1) family history of hypertension, (2) advancing age, (3) gender, male below age 50 and female above age 50, (4) black race, (5) high dietary sodium intake, (6) glucose intolerance, (7) cigarette smoking, (8) obesity, (9) heavy alcohol consumption, and (10) low dietary potassium, calcium, and magnesium intake.

Several hypotheses have been proposed to explain the onset of primary hypertension in individuals at risk. They include (1) increases in blood volume, (2) inappropriate autoregulation, (3) overstimulation of sympathetic neural fibers in the heart and vessels, (4) water and sodium retention by the kidneys, and (5) hormonal inhibition of sodium-potassium transport across cell walls in the kidneys and blood vessels. Which is the dominant hypothesis during pathogenesis of primary hypertension is uncertain.

The hemodynamic hypothesis of onset is closely related to all but the neural hypothesis. It attributes the onset of hypertension to fluid overload. According to this hypothesis, early primary hypertension consists of a series of cardiovascular adjustments to an increase in blood volume. First, cardiac output increases to handle the increased volume of blood circulating through the heart. As the systemic arteries sense the volume increase, their autoregulatory mechanisms try to slow things down by causing vasoconstriction. Because blood volume remains high, the increase in total peripheral resistance caused by the vasoconstriction leads to hypertension.

The autoregulatory hypothesis proposes that, although primary hypertension begins with increased cardiac output, it is maintained by an alteration of vascular autoregulation. The defect consists of the failure of autoregulatory mechanisms to return toward baseline following water and sodium excretion by the kidneys.

Another hypothesis about the onset of primary hypertension is that neurally stimulated vasoconstriction is the initiating event. Herein, the cardiovascular control centers in the brain overstimulate the sympathetic branch of the autonomic nervous system, which causes vasoconstriction. Because the sympathetic nervous system innervates both the heart and the vessels, sympathetic overstimulation increases cardiac output as well as peripheral resistance.

Sodium retention may initiate primary hypertension by an inherited defect of sodium excretion in the kidneys. The defect in renal sodium excretion is aggravated by dietary sodium intake of more than 50 mEq/day. Another mechanism of sodium retention is believed to be an interruption of the sodium-potassium pump. In individuals with this defect, a hormone is thought to inhibit sodium excretion from cells. This undiscovered humoral sodium-transport inhibitor would not only cause intracellular sodium to accumulate but also seems to cause increases of intracellular calcium. The presence of extra calcium in vascular smooth muscle cells increases vascular vasoconstriction and increases peripheral resistance.

Secondary hypertension is caused by any systemic disease process that raises peripheral vascular resistance or cardiac output. Fortunately, if the cause is identified and removed before permanent structural changes occur, blood pressure can return to normal.

Some Causes of Secondary Hypertension

Renal Vascular Disorders

Parenchymal disease such as acute and chronic glomerulonephritis, narrowing or stenosis of renal artery due to atherosclerosis or congenital abnormality

Endocrine Disorders

Cushing disease or syndrome increases secretion of glucocorticoids because of adrenal disease or pituitary dysfunction, primary aldosteronism may be caused by increased aldosterone secretion from an adrenal tumor, pheochromocytoma of the adrenal medulla causes increased secretion of adrenal catecholamines

Vascular Disease

Coarctation of the aorta, congenital constriction of aorta

Acute Stress

Releases epinephrine, norepinephrine, and glucocorticoids

Neurologic Disorders

Higher systemic blood pressure has to maintain perfusion

Complicated hypertension is sustained primary hypertension that causes pathologic effects in addition to hemodynamic alterations and fluid and electrolyte imbalances. Complicated hypertension compromises the structure and function of vessels, the heart, kidneys, eyes, and brain. Vascular complications include the formation, dissection, and rupture of aneurysms or outpouchings in vessel walls as well as gangrene resulting from vessel occlusion. Possible renal complications include parenchymal damage, renal arteriosclerosis, and renal insufficiency or failure. Cardiovascular complications include left ventricular hypertrophy, angina pectoris, congestive heart failure or left heart failure, coronary artery disease, myocardial infarction, and sudden death. Complications specific to the retina include retinal vascular sclerosis, exudation, and hemorrhage. Cerebrovascular complications are similar to those of other arterial beds and include transient ischemia, stroke, cerebral thrombosis, aneurysm, and hemorrhage.

Malignant hypertension is a rapidly progressive hypertension in which diastolic pressure is usually above 140 mm Hg. It can cause profound cerebral edema that disrupts cerebral function and causes loss of consciousness. High hydrostatic pressures in the capillaries cause vascular fluid to move into the interstitial space. If blood pressure is not reduced, cerebral edema and dysfunction increase until death occurs.

The early stages of hypertension have no clinical manifestations; thus, hypertension is called a silent disease. Some hypertensive individuals never have signs, symptoms, or complications; whereas others become very ill and their hypertension can cause death. Others have anatomic and physiologic damage caused by past hypertensive disease even if current blood pressure is within normal ranges. Most of the clinical manifestations of hypertensive disease are caused by complications that damage organs and tissues other than the vascular system. Besides elevated blood pressure, the signs and symptoms are specific for the organs or tissues affected. Heart disease, renal insufficiency, central nervous system dysfunction, impaired vision, impaired mobility, vascular occlusion, or edema can be caused by sustained hypertension.

Hypertension is usually managed with both pharmacologic and nonpharmacological methods. Treatment begins with reducing or eliminating risk factors. The usual dietary recommendations are to restrict sodium intake, to increase potassium intake, to restrict saturated fat intake, and to adjust caloric intake to maintain optimum weight. Physical training increases stroke volume which lowers heart rate and thus systolic blood pressure. Relaxation reduces levels of circulating catecholamines which reduce vascular tone and blood pressure. Discontinuance of cigarettes eliminates the vaso-constrictor effects of nicotine.

Four groups of drugs are used to manage hypertension. Diuretics reduce blood pressure by reducing blood volume and cardiac output. Angiotensin inhibitors reduce blood pressure by preventing the vasoconstrictive renin-angiotensin mechanism from acting upon the vascular smooth muscle. Vascular smooth muscle relaxants lower blood pressure by blocking calcium influx to smooth muscle cells; this promotes vasodilation. Adrenergic blockers prevent receptor binding with neurohumoral stimulators of increased cardiac output and vasoconstriction.

3. Define and identify the causes of orthostatic or postural hypotension.
Study text page 1011.

Orthostatic or **postural hypotension** is a drop in both systolic and diastolic arterial blood pressure on standing from a reclining position. The normal or compensatory vasoconstrictor response to standing is replaced by a marked vasodilation and blood pooling in the muscle vasculature and in the splanchnic and renal beds. Acute orthostatic hypotension may be the result of (1) anatomic variation, (2) altered body chemistry, (3) antihypertensive and antidepressant therapy, (4) prolonged immobility caused by illness, (5) starvation, (6) physical exhaustion, (7) fluid volume depletion, and (8) venous pooling.

Chronic orthostatic hypotension may be secondary to a specific disease. The diseases that may cause secondary orthostatic hypotension are adrenal insufficiency, diabetes mellitus, intracranial tumors, cerebral infarcts, and peripheral neuropathies.

4. Define aneurysm and list the types.
Study text pages 1011-1014; refer to Figures 27-5 through 27-8.

An **aneurysm** is a localized dilation or outpouching of a vessel wall or cardiac chamber. The tension on the wall increases as the vessel becomes thinner so the possibility of rupture increases. This is an example of the law of Laplace. The stretching produces infarct expansion, a weak and thin layer of necrotic muscle, and fibrous tissue that bulges with each systole. With time, the aneurysm can leak, cause pressure on surrounding organs, impair blood flow, or rupture. The aorta is particularly susceptible to aneurysm formation because of the constant stress on its vessel wall and the absence of penetrating vasa vasorum in its adventitial layer. Three-fourths of all aneurysms occur in the abdominal aorta.

True aneurysms are fusiform and circumfunctional in nature and involve all three layers of the arterial wall; there is weakening of the vessel wall.

False aneurysms or saccular aneurysms are usually the result of trauma. These aneurysms are caused by a break in the wall or a dissection of the layers of the arterial wall; blood is contained at the point of aneurysm by the adventitial layer. Treatment of aneurysms is nearly always surgical. Leaking cerebral aneurysms are treated with clot-stabilizing drugs and a number of clinical measures designed to reduce intracranial pressure and promote hemodynamic stability before surgical intervention.

5. Distinguish between a thrombus and an embolus.

Study text pages 1014-1916.

A **thrombus** is a blood clot that remains attached to a vessel wall. Thrombi tend to develop wherever intravascular conditions promote activation of the coagulation cascade. In the arteries, activation of the coagulation cascade is usually caused by roughening of the tunica intima by atherosclerosis. Infectious agents also roughen the normally smooth lining of the artery which causes platelets to adhere readily. Pooling of arterial blood within an aneurysm can stimulate thrombus formation. In the veins, thrombus formation is more often associated with inflammation. Thrombi also form on heart valves if there is inflammation of the endocardium or rheumatic heart disease.

A thrombus poses two threats to the circulation. First, the thrombus may be large enough to occlude the artery and cause ischemia in the tissue supplied by the artery. Alternatively, the thrombus may dislodge and travel through the vascular system until it occludes flow into a distal systemic or pulmonic vascular bed.

Pharmacologic treatment includes the administration of heparin and warfarin which interfere with the clotting cascade thereby slowing or stopping thrombus growth. Also, the intravenous or intraarterial administration of streptokinase can dissolve the thrombus.

Embolism is the obstruction of a vessel by an **embolus** or a bolus of matter that is circulating in the blood stream. The embolus may be a dislodged thrombus, an air bubble, or an aggregate of fat, bacteria, or cancer cells. An embolus travels in the bloodstream until it reaches a vessel through which it cannot pass; an embolus will eventually lodge in a systemic or pulmonary vessel. Pulmonary emboli originate mostly from the deep veins of the legs or in the heart. Systemic emboli most commonly originate in the left heart and are associated with thrombi after myocardial infarction, valvular disease, left heart failure, endocarditis, and dysrhythmias.

Pulmonary artery embolism from the right heart causes chest pain and dyspnea. The systemic emboli passing through the left heart have varied effects. Renal artery embolism causes abdominal pain and oliguria. Mesenteric artery embolism causes abdominal pain and a paralytic, ischemic bowel. Embolism of a coronary or cerebral artery is an immediate threat to life if the embolus severely obstructs these important major vessels. Occlusion of a coronary artery will cause a myocardial infarction; whereas occlusion of a cerebral artery will cause a stroke or CVA.

6. Distinguish between arterial and venous occlusive disease.

Study text pages 1016-1018; refer to Figure 27-9.

Thromboangiitis obliterans, or Buerger disease, tends to occur in young men who are heavy cigarette smokers. It is an inflammatory disease of the peripheral arteries. Inflammation, thrombus formation, and vasospasm can eventually occlude and obliterate portions of small and medium-sized arteries in the feet and sometimes in the hands. The pathogenesis of thromboangiitis obliterans is unknown.

The chief symptom of thromboangiitis obliterans is pain and tenderness of the affected part. Clinical manifestations are caused by sluggish blood flow and include rubor caused by dilated capillaries under the skin and cyanosis caused by blood that remains in the capillaries after its oxygen has diffused into the interstitium. The most important part of treatment is cessation of cigarette smoking. Vasodilators may alleviate vasospasm. If vasospasm persists, sympathectomy may be performed and gangrene necessitates amputation.

Raynaud phenomenon and **Raynaud disease** are characterized by attacks of vasospasm in the small arteries and arterioles of the fingers and, less commonly, the toes. Raynaud phenomenon is secondary to systemic diseases such as collagen vascular disease, pulmonary hypertension, thoracic outlet syndrome, myxedema trauma, serum sickness, or long-term exposure to environmental conditions like cold or vibrating machinery in the workplace. Raynaud disease is a primary vasospastic disorder of unknown origin tending to affect young women. It consists of vasospastic attacks triggered by brief exposure to cold or by emotional stress. Genetic predisposition may play a role in its development.

The vasospastic attacks of either disorder cause changes in skin color and sensation because of ischemia. Vasospasm occurs with varying frequency and severity and causes pallor, numbness, and the sensation of cold in the digits. Also, sluggish blood flow resulting from ischemia may cause the skin to appear cyanotic. Rubor follows as vasospasm ends and the capillaries become engorged with oxygenated blood.

Treatment for Raynaud phenomenon consists of removing the stimulus or treating the primary disease process. Treatment of Raynaud disease is limited to prevention or alleviation of vasospasm itself. Cold, emotional stress, and cigarette smoking are avoided. Exercises that build centrifugal force in the extremities are also helpful in the early stages of vasospasm for either entity.

A **varicose vein** is a vein in which blood has pooled. Varicose veins are distended, tortuous, and palpable. Varicose veins in the legs are caused by trauma to the saphenous veins that damages one or more valves or by venous distention from a combination of standing for long periods and the action of gravity on blood within the legs. If a valve is damaged and permits backflow, a section of the vein is subjected to the pressure exerted by a larger volume of blood under the influence of gravity. The vein swells as it becomes engorged and surrounding tissue becomes edematous because increased hydrostatic pressure pushes plasma through the stretched vessel wall.

Varicose veins and valvular incompetence can progress to **chronic venous insufficiency** (CVI). This condition is characterized by chronic pooling of blood in the veins of the lower extremities and leads to hyperpigmentation of the skin over the feet and ankles. Edema of the feet and ankles may progress proximally to the knees. Any trauma or pressure lowers the oxygen supply by further reducing blood flow into the area. Cell death occurs and necrotic tissue develops into **venous stasis ulcers**. Persistent ulceration develops because the high metabolic demands of healing tissue cannot be met by the existing compromised circulation.

Venous thrombi are more common than arterial thrombi because flow and pressure are lower in the veins than in the arteries. With aging, the deep veins in the lower extremities become especially susceptible to thrombus formation. This is notable in individuals with long-term bedrest or those wearing constrictive clothing. The inflammatory response triggered by the clotting cascade causes extreme tenderness, swelling, and redness in the area of thrombus formation. With venous occlusion, the skin is discolored rather than pale, edema is prominent, and pain is most marked at the site of occlusion. Treatment of varicose veins and chronic venous insufficiency begins with the individual wearing antiembolism stockings and avoiding standing and constrictive clothing. If conservative treatment is ineffective, saphenous vein stripping may be performed.

Superior vena cava syndrome (SVCS) is a progressive occlusion of the superior vena cava (SVC) that leads to venous distention in the upper extremities and head. The leading cause of SVCS is bronchogenic cancer, followed by lymphomas and metastasis of other cancers. The SVC is a relatively low-pressure vessel that lies in the closed thoracic compartment; therefore, tissue expansion within the thoracic compartment can easily compress the SVC.

Clinical manifestations of SVCS include edema and venous distension in the upper extremities and face including the ocular beds. Cerebral and central nervous system edema may cause headache, visual disturbance, or impaired consciousness. Respiratory distress may be present because of edema of the bronchial structures or compression of the bronchus by a carcinoma. SVCS is generally not a vascular emergency but rather is an oncologic problem. Treatment consists of radiotherapy for the neoplasm and the administration of diuretics, steroids, and anticoagulants.

7. **Characterize coronary artery disease; distinguish between myocardial ischemia and myocardial infarction and list complications of each.**

   Study text pages 1018-1031, refer to Figures 27-10 through 27-15 and Tables 27-5 through 27-7.

Coronary artery disease, myocardial ischemia, and **myocardial infarction** all impair the pumping ability of the heart by depriving the heart muscle of oxygen and nutrients. **Coronary artery disease** (CAD) diminishes the myocardial blood supply until deprivation impairs myocardial metabolism. The myocardial cells remain alive but are unable to function normally. Persistent ischemia or the complete occlusion of a coronary artery causes infarction or death of the deprived myocardial cells and tissues.

In the United States, coronary artery disease is responsible for nearly 50 percent of all deaths and one-third of deaths in persons between 35 and 65 years of age. The risk factors for CAD are classified as either modifiable or nonmodifiable. The nonmodifiable risk factors are variables that cannot be altered by persons wishing to decrease their risk of cardiovascular disease. These include advanced age, male gender until age 60, black or oriental race, genetic predisposition, and diabetes mellitus type I. The modifiable risk factors include hyperlipidemia, hypertension, cigarette smoking, diabetes mellitus type II, obesity, sedentary lifestyle, psychosocial stress, postmenopausal hormone therapy, and heavy alcohol consumption.

The most common cause of **myocardial ischemia** is atherosclerosis. The growing mass of plaque, platelets, fibrin, and cellular debris can eventually narrow the coronary artery lumen enough to impede blood flow. Platelet aggregations are known to release a prostaglandin which is a potent vasoconstrictor capable of causing spasm of the coronary arteries. This prostaglandin, thromboxane A_2, also promotes platelet aggregation so that a vicious positive feedback cycle of vasoconstriction and platelet buildup occur in the vessel walls.

Imbalances between blood supply and myocardial demand cause myocardial ischemia. Supply is reduced by increased resistance in coronary vessels, hypotension, decreased blood volume, valvular incompetence, or anemia. Demand is increased by high systolic blood pressure, increased ventricular volume, left ventricular hypertrophy, increased heart rate, and hyperviscosity of the blood. Ischemia occurs whenever demand exceeds supply.

Myocardial cells become ischemia within 10 seconds of coronary occlusion. After several minutes, the heart cells lose their ability to contract. Anaerobic processes take over and lactic acid accumulates. Cardiac cells remain viable for approximately 20 minutes under ischemic conditions. If blood flow is restored, aerobic metabolism resumes, and contractility is restored. If the coronary arteries cannot compensate for lack of oxygen, **myocardial infarction** occurs.

Myocardial Ischemia/Infarction

Angina Pectoris	Unstable Angina	Prinzmetal Angina	Infarction
Cause			
Temporary ischemia, exertion	Advanced ischemia, occurs at rest	Vasospasm, occurs at night and at rest	Irreversible ischemia, cellular necrosis with repair or scarring
Electrocardiography			
Normal, transient ST depression and T wave inversion	Normal, transient ST depression and T wave inversion	Transient ST elevation	Irreversible abnormal, pronounced Q waves
Plasma Enzyme Levels			
Negative	Negative	Negative	CPK-MB fraction, LDH, and SGOT or AST elevation
Pain Relief and Treatment			
Rest and nitroglycerin, beta blockers, calcium antagonists	Rest and nitroglycerin ineffective, beta blockers, calcium antagonists	Nitroglycerin, beta blockers, calcium antagonists	Narcotics, anticoagulant therapy, beta blockers

Note: The first symptom of myocardial ischemia or infarction is usually sudden, severe chest pain. The pain of infarction is more severe and persistent than the pain of ischemia; it may be heavy and crushing and radiating to neck, jaw, back, shoulder, or left arm.

The number and severity of postinfarction complications depend on the location and extent of necrosis, the individual's physiologic condition before the infarction, and the therapeutic intervention. **Dysrhythmias** or arrhythmias, which are disturbances of cardiac rhythm, are the most common complication of acute myocardial infarction and affect more than 90 percent of individuals. Sudden death resulting from cardiac arrest is often caused by dysrhythmias, particularly ventricular fibrillation. Acute myocardial infarction is usually accompanied by left ventricular failure characterized by pulmonary congestion, reduced myocardial contractility, and abnormal heart wall motion. Inflammation of the pericardium, or pericarditis, is a frequent complication of acute myocardial infarction. Dressler's postinfarction pericarditis syndrome is thought to be an antigen-antibody response to the necrotic myocardium. Pain, fever, friction rub, pleural effusion, and arthralgias may accompany this syndrome. Transient ischemic attacks or an outright cerebrovascular accident may result from thromboemboli that have broken loose from coronary arteries or cardiac valves to occlude cerebral vessels. Pulmonary emboli are especially common. Rupture of the wall of the infarcted ventricle may be a consequence of aneurysm formation because of decreased muscle mass at the infarcted site.

8. Characterize the terms associated with pericardial disease.

Study text pages 1032-1034; refer to Figures 27-16 through 27-18.

Pericardial disease is often a localized manifestation of another disorder. Infection, trauma or surgery, neoplasms, or metabolic, immunologic, or vascular disorders can elicit a pericardial response. Pericarditis, pericardial effusion, or constrictive pericarditis are the consequences of the response.

Acute pericarditis, although idiopathic, is commonly caused by infection, connective tissue disease, or radiation therapy. The pericardial membranes become inflamed and roughened and an exudate may develop. Symptoms include sudden onset of severe chest pain that worsens with respiratory movements. Individuals with acute pericarditis may also report dysphagia, restlessness, irritability, anxiety, weakness, and malaise. Friction rub or a short, scratchy, grating sensation similar to the sound of sandpaper may be heard at the cardiac apex and left sternal border and is pathognomonic for pericarditis. Treatment for uncomplicated acute pericarditis consists of relieving symptoms. Analgesics are given to relieve pain and salicylates and nonsteroidal anti-inflammatory drugs are used to reduce inflammation.

Pericardial effusion is the accumulation of fluid in the pericardial cavity and is possible with all forms of pericarditis. The fluid may be a transudate or an exudate. Pericardial effusion indicates an underlying disorder. If the fluid creates sufficient pressure to cause cardiac compression, it becomes a serious condition known as **tamponade**. The danger of tamponade is that pressure exerted by the pericardial fluid will eventually equal diastolic pressure within the heart chambers. The first structures to be affected by tamponade are the right atrium and ventricle as diastolic pressures are normally lowest. Subsequent decreased atrial filling leads to decreased ventricular filling, decreased stroke volume, and reduced cardiac output. Life-threatening circulatory collapse may develop.

The most significant clinical finding in tamponade is pulsus paradoxus. In this circumstance, arterial blood pressure during expiration exceeds arterial pressure during inspiration by more than 10 mm Hg. There is impairment of diastolic filling of the left ventricle plus reduction of blood volume within all cardiac chambers. Treatment of pericardial effusion or tamponade generally consists of aspiration of the excessive pericardial fluid. The fluid may be analyzed to identify the cause of the effusion so the underlying cause of tamponade may be corrected.

Constrictive pericarditis is either idiopathic or associated with radiation exposure, rheumatoid arthritis, uremia, or coronary artery bypass graft. In constrictive pericarditis, fibrous scarring with occasional calcification of the pericardium causes the visceral and parietal pericardial layers to adhere; thus, there is obliteration of the pericardial cavity. Like tamponade, constrictive pericarditis compresses the heart and eventually reduces cardiac output. Unlike tamponade, however, constrictive pericarditis always develops gradually.

Symptoms are exercise intolerance, dyspnea on exertion, fatigue, anorexia, weight loss, edema, distention of the jugular vein, and hepatic congestion. Chest x-ray films frequently show prominent pulmonary vessels and calcification of the pericardium. Initial treatment for constrictive pericarditis involves digitalis glycosides, diuretics, and sodium restriction. Surgical removal of the pericardium may be indicated since its removal does not compromise cardiac function.

9. Compare the cardiomyopathies.

Study text pages 1034-1038; refer to Figure 27-19 through 27-21 and Tables 28-8 and 28-9.

The **cardiomyopathies** are a diverse group of diseases that primarily affect the myocardium itself and are not secondary to the usual cardiovascular disorders such as coronary artery disease, hypertension, or valvular dysfunction. They may be secondary to infectious disease, exposure to toxins, systemic connective tissue disease, infiltrative and proliferative disorders, or nutritional deficiencies; most cases of cardiomyopathy are idiopathic.

Characteristics of Cardiomyopathies

	Dilated	*Hypertrophic*	*Restrictive*
Hemodynamic changes			
Cardiac output	Decreased	Normal	Normal or decreased
Stroke volume	Decreased	Normal or increased	Normal or decreased
Ventricular filling pressure	Increased	Normal or increased	Increased
Ejection fraction	Decreased	Increased	Decreased
Structural changes	Biventricular dilatation, chamber size increased, decreased mitral valve competence	Marked hypertrophy of left ventricle, occasionally of right ventricle, possible disproportionate hypertrophy of septum, chamber size normal or decreased, decreased mitral valve competence	Reduced ventricular compliance, infiltration of myocardium with amyloid or hemosiderin or glycogen deposits, chamber size decreased, decreased mitral valve competence

10. Identify the causes and manifestations of valvular dysfunction.

Study text pages 1038-1043; refer to Figures 27-22 through 27-25 and Table 27-10.

In **valvular stenosis**, the valve orifice is constricted or narrowed. This impedes the forward flow of blood and increases the workload of the cardiac chamber "in front" of or before the diseased valve. Increased volume and pressure cause the myocardium to work harder and myocardial hypertrophy develops.

In **valvular regurgitation**, known also as insufficiency or incompetence, the valve leaflets or cusps fail to close completely. This permits blood flow to continue even when the valve should be closed. During systole, some blood leaks back into the atrial "upstream" chamber. This increases the workload of both atrium and ventricle. Increased volume leads to chamber dilatation; increased workload leads to hypertrophy. Although all four heart valves may be affected, those of the left heart are more commonly affected than those of the right heart.

Valvular Stenosis and Regurgitation

	Cause	*Manifestation*
Aortic stenosis	Rheumatic heart disease, congenital malformation, calcification degeneration	Decreased stroke volume, left ventricular failure, dyspnea, angina, systolic murmur
Mitral stenosis	Acute rheumatic heart fever, bacterial endocarditis	Decreased stroke volume, right ventricular failure, chest pain, orthopnea, pulmonary hypertension, dysrhythmia, palpitations, induced thrombi, ascites, chest pain, diastolic murmurs
Aortic regurgitation	Bacterial endocarditis, hypertension, connective disease disorders	Congestive left heart failure, dyspnea, throbbing peripheral pulse, palpitations, chest pain, diastolic and systolic murmurs
Mitral regurgitation	Rheumatic heart disease, mitral valve prolapse, CAD, infective endocarditis, connective tissue disorders	Left heart failure, pulmonary hypertension, dyspnea, hemoptysis, palpitations, murmur throughout systole
Tricuspid regurgitation	Congenital, high blood pressure in pulmonary circulation or right ventricle	Right heart failure, peripheral edema, ascites, hepatomegaly, murmur throughout systole

11. Distinguish between rheumatic heart disease and infective endocarditis.

Study text pages 1043-1048; refer to Figures 27-26 and 27-27 and Table 27-11.

Rheumatic Heart Disease and Infective Endocarditis

Cause	Pathophysiology	Manifestations	Treatment
RHD Sequel to pharyngeal infection with group A beta-hemolytic streptococci, immune response to streptococcal cell membrane antigens	Carditis of all three layers of heart wall, endocardial inflammation and vegetative growth on valves, valvular stenosis, Aschoff bodies	Fever, lymphadenopathy, acute migratory polyarthritis, chorea, erythema marginatum or truncal rash, history of streptococcal pharyngeal infection, high anti-streptolysin O titer, ECG abnormalities	Oral penicillin or erythromycin, salicylates, surgical repair of damaged valves
Infective endocarditis Streptococci or staphylococci, viruses, fungi, rickettsiae	Prior endothelial damage to valves, mitral valve prolapse, prosthetic valves, septal defects, blood-borne microbial colonization to damaged valve, adhered microbes multiply and form endocardial vegetations	Fever, cardiac murmur, petechial lesions of skin and mucosa, positive blood cultures, ECG abnormalities	Long-term antimicrobial therapy - penicillin and streptomycin, prophylactic antibiotics for procedures increasing risk of transient bacteremia

12. Discuss altered contractility and ratio of oxygen supply and demand as mechanisms for heart failure.

Study text pages 1048-1055; refer to Figures 27-28 and 27-29.

According to the Frank-Starling law of the heart, contractility is optimal within a certain range of myocardial cell lengths; the more the myocardium is stretched, the harder it contracts. Normally, an increase of diastolic stretch results in a larger systolic ejection force and a larger stroke volume. Increases of preload increase myocardial oxygen consumption by requiring a greater force of contraction to accomplish systole. The increased force of cardiac contraction is accompanied by increased metabolic demand in the myocardium and more oxygen is required to support myocardial metabolism. Unfortunately, increased myocardial stretch decreases myocardial capillary perfusion by mechanically narrowing coronary capillary lumina. Also, if pre-load increases beyond the ventricle's ability to empty, the coronary artery blood supply will drop as the ejection fraction decreases. These two factors will cause the overworked and overstretched myocardium to become hypoxic. Afterload is the force or pressure against which a cardiac chamber must eject blood during systole. Increased afterload is associated with increased systemic vascular resistance or pulmonary vascular resistance such as occurs in systemic or pulmonary hypertension. To maintain cardiac output, the ventricles must eject the same amount of blood during the same amount of time into an area of higher resistance. Therefore, the ventricular myocardium must use greater force during ejection and consume more oxygen with each contraction. To maintain blood pressure, the ventricles must contract with more force to raise the ejection fraction. The ventricular myocardium will also require more oxygen as the force of contraction increases. The myocardial need for oxygen is affected by heart rate, force of contraction, and metabolic rate. Dysrhythmias alter filling times, preloads, afterloads, oxygen demand, and cardiac output. These abnormal heart rhythms contribute to heart failure as the demands are always in states of flux.

13. Characterize dysrhythmias of the heart.
    Study text page 1048; refer to Tables 27-12 and 27-13.

Dysrhythmias or arrhythmias can be caused by either an abnormal rate of impulse generation or an abnormal conduction of impulses. Dysrhythmias can impair the pumping of the heart and cause heart failure. One kind of dysrhythmia is a **heart block.** In AV node block, impulses are prevented from reaching the ventricular myocardium; the ventricles contract at a slower rate than normal.

Bradycardia is a slow heart rhythm below 50 beats per minute. Slight bradycardia is normal during sleep and in conditioned athletes. Abnormal bradycardia can result from improper autonomic nervous control of the heart or from a damaged SA node. Pacemakers can assist in blocks and bradycardia.

Tachycardia is a very rapid heart rhythm over 100 beats per minute. Tachycardia is normal during and after exercise and during the stress response. Abnormal tachycardia results with improper autonomic control mechanisms of the heart, blood loss or shock, the action of drugs and toxins, and fever.

Sinus arrhythmia is a variation in heart rate during breathing. Typically, the rate increases during inspiration and decreases during expiration. The causes of sinus arrhythmia are unknown. This phenomenon is common in young people and infrequently requires treatment.

Premature contractions or extrasystoles are contractions that occur before the next expected contraction. For example, premature atrial contractions may occur shortly after the ventricles contract. Premature contractions may occur with inadequate sleep, too much caffeine or nicotine, or alcoholism, or because of heart damage. Frequent premature contractions can lead to fibrillation during which cardiac muscle fibers contract out of sequence with each other. In fibrillation, the affected heart chambers do not effectively pump blood so tissue and organ perfusion is impaired. **Atrial fibrillation** occurs frequently in mitral stenosis, rheumatic heart disease, and infarction of the atrial myocardium. This condition can be treated with drugs such as digoxin or by defibrillation, which electrically shocks cardiac muscle fibers to contract in unison. **Ventricular fibrillation** is a life-threatening condition as the ventricle cannot fill or eject blood to vital tissues since contractions are so rapid. If fibrillation is not corrected immediately by defibrillation or some other method, death may occur within minutes.

14. Summarize the causes of heart failure.
    Study text pages 1056-1062.

Causes of Heart Failure

Impaired cardiac function	*Excessive demands*

Myocardial disease
    Coronary artery disease
    Myocardial infarction
    Myocarditis
    Cardiomyopathies
	Increased pressure
	    Systemic hypertension
	    Pulmonary hypertension

Valvular heart disease
    Stenotic valves
    Regurgitant valves
	Increased volume
	    Excessive intravenous fluid

Severe pericardial effusion
Pericarditis
Congenital heart defects
	Increased perfusion
	    Thyrotoxicosis
	    Anemia
	    Septicemia

15. Compare the pathophysiology, manifestations, and treatment of right and left side heart failure.

Study text pages 1056-1062; refer to Figures 27-31 through 27-36.

Right Heart Failure

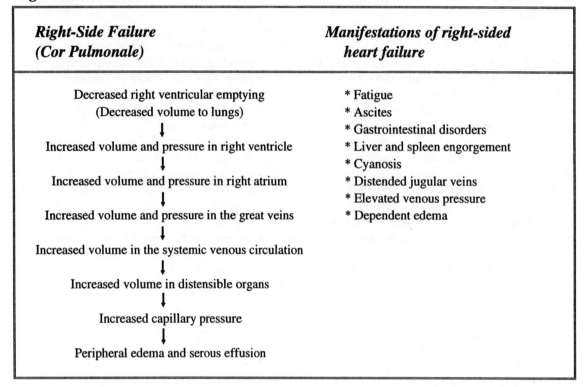

Right-Side Failure (Cor Pulmonale)	Manifestations of right-sided heart failure
Decreased right ventricular emptying (Decreased volume to lungs) ↓ Increased volume and pressure in right ventricle ↓ Increased volume and pressure in right atrium ↓ Increased volume and pressure in the great veins ↓ Increased volume in the systemic venous circulation ↓ Increased volume in distensible organs ↓ Increased capillary pressure ↓ Peripheral edema and serous effusion	* Fatigue * Ascites * Gastrointestinal disorders * Liver and spleen engorgement * Cyanosis * Distended jugular veins * Elevated venous pressure * Dependent edema

Note: Treatment for right heart failure begins with treatment of the underlying left heart failure or pulmonary disease. Diuretics and restricted water and sodium intake are used to reduce venous blood volume or preload. Myocardial contractility is enhanced with digoxin or other cardiotonic medications.

Left Heart Failure

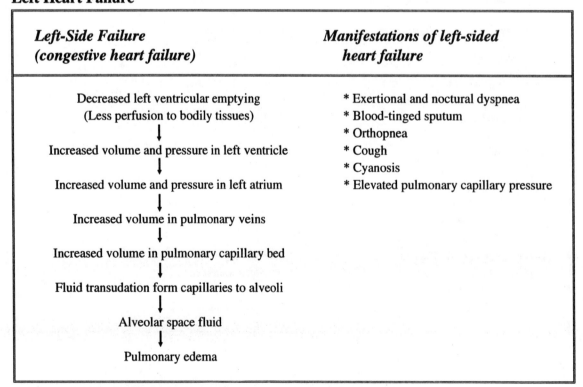

Left-Side Failure (congestive heart failure)	Manifestations of left-sided heart failure
Decreased left ventricular emptying (Less perfusion to bodily tissues) ↓ Increased volume and pressure in left ventricle ↓ Increased volume and pressure in left atrium ↓ Increased volume in pulmonary veins ↓ Increased volume in pulmonary capillary bed ↓ Fluid transudation form capillaries to alveoli ↓ Alveolar space fluid ↓ Pulmonary edema	* Exertional and noctural dyspnea * Blood-tinged sputum * Orthopnea * Cough * Cyanosis * Elevated pulmonary capillary pressure

Note: Treatment for left heart failure is to correct the underlying cause. Valvular dysfunction may require surgery. Vasodilators can improve coronary artery perfusion. The hypotension associated with left ventricular failure is usually treated with a cardiotonic antihypotensive. Oxygen is administered continuously to increase the supply of oxygen to the myocardium. Diuretics are given to decrease pulmonary edema and blood volume and sodium and fluid intake are restricted. Morphine sulfate dilates the pulmonary and systemic vessels, which decreases pulmonary and systemic capillary hydrostatic pressure. Also, morphine sulfate is an analgesic and an opiate, which improves the emotional state of the individual and may limit the cerebrally mediated release of epinephrine.

16. Classify the different types of shock by etiology.

Study text pages 1062-1069; refer to Figures 27-37 through 27-41.

Shock is a condition in which the cardiovascular system fails to perfuse the tissues adequately. This failure results in widespread impairment of cellular metabolism. Any factor that alters heart function, blood volume, or blood pressure can cause shock.

Ultimately, shock, irrespective of its cause, progresses to organ failure and death unless compensatory mechanisms or clinical intervention reverse the process. Shock causes many diverse signs and symptoms. The individual may feel sick, weak, cold, hot, nauseated, dizzy, confused, afraid, thirsty, and short of breath. Blood pressure, cardiac output, and urinary output are usually decreased. Respiratory rate is usually increased.

Types of Shock

Type	*Causes*
Cardiogenic (heart failure)	Myocardial ischemia, myocardial infarction, congestive heart failure, myocardial or pericardial infections, drug toxicity
Hypovolemic (insufficient intravascular fluid volume)	Loss of whole blood plasma or extracellular fluid, fluid sequestration
Neurogenic (neural alterations of vascular smooth muscle tone)	Loss of sympathetic motor tone to vascular smooth muscle with vasodilation
Anaphylactic (immunologic alterations)	Hypersensitivity leads to vasodilation and peripheral pooling
Septic (infectious processes)	Bacteremia, endotoxins, interleukins (IL), tumor necrosis factor (TNF), platelet-activity factor (TAF), and myocardial depressant substance (MDS) all promote the inflammatory process and vasodilation, reduced cardiac output and tissue perfusion, impaired cellular metabolism

17. Briefly diagram the common events found in all types of shock and relate the events to the signs and symptoms of shock.
   Refer to Figures 27-37 through 27-41.

Events, Signs, and Symptoms of Shock

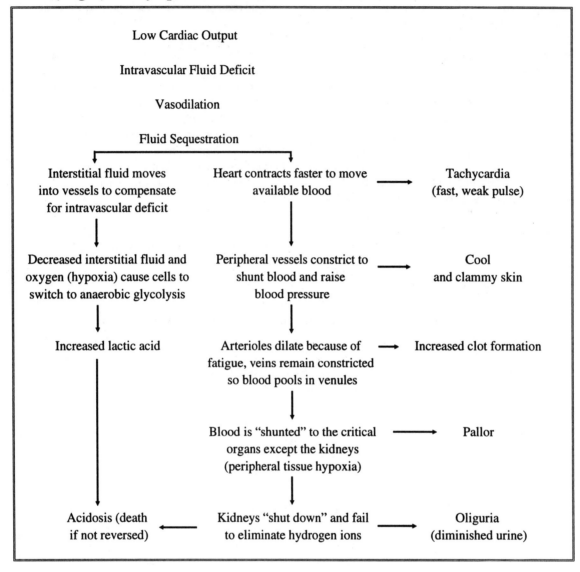

18. Illustrate the pathogenic sequence of multi-system organ failure in shock; identify organ/tissue abnormalities with their manifestations and characterize impaired cellular metabolism because of shock.

Study text pages 1069-1076; refer to Figures 27-42 and 27-43 and Table 27-15.

Pathogenesis of Multisystem Organ Failure

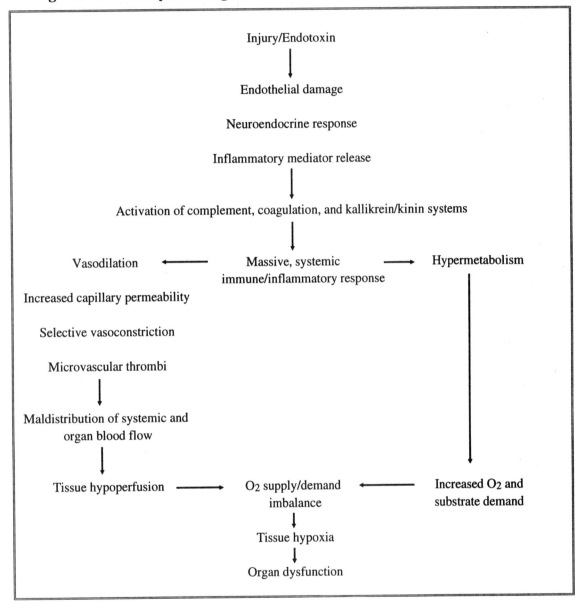

Injury/Endotoxin

Endothelial damage

Neuroendocrine response

Inflammatory mediator release

Activation of complement, coagulation, and kallikrein/kinin systems

Vasodilation ← Massive, systemic immune/inflammatory response → Hypermetabolism

Increased capillary permeability

Selective vasoconstriction

Microvascular thrombi

Maldistribution of systemic and organ blood flow

Tissue hypoperfusion → O₂ supply/demand imbalance ← Increased O₂ and substrate demand

Tissue hypoxia

Organ dysfunction

Organ Clinical Abnormalities Seen in Shock

Organ/Tissue	Symptoms and signs
Brain	Sleep abnormalities, confusion, stupor
Kidneys	Salt and water retention, azotemia, hyponatremia, impaired drug excretion, oliguria, edema, acidosis
Lungs	Dyspnea, orthopnea, pulmonary edema, tachypnea, rales, pleural effusions
Liver	Jaundice, abdominal distention, muscle wasting, bleeding, enlargement, tenderness, ascites
Skeletal muscle	Fatigue, tiredness, decreased aerobic capacity, acidosis, tachypnea
Skin	Cold, pale, cyanotic, perspiring extremities, impaired heat loss, dependent pitting edema
Gut	Ascites, poor absorption, anorexia, constant fullness, diarrhea, constipation, pancreatitis

Shock's Impairment of Cellular Metabolism

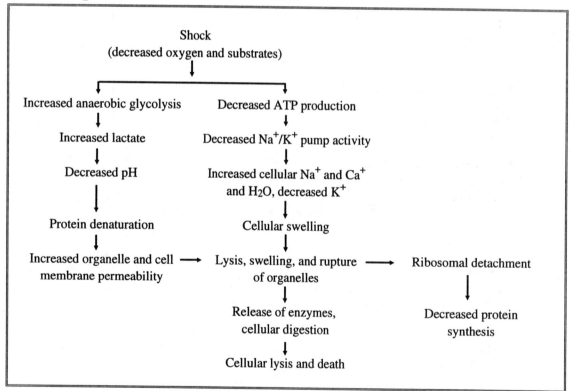

Practice Examination

1. Arteriosclerosis raises the systolic blood pressure by
   a. increasing arterial distensibility and vessel lumen radius or diameter.
   b. increasing arterial distensibility and decreasing vessel lumen radius or diameter.
   c. decreasing arterial distensibility and increasing vessel lumen radius or diameter.
   d. decreasing arterial distensibility and lumen diameter.
   e. None of the above is correct.

2. Events in the development of atherosclerotic plaque include all except
   a. accumulation of LDL (low-density lipoprotein).
   b. smooth muscle proliferation.
   c. calcification.
   d. decreased elasticity.
   e. complement activation.

3. G.P. is a 50-year-old male who was referred for evaluation of blood pressure. If he had a high diastolic blood pressure, which of the following readings belongs to G.P.?
   a. 140/82 mm Hg
   b. 160/72 mm Hg
   c. 130/95 mm Hg
   d. 95/68 mm Hg
   e. 140/72 mm Hg

4. The complications of uncontrolled hypertension include all except
   a. cerebrovascular accidents.
   b. anemia.
   c. renal injury.
   d. cardiac hypertrophy.
   e. All of the above are complications.

5. Primary hypertension
   a. is essentially idiopathic.
   b. can be caused by renal disease.
   c. can be caused by hormone imbalance.
   d. results from arterial coarctation.
   e. b, c, and d are correct.

6. Orthostatic hypotension is caused by all except
   a. increased age.
   b. increased blood volume.
   c. autonomic nervous system dysfunction.
   d. bed rest.
   e. severe varicose veins.

7. Localized outpouching of a vessel wall or heart chamber is a/an
   a. thrombus.
   b. embolus.
   c. thromboembolus.
   d. aneurysm.
   e. vegetation.

8. Which is a possible cause of varicose veins?
   a. gravitational forces on blood
   b. long periods of standing
   c. trauma to the saphenous veins
   d. Both b and c are correct.
   e. a, b, and c are correct.

9. A 76-year-old male came to the emergency room after experiencing chest pain while shoveling snow. Laboratory tests revealed essentially normal blood levels of SGOT or AST, CPK, and LDH enzymes. The chest pain was relieved following bedrest and nitroglycerin therapy. The most probable diagnosis is
   a. myocardial infarct.
   b. emphysema.
   c. angina pectoris.
   d. hepatic cirrhosis.
   e. acute pancreatitis.

10. Complications of an infarcted myocardium could likely include
   1. emphysema.   a. 1, 2, 3
   2. heart failure.   b. 2, 4, 5
   3. endocarditis.   c. 2, 3, 5
   4. death.   d. 1, 2, 4, 5
   5. shock.   e. 1, 3, 5

11. In pericardial effusion,
   a. fibrotic lesions obliterate the pericardial cavity.
   b. there is associated rheumatoid arthritis.
   c. tamponade compresses the right heart before affecting other structures.
   d. arterial blood pressure during expiration exceeds that during inspiration.
   e. Both c and d are correct.

12. Biventricular dilation is observed in _____ cardiomyopathy.
   a. congestive
   b. hypertrophic
   c. restrictive
   d. Both a and b are correct.
   e. a, b, and c are correct.

Match the valvular dysfunction with its appropriate characteristic.

13. aortic stenosis   a. right ventricular hypertrophy
14. tricuspid regurgitation   b. left ventricular hypertrophy
15. mitral stenosis   c. right atrial hypertrophy
16. mitral regurgitation   d. left atrial hypertrophy
                                     e. left atrial/right ventricular hypertrophy
                                     f. right and left ventricular/left atrial hypertrophy
                                     g. hypertrophy of all chambers

17. Rheumatic heart disease
   1. is caused by staphylococcal infections.   a. 1, 4
   2. is caused by hypersensitivity/immunity to streptococci.   b. 2, 4
   3. damages the tricuspid valve most often.   c. 2, 3
   4. usually damages a mitral valve.   d. 1, 3
   5. usually causes tricuspid stenosis.

18. Which is not an expected finding in acute rheumatic fever?
   a. elevated ESR (erythrocyte sedimentation rate)
   b. elevated ASO titer (antistreptolysin O)
   c. leukopenia
   d. fever

19. Bacterial (or infective) endocarditis differs from rheumatic heart disease because bacterial endocarditis
   1. is an infection of the heart, endocardium, and valves.   a. 1, 2
   2. always follows rheumatic fever.   b. 1, 3
   3. may occur following dental or other surgical procedures.   c. 2, 3
   4. commonly involves the vena cava valve.   d. 2, 4
   5. is caused by a type III hypersensitivity.   e. 5

20. Patients with only left-sided heart failure would exhibit
    1. hepatomegaly.   a. 1, 3
    2. dyspnea.   b. 1, 3, 5
    3. ankle swelling.   c. 2, 4
    4. pulmonary edema.   d. 4
    5. peripheral edema.   e. 5

21. In congestive heart failure, the pump or myocardium itself fails because of
    1. loss of contractile force of the heart.   a. 1, 2
    2. hypertension.   b. 2, 3
    3. cardiac dysrhythmias.   c. 3, 4
    4. intermittent claudication from occlusive   d. 1, 2, 3, 4, 5
       vascular disease.   e. 1, 2, 3

22. Shock is a complex pathophysiological process involving all of the following events except
    a. decreased blood perfusion to kidneys.
    b. acidosis.
    c. rapid heart rate.
    d. hypertension.
    e. anaerobic glycolysis.

23. Septic shock is the result of
    a. anesthetics.
    b. toxins from bacteremia.
    c. massive loss of body fluid.
    d. emotional stress causing collapse of blood vessel tone.
    e. pump failure.

24. Select the incorrect statement concerning hypertension.
    a. Malignant hypertension is characterized by a diastolic pressure of over 140 mm Hg.
    b. Approximately 90 percent of cases are of the essential or primary type.
    c. Headache is the most reliable symptom.
    d. When left untreated, the major risks include CVAs and cardiac hypertrophy.

25. A 53-year-old male was admitted to the emergency room after experiencing shortness of breath, weakness, cardiac dysrhythmias, and chest pain which did not subside following nitroglycerine therapy. Laboratory tests revealed the patient had an elevated serum CPK and SGOT or AST level. EKG tracings revealed a prominent Q-wave and an elevated ST segment. The most probable diagnosis is
    a. a transient ischemic attack.
    b. an acute myocardial infarct.
    c. an attack of unstable angina pectoris.
    d. Prinzmetal angina.
    e. coronary artery vasospasm.

Case Study

W.S., a 51-year-old white male, was assisting in the launching of his best friend's water ski boat from a faulty boat trailer when he began to experience chest discomfort. At first, he believed his discomfort was because of the extreme July heat. Gradually, the discomfort became a crushing pain in his sternal area that radiated into his left arm and lower jaw. His friend suspected an ensuing heart attack and convinced W.S. to check into an emergency room. During the drive down a canyon with steep, winding curves, W.S. collapsed and became unconscious.

On arrival at the emergency room, W.S. was unconscious. His skin was cool, clammy, and very pale. His blood pressure was so low that it had to be palpated and his pulse was weak and irregular. Established resuscitation procedures were followed. After his return to consciousness, an electrocardiogram showed evidence of anterior myocardial injury and blood was drawn to check enzyme and electrolyte levels. When history could be obtained, W.S. stated he was a harassed advertising executive and denied significant illnesses.

However, he was being treated for essential or primary hypertension. He acknowledged smoking three packs of cigarettes a day for 30 years. His father died of a heart attack at the age of 47.

W.S.'s subsequent electrocardiograms and serum levels of CPK, LDH, and SGOT or AST verified myocardial infarction. Also, the area of infarction was in the anterior myocardium.

Knowing the diagnosis, identify W.S.'s risk factors, the early causes and precipitating events of his infarction, and the justification for using anticoagulant therapy.

Alterations of Cardiovascular Function in Children

Prerequisite Objectives

a. Describe the embryologic development of the cardiovascular system.
   Review text pages 1086-1087; refer to Figures 28-1 and 28-2.

Remember!

- The heart arises from the mesenchyme and begins its development as an enlarged blood vessel with a large lumen and muscular wall. The midsection of this tube begins to grow faster than its ends so the tube bulges and twists until both ends of the tube come together and fuse. The superior part of the tube is the truncus arteriosus, which divides longitudinally into the pulmonary artery and aorta. The lower part of the tube becomes the superior and inferior vena cavae. The development of the cardiac septa that eventually divides the four chambers is an intricate process. If development of the septa proceeds normally, the four-chambered heart will be present by the sixth or seventh week of gestation.

---

b. Describe the flow of blood through the fetal circulation.
   Review text pages 1087-1088; refer to Figure 28-3.

Remember!

- Blood for the fetus is oxygenated in the placenta and returns to the fetus through the umbilical vein. Part of this blood passes through the liver, but about half the flow is diverted from the liver through the ductus venosus, a connection between the hepatic vessels and the inferior vena cava, into the inferior vena cava. This blood flows into the heart and passes through the foramen ovale, an opening between the right and left atria, through the left ventricle, and into the aorta. From there it flows to the head and upper extremities. Blood returning from the upper body collects in the superior vena cava. A small portion of this blood flows into the right ventricle and out through the pulmonary artery. A small amount of this blood enters the lungs. The largest amount, however, flows through the ductus arteriosus, a connection between the pulmonary artery and the aorta, into the descending aorta, to the body, and then back to the placenta vein through the two umbilical arteries.

---

c. Describe the events involved in the change from fetal to independent circulation that takes place immediately after birth.

> Review text pages 1088-1089; refer to Figure 28-4.

Remember!

- After birth, systemic resistance rises and pulmonary resistance falls. Pulmonary vascular resistance drops suddenly at birth because the lungs expand and the pulmonary vessels dilate. It continues to decrease gradually over the first six to eight weeks after birth. Decreased resistance causes the right myocardium to thin. Systemic vascular resistance increases markedly at birth because severance of the umbilical cord removes the low resistance placenta from the systemic circulation. Increased systemic resistance causes the right myocardium to thicken. Changes in resistance cause the fetal connections between the pulmonary and systemic circulatory systems to disappear. The foramen ovale closes functionally at birth and anatomically several months later. The ductus arteriosus closes functionally 15 to 18 hours after birth and anatomically within 10 to 21 days. The ductus venosus closes within one week after birth.

Objectives

After successful study of this chapter, the learner will be able to:

1. Identify the most common congenital defects of ventricular outflow and describe their pathophysiology.

> Study text pages 1093-1096; refer to Figures 28-5 through 28-8 and Tables 28-2 through 28-4.

Pulmonary stenosis is caused by the restriction or thickening of the leaflets of the pulmonary valve. Outflow is restricted from the right ventricle resulting in increased afterload and, if severe, may cause right ventricular hypertrophy and dilation. If pressures are high enough, the foramen ovale may reopen resulting in a right-to-left shunt and cyanosis. Mild cases result in little or no symptomatology while severe cases may require surgical correction. As with all congenital defects, evaluation is by electrocardiogram (ECG), chest x-ray, angiography, or echocardiogram.

Coarctation of the aorta is caused by a narrowing of the aorta anywhere between the origin of the aortic arch and the abdominal bifurcation, although 98 percent occur in the aortic arch just below the left subclavian artery. This defect may be considered in terms of its proximity to the ductus arteriosus. **Postductal coarctation** consists of a narrowed aorta distal to the ductus arteriosus. With complete closure of the ductus after birth, blood may no longer flow through this immature pathway, resulting in increased blood flow to the head and upper extremities and decreased blood flow to the lower extremities. In more severe cases, brachial pulses will be increased and femoral pulses will be decreased. A murmur will be present because of turbulent blood flow around the coarctation. In order to compensate, somewhat, for this process, small arteries may begin to branch off from the subclavian arteries and joint the intercostal arteries. These vessels give a "notched" appearance to the ribs on chest x-ray as they pass over them. In severe cases, cardiac failure may result. **Preductal coarctation** results if the aortic narrowing occurs proximal to the ductus arteriosus. A shunt is created between the aorta and pulmonary artery if the ductus remains open and pressures differ between systemic and pulmonary circulation. If systemic pressure is greater, blood will flow from the aorta to the pulmonary artery across the ductus arteriosus in a left-to-right direction. The reverse is true if pulmonary pressures are greater. As in postductal coarctation, congestive heart failure is a danger.

Evaluation includes ECG and cardiac imaging. Surgical correction includes resection of the affected site on the aorta with various grafts and closure of the ductus. High-flow oxygen is avoided prior to correction because the ductus responds to high oxygen concentration by constricting, thereby worsening the pathophysiology caused by the coarctation.

2. Describe the major acyanotic defects with increased pulmonary blood flow and describe their pathophysiology and treatment.

> Study text pages 1096-1100; refer to Figures 28-9 through 28-11 and Table 28-5.

Ventricular septal defect (VSD) is essentially a defect in the intraventricular septum leading to blood flow between the chambers of the heart. Small defects have very little associated pathology and often close on their own with the shunt usually flowing left-to-right. Large defects are a different matter. In a large VSD, pressures may become equal in both chambers with blood flow again being left-to-right due to higher systemic pressures. In this case, large amounts of blood flow into the lungs through the pulmonary artery and back to the left heart causing a great deal of left ventricular stress. Heart failure may eventually result. A related physiologic event is a constriction of the pulmonary blood vessels in an effort to limit pulmonary blood flow. If this process is too prolonged or severe, pulmonary pressures increase above systemic pressures and a right-to-left shunt results. This cyanotic event is known as **Eisenmenger syndrome** and is usually a fatal complication of VSD. Clinical presentation includes a holosystolic murmur, usually heard best at the left sternal border. In this instance, the louder the murmur, the smaller the defect. X-ray and ECG are usually normal unless left ventricular stress is present. Echocardiography illustrates flow across the defect. Treatment ranges from observation in mild cases to surgical correction in more serious cases.

Patent ductus arteriosus (PDA) results from the failure of the ductus arteriosus to close by 10 to 21 days of life. This process comprises approximately 10 percent of congenital heart defects and is of unknown etiology. Hemodynamic effects are dependent on the size of the ductus and are generally similar to VSD, as are the potential complications. Infants are usually asymptomatic at birth. Symptoms tend to present between two and six weeks of age as pulmonary and systemic pressures approach mature values causing a left-to-right shunt. Complications include congestive heart failure. Clinical manifestations include a "machinery" murmur, cardiomegaly, and accented pulmonary vascular marking on chest x-ray. Echocardiography demonstrates the abnormal blood flow. Treatment is usually by surgical ligation.

Atrial septal defects (ASDs) are abnormal communications across the interatrial septum that behave much like VSDs. The size of the ASD determines the direction of flow. If small, the shunt is left-to-right; if large, the pressures in the atria are equal and shunt direction is determined by resistance of the ventricles. At birth, atrial size and resistance are generally equal; but as the infant grows, the left ventricle thickens and systemic pressure rises causing a left-to-right shunt. These defects may be so mild that they go undetected until preschool age. A soft murmur is often heard at the second intercostal space and a fixed splitting of the second heart sound also may be heard. This finding is indicative of right ventricular overload. X-ray may demonstrate cardiomegaly and pulmonary vascular congestion. ECG may demonstrate ventricular stress. Echocardiography or cardiac catheterization will demonstrate the defect. Treatment is generally surgical correction.

3. Describe the major cyanotic cardiac defects with increased pulmonary blood flow.

Study text pages 1100-1105; refer to Figures 28-12 through 28-14 and Table 28-5.

Complete transposition of the great vessels results in the effective switching of the aorta and pulmonary arteries so that pulmonary circulation empties into the left heart and systemic circulation empties into the right heart. This creates two separate circulatory systems and is generally a fatal defect without rapid intervention. Infants born with transposition of the great vessels may survive for a time if they have an associated PDA or VSD which allows oxygenated and unoxygenated blood to mix. Infants with both defects usually become cyanotic within 24 hours of birth. Chest x-ray often shows a cardiac shadow that is somewhat eggshaped and also demonstrates vascular congestion. ECG is usually normal in a child who is not in failure. Echocardiography will demonstrate the lesion, and cardiac catheterization may be used to palliate the defect by enlarging the foramen ovale to permit more mixture of blood. Surgical repair is accomplished by special procedures.

Total anomalous pulmonary venous connection (TAPVC) is a disorder in which the pulmonary circulation enters the right atrium instead of the left. TAPVC has four different variations with the same resultant pathophysiology, all of which are associated with ASD. The most common forms of this anomaly are (1) drainage of the pulmonary veins into the superior vena cava and right atrium through the right anterior cardinal vein, (2) drainage into the right atrium through the coronary sinus through a remnant of the left anterior cardinal vein, (3) attachment of the four pulmonary veins directly into the right atrium, and (4) drainage into the right atrium through the common pulmonary vein through the portal system into the inferior vena cava and right atrium. Pulmonary venous obstruction is common in all forms of TAPVC but is most common in the fourth form. Pulmonary venous obstruction limits blood return to the heart and results in pulmonary engorgement and pulmonary edema. TAPVC in any form results in a mixture of oxygenated and unoxygenated blood being pumped to the systemic circulation. Because pulmonary venous obstruction causes continuation of high pulmonary vascular resistance, the shunt is usually right-to-left. The amount of cyanosis generated by this anomaly is dependent on the mixture of unoxygenated and oxygenated blood which is a phenomenon driven by pulmonary vascular resistance. Thus, the greater the pulmonary vascular resistance, the greater the cyanosis. Infants with this problem generally present cyanosis, tachypnea, and poor feeding. Congestive heart failure is a frequent complication. X-rays usually show a normal cardiac shadow and findings of pulmonary edema. Echocardiography demonstrates the anomalous blood flow, and cardiac catheterization reveals equally low oxygen saturations in all chambers of the heart and will indicate the amount of pulmonary hypertension. Most infants die by two months of age without surgical correction.

4. Describe tetralogy of Fallot or major cyanotic heart defect with decreased pulmonary blood flow.

Study text pages 1105-1107; refer to Figure 28-15.

Tetralogy of Fallot is a syndrome of four defects and is the most common cyanotic heart anomaly. It is frequently associated with Down syndrome, first trimester rubella, and Noonan syndrome. It accounts for 10 percent of all congenital heart defects and has a recurrence rate of 3 percent in affected families. The associated defects that comprise tetralogy are (1) a VSD that is usually large and placed high on the septum, (2) an overriding aorta that straddles the VSD, (3) pulmonary stenosis, and (4) right ventricular hypertrophy due to obstruction of blood flow from the right ventricle. The pathophysiology associated with tetralogy may be complex and is dependent on the degree of pulmonary stenosis as well as the size of the VSD and pulmonary and systemic pressures. Depending on these factors, the shunt may be either left-to-right or right-to-left. In any event, these defects result in hypoxemia in the systemic circulation while the body attempts to compensate by increasing red cell production and increasing blood flow to the lungs through collateral bronchial vessels. Pulmonary blood flow in the infant may remain adequate if the ductus arteriosus remains patent. In the event that the ductus closes, cyanosis usually occurs. Exertion or high environmental temperatures may exacerbate the problem. The "tetralogy spell" in older infants and children is often seen in the early morning or afternoon on exertion and with high temperatures. These episodes consist of cyanosis with the child assuming a characteristic "squat" position. Infants cannot squat but assume a knee-chest position. Episodes may also be accompanied by syncope or seizures due to hypoxia. Congestive heart failure is usually not a feature of this anomaly because blood can exit the right heart through the overriding aorta without a build-up of afterload.

The murmur of tetralogy is usually a systolic ejection murmur. Enlargement of the left chest because of an enlarged right ventricle and a "heave" may be noted. ECG demonstrates right ventricular stress, and a characteristic "boot-shaped" cardiac shadow is noted on x-ray. Pulmonary ventricular markings are decreased. Cardiac catheterization and echocardiography demonstrate the defect. Without surgical treatment, the life expectancy of most affected children is approximately 12 years. Surgical treatment is usually accomplished in two stages by various surgical shunting procedures.

5. Describe the etiology and pathophysiology of rheumatic heart disease.

Study text pages 1110-1111.

Rheumatic heart disease, accounting for nearly 40 percent of heart disease in the 1920s, dwindled to an incidence of approximately two cases per 1000 in the 1970s. Lately, however, it has made a dramatic comeback in various areas of the United States such as the Intermountain West, Texas, Ohio, and Hawaii. The initiating factor in rheumatic fever is infection with group A beta-hemolytic streptococcus, so it is not surprising that the usual age of onset of this disease is between five and 10 years of age. The most accepted hypothesis is that rheumatic fever is an autoimmune response which is triggered by a hypersensitive reaction to a toxin from the microbial organism. Rheumatic fever does not occur during the acute infection but follows some days later.

6. Describe the pathophysiology related to Kawasaki disease.

Study text pages 1111-1112.

Kawasaki disease is an acute, self-limiting vasculitis that may result in cardiac sequelae. Eighty percent of cases occur in children younger than five years of age; a peak incidence is in toddlerhood. Currently, it is the leading cause of pediatric acquired heart disorders in the United States. This disease tends to cluster in miniepidemics and may be related to an infectious process with an autoimmune component. The disease process progresses through four clinical stages:

Stage 1 - onset to 12 days: Small venules, arterioles, and the heart become inflamed.

Stage 2 - 12 to 25 days: Inflammation of larger vessels occurs and coronary artery aneurysms appear.

Stage 3 - 26 to 40 days: Medium-sized arteries begin granulation and inflammation subsides in the microcirculation.

Stage 4 - day 40 and beyond: The vessels develop scarring, thickening of the intima, calcification, and formation of thrombi; arteritis is most frequent in the coronaries but may occur in a variety of arteries; 10 to 20 percent of children develop aneurysms in this process.

Diagnosis is made by evaluating six major findings, five of which must be present for diagnosis. These findings include (1) fever greater than 104° F, (2) bilateral conjunctivitis, (3) erythema of the oral mucosa, (4) erythema with desquamation of the palms and soles, (5) polymorphous erythematous rash, and (6) cervical lymphadenopathy. These may be accompanied by arthritis and abdominal pain. Later complications include coronary thrombosis. Echocardiography may monitor the disease in the coronary arteries. Treatment is nonspecific and supportive.

Practice Examination

True/False

____ 1. Shunts are usually independent of systemic or pulmonary pressures and are due solely to defects within the heart.

____ 2. A patent ductus arteriosus or VSD is sometimes desirable when it is associated with other cardiac defects.

____ 3. VSD always requires surgical closure.

____ 4. In ASD or VSD, louder murmurs indicate smaller defects.

____ 5. Cyanosis is not a major finding in transposition of the great vessels due to the fact that the blood is free to travel normally to the lungs.

Fill-in-the-Blank

6. Abnormal blood flow within the heart is usually referred to as a _____.

7. In VSD, the shunt is generally _____-to-_____.

8. Cyanotic defects usually shunt _____-to-_____.

9. Cyanosis due to cardiac defects is usually due to mixture of _____ and _____ blood.

10. Some cardiac defects are not obvious at birth due to the fact that systemic and pulmonary pressures are nearly _____ at that point.

11. The ductus arteriosus responds to high oxygen concentrations by _____.

12. The ductus arteriosus should be totally closed by _____ of age.

13. Thickening or restriction of the valve from the right ventricle is known as _____.

14. Defects that obstruct outflow from the ventricles tend to cause increased _____ which may lead to

_____.

15. Narrowing of the great vessel leading to the systemic circulation is known as

_____.

Match the description with the alteration. More than one answer may apply.

16. associated with group A beta-hemolytic streptococci
17. likely associated with an infectious etiology and an autoimmune response
18. vasculitis associated with aneurysm
19. if mild, often self-correcting
20. knee-chest position with acute cyanosis and dyspnea
21. ASD, overriding aorta, pulmonary stenosis, right ventricular hypertrophy
22. death by 12 years of age without surgical correction
23. immediate cyanosis and distress after birth
24. two separate circulatory systems
25. may be associated with coronary thrombosis

a. Kawasaki disease
b. VSD
c. tetralogy of Fallot
d. transposition of the great vessels
e. rheumatic fever

Case Study

David M. is a 7-year-old boy requiring a routine physical examination at the nurse practitioner's office. David's past medical and family history is not unusual. His activity level is normal and his mother assumes that he is quite healthy.

David's physical examination is normal until the cardiovascular system is evaluated. Then, he is noted to have a systolic ejection murmur which is best heard at the base of the heart and radiates posteriorly. There are also bounding brachial pulses and severely decreased pulses in the lower extremities. The lungs are clear to auscultation. Chest x-ray is within normal limits as is the ECG. A pediatric cardiology consultation is requested.

What cardiac defect causes such a striking discrepancy in blood flow to the upper and lower extremities?

Structure and Function of the Pulmonary System

Objectives

After successful study of this chapter, the learner will be able to:

1. **Identify the sequence of structures of the pulmonary system as air moves into and out of the gas-exchange portions of the lungs; list the defense mechanisms of the pulmonary system.**
   Review text pages 1120-1127; refer to Figures 29-1 through 29-6 and Table 29-1.

2. **Describe lung volumes and capacities.**
   Review text page 1131; refer to Figure 29-12.

3. **Relate changes in the thoracic volume to contractions, alveolar surface tension, elastic properties of the lungs and chest wall, and conducting airway resistance.**
   Review text pages 1131-1135; refer to Figures 29-13 through 29-15.

4. **Describe the neural and chemical control of ventilation.**
   Review text pages 1135-1137; refer to Figure 29-16.

5. **Describe the alveolocapillary membrane and the diffusion of oxygen and carbon dioxide across it.**
   Review text pages 1126-1128; refer to Figures 29-8, 29-9, and 29-19.

6. **Identify the factors in the transport of oxygen to the cells of the body and describe oxyhemoglobin association and disassociation; identify the factors in the transport of carbon dioxide from the cells.**
   Refer to Figures 29-17, 29-18, and 29-20.

7. **Identify the normal values for arterial and venous blood gases and their significance.**
   Refer to Table 29-4.

8. **Note the pulmonary changes that occur with normal aging.**
   Review text page 1145.

Practice Examination

1. Considering the sequence of structures through which air enters the pulmonary system, the larynx is to the trachea as the
   a. bronchioles are to the segmental bronchi.
   b. alveoli are to the alveolar ducts.
   c. alveolar ducts are to respiratory bronchioles.
   d. respiratory bronchioles are to the alveolar ducts.
   e. All of the above are correct.

2. The cilia of the bronchial wall
   a. ingest bacteria.
   b. trigger the sneeze reflex.
   c. trap and remove bacteria.
   d. propel mucus and trapped bacteria toward the oropharynx.
   e. Both a and c are correct.

3. As the terminal bronchioles are approached distally,
   a. the epithelium becomes thicker.
   b. mucus-producing glands increase.
   c. ciliated cells become fewer.
   d. cartilaginous support increases.
   e. the smooth muscle layer thickens.

4. The left bronchus
   a. is shorter and wider than the right.
   b. is symmetrical to the right.
   c. has a course more vertical than the right's.
   d. is more angled than the right.
   e. has more bronchial wall layers.

5. The acinus has
   a. cilia.
   b. bronchiolar arteries and veins.
   c. goblet cells and alveoli.
   d. respiratory bronchioles and alveoli.
   e. All of the above are correct.

6. Alveoli are excellent gas exchange units because of
   a. their large surface area.
   b. a very thin epithelial layer.
   c. extensive vascularization.
   d. Both b and c are correct.
   e. a, b, and c are correct.

7. Surfactant
   a. facilitates O_2 exchange.
   b. produces nutrients for the alveoli.
   c. permits air exchange between alveolar ducts.
   d. facilitates alveolar expansion during inspiration.
   e. All of the above are correct.

8. For gas at a constant temperature, which relationship is true?
   a. As the volume decreases, the number of molecules of the gas increases.
   b. As the pressure increases, the number of molecules of the gas increases.
   c. As the volume decreases, the pressure increases.
   d. As the partial pressure increases, less gas will dissolve in a liquid.

9. When the diaphragm and external intercostal contract,
   a. the intrathoracic volume increases.
   b. the intrathoracic pressure increases.
   c. the intrathoracic volume decreases.
   d. None of the above is corect.

Match the following with the best description or example.

10. inspiratory reserve volume   a. amount of air remaining in lungs after a forced expiration
11. vital capacity   b. taking an extra deep breath of air just before diving
       c. includes sum of tidal, expiratory reserve, and inspiratory reserve volumes
       d. the extra air pushed out during a forced exhalation

12. Oxygen diffusion from the alveolus to the alveolar capillary occurs because
   a. the pO_2 is less in the capillary than in the alveolus.
   b. the pO_2 is greater in the atmosphere than in the arterial blood.
   c. oxygen diffuses faster than CO_2.
   d. the pO_2 is higher in the capillary than in the alveolus.

13. A shift to the right in the oxyhemoglobin dissociation curve
   a. prevents oxygen release at the cellular level.
   b. causes oxygen to bind tighter to hemoglobin.
   c. improves oxygen release at the cellular level.
   d. Both a and b are correct.
   e. None of the above is correct.

14. In which of the following sequences does pO_2 progressively decrease?
   a. blood in aorta, atmospheric air, body, and tissues
   b. body tissues, arterial blood, alveolar air
   c. body tissues, alveolar air, arterial blood
   d. atmospheric air, blood in aorta, body tissues

15. Most O_2 is carried in the blood _____; whereas most CO_2 is carried _____.
   a. dissolved in plasma / associated with salt or an acid
   b. bound to hemoglobin / associated with bicarbonate/carbonic acid
   c. combined with albumin / associated with carbonic acid and hemoglobin
   d. bound to hemoglobin / bound to albumin

16. Alveoli are well-suited for diffusion of respiratory gasses because
   a. they are small and thus have a small total surface area.
   b. vascularization is minimal, allowing greater air circulation.
   c. they contain four thick layers, preventing air leakage.
   d. they contain surfactant which helps prevent alveolar collapse.

17. Which of the following ordinarily brings about the greatest increase in the rate of respiration?
   a. hypercapnia (excess carbon dioxide)
   b. increased O_2
   c. increased arterial pH
   d. sudden rise in blood pressure

18. Given that the oxygen content of blood equals (1.34 ml of O_2 per gram of hemoglobin) times arterial oxygen saturation percent, if hemoglobin concentration is 15 gms/dL and arterial saturation is 98 percent, what is the arterial oxygen content?
   a. 13.2 ml/dL of blood
   b. 19.7 ml/dL of blood
   c. 14.7 ml/dL of blood
   d. None of the above is correct.

19. Giving an individual oxygen _____ the partial pressure of oxygen in his/her alveoli, so _____ oxygen will dissolve into the individual's blood.
   a. increases / less
   b. increases / more
   c. decreases / more
   d. decreases / less

20. The Hering-Brewer reflex
   a. involves stretch receptors.
   b. inhibits the inspiratory and apneustic areas.
   c. causes expiration.
   d. prevents lung overinflation.
   e. All of the above are correct.

21. Which of the following increases the respiratory rate?
   a. increased pCO_2, decreased arterial pressure, decreased pH, decreased pO_2
   b. increased pCO_2, decreased arterial pressure, increased pH, decreased pO_2
   c. decreased pCO_2, decreased arterial pressure, decreased pH, increased pO_2
   d. decreased pCO_2, decreased arterial pressure, decreased pH, decreased pO_2

22. The pneumotaxic center
   a. shortens inspiration.
   b. prolongs inspiration.
   c. facilitates expiration.
   d. None of the above is correct.
   e. Both a and c are correct.

Match the normal range of blood gases with its arterial or venous state.

23. pCO_2 of 35-45 mm Hg
24. oxygen saturation of 70-75%
25. oxygen content of blood of 19-20 ml/dl

a. arterial blood
b. mixed venous blood

CHAPTER 30

Alterations of Pulmonary Function

Prerequisite Objectives

a. Compare the structures of the lower airway as the generations of division move toward the alveoli.
   Refer to Figures 29-1 through 29-7.

> ## Remember!
>
> - The trachea and mainstem bronchi are composed mainly of cartilage with a lining of mucous membrane. When the bronchi enter the lungs, they branch further. Instead of cartilaginous rings, smooth muscle encircles the bronchi with cartilage interspersed among the muscle bundles. By the time the bronchioles are reached, supportive cartilage is no longer present. The bronchioles are capable of constriction because of their layer of smooth muscle. Smooth muscle becomes thinner in the terminal bronchioles. The epithelium changes from pseudostratified and ciliated columnar in the bronchi to nonciliated cuboidal in the terminal bronchiales and finally to squamous in alveoli. Macrophages must remove any debris that reaches the respiratory bronchioles and alveoli because of the absence of cilia.

b. Define the measurements of lung volume.
   Review text page 1131; refer to Figure 29-12.

> ## Remember!
>
> - Tidal volume (TV) is the amount of gas inspired and expired during normal breathing. Inspiratory reserve volume (IRV) is the amount of gas that can be inspired in additional to the tidal volume. Expiratory reserve volume (ERV) is the amount of gas that can be expired after a passive or relaxed expiration. Residual volume is the volume of gas that cannot be expired and is always present in the lungs.
>
> - Total lung capacity (TLC) is the total gas volume in the lung when the lung is maximally inflated. It is made up of RV, ERV, TV, and IRV. Vital capacity (VC) is the maximum amount of gas that can be expired from the lung. It includes IRV, TV, and ERV. Functional residual capacity (FRC) is the amount of gas remaining in the lung at the end of a passive expiration or RV and ERV. Inspiratory capacity (IC) is the amount of gas that can be inspired after a passive expiration from FRC. It includes TV and IRV. The lung capacities are always the sum of two or more volumes. Normal values for volumes and capacities are based on age, sex, and height.

(Continued)

- With each breath, a portion of the tidal volume remains in the conducting airways. This is the anatomical dead space. In certain disease conditions, some of the respiratory bronchioles and alveoli receive adequate ventilation but do not participate in gas exchange because they are not perfused by the pulmonary circulation. The volume of gas in unperfused alveoli is known as alveolar dead space.

c. Describe the diaphragmatic movement in inspiration and expiration; indicate other factors involved in the mechanism of breathing.

   Review text pages 1131-1135; refer to Figures 29-14 and 29-15.

Remember!

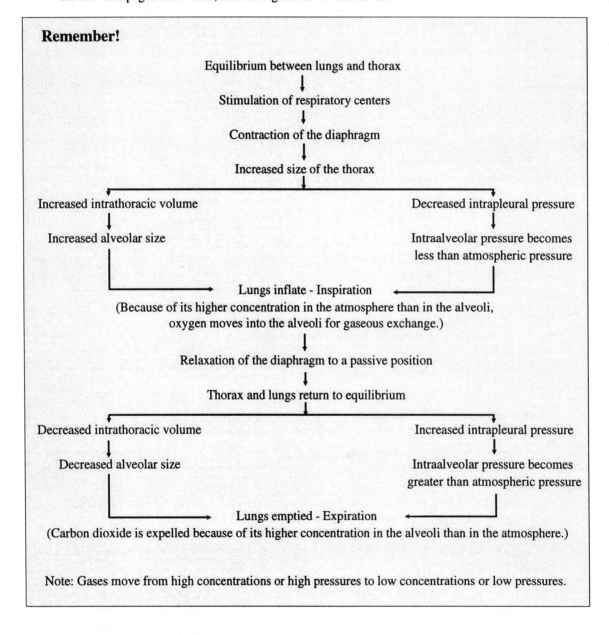

Equilibrium between lungs and thorax
↓
Stimulation of respiratory centers
↓
Contraction of the diaphragm
↓
Increased size of the thorax

Increased intrathoracic volume   Decreased intrapleural pressure
↓   ↓
Increased alveolar size   Intraalveolar pressure becomes
                                   less than atmospheric pressure

Lungs inflate - Inspiration
(Because of its higher concentration in the atmosphere than in the alveoli,
oxygen moves into the alveoli for gaseous exchange.)
↓
Relaxation of the diaphragm to a passive position
↓
Thorax and lungs return to equilibrium

Decreased intrathoracic volume   Increased intrapleural pressure
↓   ↓
Decreased alveolar size   Intraalveolar pressure becomes
                                   greater than atmospheric pressure

Lungs emptied - Expiration
(Carbon dioxide is expelled because of its higher concentration in the alveoli than in the atmosphere.)

Note: Gases move from high concentrations or high pressures to low concentrations or low pressures.

- Other factors involved in the mechanics of breathing include alveolar surface tension, elasticity of the lungs and chest wall, and resistance to air flow through the conducting airways. Surface tension occurs at any gas-liquid interface and is the tendency for liquid molecules exposed to air to adhere to one another. This phenomenon decreases the surface area exposed to the air. According to the law of Laplace, the pressure (P) required to inflate a sphere is equal to two times the surface tension (T) divided by the radius (r) of the sphere, or $P = 2T/r$. As the radius of the sphere or alveolus becomes smaller and the surface tension increases, more pressure is required to inflate it.

- Surfactant in the alveoli has a detergent-like effect that separates the liquid molecules, thus decreasing alveolar surface tension. Surfactant reverses the law of Laplace. The alveoli are much easier to inflate at low lung volumes after expiration than at high volumes after inspiration. The decrease in the surface tension caused by surfactant also is responsible for keeping the alveoli free of fluid. In the absence of surfactant, the surface tension tends to attract fluid into the alveoli.

- The lung and chest wall have elastic properties that permit expansion during inspiration and relaxation to original dimension during expiration. Elasticity can be expressed as the change in pressure divided by the change in volume, or $E = \Delta P/\Delta V$. During inspiration, the diaphragm and intercostal muscles contract, air flows into the lungs, and the chest wall expands. Muscular effort is needed to overcome the resistance of the lungs to expansion. During expiration, the muscles relax and the elastic recoil of the lungs causes the thorax to decrease in volume until balance between the chest wall and lung recoil forces is reached.

- Compliance is the measure of lung and chest wall distensibility. It represents the relative ease with which these structures can be stretched. Compliance is, therefore, the reciprocal of elasticity. Compliance is determined by alveolar surface tension and the elastic recoil of the lung and chest wall and can be expressed by the change in volume divided by change in pressure, or $C = \Delta V/\Delta P$. An increase in compliance indicates that the lungs and/or chest wall are abnormally easy to inflate and have lost some elastic recoil. A decrease indicates that the lungs and/or chest wall are abnormally stiff or difficult to inflate.

- Airway resistance is determined by the length, radius, and cross-sectional area of the airways and density, viscosity, and velocity of the gas. Resistance is computed by dividing change in pressure (P) by rate of flow (F), or $R = P/F$. Resistance is inversely proportional to the fourth power of the radius; thus, anything decreasing the radius of the airways increases airway resistance.

Objectives

After successful study of this chapter, the learner will be able to:

1. Define the terms used in describing the signs and symptoms of pulmonary disease.
Study text pages 1149-1152.

Dyspnea is the subjective sensation of uncomfortable breathing. It is often described as breathlessness, air hunger, shortness of breath, or labored breathing. Dyspnea occurs if increased airway resistance or decreased compliance cause respiratory effort greater than appropriate for the ventilation achieved. The signs of dyspnea include flaring of the nostrils, use of accessory muscles of respiration, and retraction of the intercostal spaces.

Orthopnea is experienced in the horizontal position. This position redistributes body water and causes the abdominal contents to exert pressure on the diaphragm, which decreases its efficiency of contraction and causes dyspnea.

Paroxysmal nocturnal dyspnea is seen in individuals with left ventricular failure who wake up at night gasping for air and have to sit up or stand to relieve the dyspnea. This dyspnea results from redistribution of body water into the lungs while the individual is recumbent.

Strenuous exercise or metabolic acidosis induces **Kussmaul respiration** or **hyperpnea.** Kussmaul respiration is characterized by a slightly increased ventilatory rate, effortless tidal volumes, and no expiratory pause.

Cheyne-Stokes respirations are characterized by alternating periods of deep and shallow breathing. Apnea, cessation of breathing lasting from 15 to 60 seconds, is followed by increased ventilation after which ventilation decreases again to apnea. Cheyne-Stokes respirations occur in any condition that slows the blood flow to the brain stem or slows impulses to the respiratory centers of the brain stem.

Hypoventilation is inadequate alveolar ventilation in relation to metabolic demands. It is caused by alterations in pulmonary mechanics or in the neurologic control of breathing. With hypoventilation, CO_2 removal does not keep up with production and CO_2 rises in the blood causing **hypercapnia.**

Hyperventilation is alveolar ventilation that exceeds metabolic demands. The lungs remove CO_2 at a faster rate than it is produced which results in **hypocapnia** or low levels of CO_2 in the blood**.**

Coughing is a protective reflex that cleanses the lower airways by an explosive expiration that removes inhaled particles, accumulated mucus, or foreign bodies. Stimulating the irritant receptors in the airway initiates the cough.

Hemoptysis is coughing up blood or bloody secretions. Hemoptysis indicates a localized infection or inflammation that has damaged the bronchi or the lung parenchyma.

Cyanosis is a bluish discoloration of the skin and mucous membranes caused by increasing amounts of desaturated or reduced hemoglobin in the blood. Cyanosis can result from decreased arterial oxygenation or decreased cardiac output.

Pain is caused by pulmonary disorders that originate in the pleurae, airways, or the chest wall. Infection and inflammation of the parietal pleura cause pain when the pleura stretches during inspiration. Pain that is pronounced after coughing occurs in individuals with infection and inflammation of the trachea and/or bronchi. Pain in the chest wall occurs with excessive coughing which makes the muscles sore.

Clubbing is the selective bulbous enlargement of the end of a finger or toe. Its pathogenesis is unknown but is associated with diseases that interfere with oxygenation.

An **abnormal sputum** is seen with different pulmonary disorders. A distinctive color or odor may indicate infection by a specific microorganism. Changes in the amount and consistency of sputum provide information about the progression of disease and the effectiveness of therapy.

2. Characterize lung conditions that are secondary to pulmonary disease or injury.
    Study text pages 1152-1162; refer to Figures 30-2 through 30-7 and Tables 30-1 and 30-2.

Conditions Caused by Pulmonary Disease or Injury

	Pathology	*Cause*
Hypoxemia	Reduced oxygenation of arterial blood	Decreased oxygen content of inspired gas, hypoventilation diffusion abnormalities in emphysema, abnormal ventilation/ perfusion ratios in bronchitis, right-to-left shunts in RDS or atelectasis
Pulmonary edema	Excess water in lungs	Heart disease increases pulmonary capillary hydrostatic pressure so fluid moves into interstitium, ARDS or inhalation of toxic gases injures capillaries and increases permeability, blockage of lymphatic vessels by CHF, edema, or tumors
Aspiration	Passage of fluid and solids into lungs, obstruction of airway, localized inflammation, noncompliance, edema, collapse	Decreased levels of consciousness, CNS abnormalities

(Continued)

Conditions Caused by Pulmonary Disease or Injury *(cont'd)*

	Pathology	*Cause*
Atelectasis	Collapse of lung tissue	External pressure from tumor or fluid or air in pleural space, abdominal distension, bronchi obstruction, inhalation of concentrated oxygen or anesthetics
Bronchiectasis	Persistent abnormal dilation of bronchi	Obstruction of airway, atelectasis, infection, cystic fibrosis, tuberculosis, weakness of bronchial wall
Bronchiolitis	Inflammatory obstruction of bronchioles	Chronic bronchitis, infection, inhalation of toxic gases
Pneumothorax	Air or gas in pleural space collapses the lung partially or totally	Rupture of pleura or chest wall
Pleural effusion	Fluid in the pleural space collapses the lung partially or totally	Fluid from blood or lymphatic vessels from CHF, hypoproteinemia, infections or malignancies cause mast cell release of capillary permeability mediators, trauma that damages blood vessels
Empyema	Pus in pleural space	Bacterial pneumonia
Pleurisy	Inflammation of the pleura, exudate of lymph, fibrin, and cells cause a friction rub	Respiratory infection
Abscess	Circumscribed area of suppuration of lung parenchyma	Aspiration pneumonia
Fibrosis	Fibrous or connective tissue in lung	Scar tissue following ARDS, tuberculosis, or inhalation of dust or asbestos
Chest wall restriction	Compromised ventilation	Grossly obese, lateral bending and rotation of spine, arthritis of spine, depression of the sternum, neuromuscular disease
Flail chest	Compromised ventilation	Fracture of ribs or sternum
Toxic gas exposure	Inflammation of airways, alveolar and capillary damage, pulmonary edema	Inhalation of smoke, ammonia, hydrogen chloride, sulfur dioxide, chlorine, phosgene, and nitrogen dioxide; prolonged levels of high concentrations of oxygen

(Continued)

Conditions Caused by Pulmonary Disease or Injury *(cont'd)*

	Pathology	*Cause*
Pneumoconiosis	Fibrous tissue or nodules in lungs	Silicosis - inhalation of silica, anthracosis- inhalation of coal dust, asbestosis - inhalation of asbestos
Allergic alveolitis	Lung inflammation or pneumonitis	Inhalation of allergens - grains, silage, bird droppings, feathers, cork dust, animal pelts, molds, mushroom compost

3. In a diagrammatic scheme, interrelate the pathogenic factors in adult respiratory distress syndrome.
   Study text pages 1162-1165; refer to Figure 30-8.

ARDS Pathophysiology

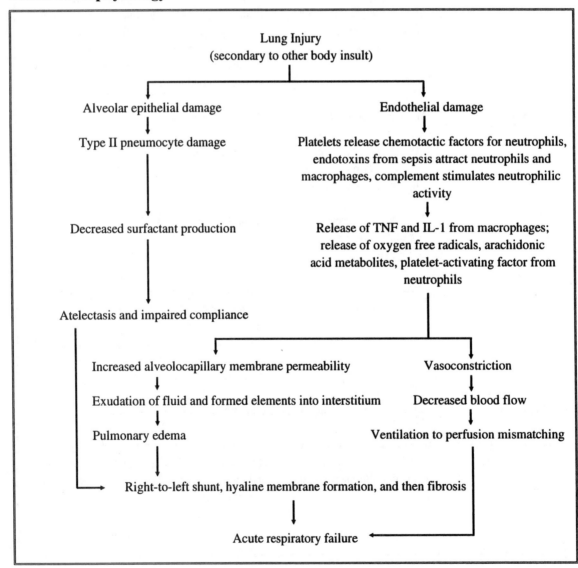

4. Compare and contrast the obstructive pulmonary diseases.

Study text pages 1165-1172; refer to Figures 30-9 through 30-14 and Table 30-3.

Obstructive pulmonary disease is characterized by difficult expiration. More force or the use of accessory muscles of expiration is required to expire a given volume of air. The most common obstructive diseases are asthma, chronic bronchitis, and emphysema. Since many individuals have both chronic bronchitis and emphysema, these diseases are grouped together and are called obstructive pulmonary disease (COPD). Asthma is more acute and intermittent than COPD but it also can be chronic.

Obstructive Pulmonary Diseases

	Asthma	*Emphysema*	*Chronic Bronchitis*
Cause of airway obstruction	Thick mucus, mucosal edema, smooth muscle spasm	Enlargement and destruction of alveoli, loss of elasticity, trapping of air	Inflammation and thickening of mucus membrane, ciliary impairment, accumulation of mucus and pus
Precipitating causes	**Extrinsic:** Environmental antigens or allergens, IgE-mast cell complex releases inflammatory mediators **Intrinsic:** Respiratory infections, drugs, air pollutants, cold and dry air, exercise and emotional stress (parasympathetic dominance causes bronchospasm)	Alpha -1- trypsin deficiency, cigarette smoke	Cigarette smoke, air pollutants, infections
Manifestations	Dyspnea, wheezing, nonproductive cough early but later mucoid, prolonged expiration, tachycardia, tachypnea	Marked dyspnea, no cough early but later, tachypnea with prolonged expiration, uses accessory muscles for ventilation, barrel chest, normal hematocrit, late cor pulmonale	Exercise intolerance, late dyspnea, wheezing, productive cough, marked hypoxemia leading to polycythemia and cyanosis, early cor pulmonale, CHF
Treatment	Anti-inflammatory agents, bronchodilators	Prophylactic antibiotics, relief of dyspnea, cautious oxygen administration	Bronchodilators, expectorants, postural drainage, percussion, anti-inflammatory agents

5. Define pneumonia and describe its causes, manifestations, and treatment.

Study text pages 1172-1174; refer to Figure 30-15.

Pneumonia is an acute infection of the lung caused by bacteria, bacteria-like microbes, or viruses. Resistant organisms, newly discovered organisms, and increasing numbers of immune compromised hosts have increased the etiological possibilities for pneumonia. The most common causal microbes are the following:

Gram-Positive Bacteria	*Gram-Negative Bacteria*	*Nonbacterial Organisms*
Streptococcus pneumoniae	*Escherichia coli*	*Pneumocystis carinii*
Staphylococcus aureus	*Pseudomonas aeruginosa*	*Mycoplasma pneumoniae*
Streptococcus pyogenes	*Klebsiella pneumoniae*	Fungi
	Proteus	Viruses
	Bacteroides species	
	Haemophilus species	
	Legionella species	

Fungi infrequently cause pneumonia but **fungal pneumonia** can be caused in immunosuppressed individuals by *Candida, Mucor,* and *Aspergillus.* The most common cause of community-acquired pneumonia is *Streptococcus pneumoniae. Mycoplasma pneumoniae* is the next most common cause of community-acquired pneumonia. *Staphylococcus aureus* and *Klebsiella pneumoniae* cause some community-acquired disease usually in individuals with other health problems such as COPD or alcoholism or those individuals with a primary viral illness. Viral pneumonia is usually caused by influenza viruses.

Most nosocomial or hospital-acquired pneumonias are caused by gram-negative bacteria such as *Escherichia coli, Klebsiella pneumoniae,* and *Pseudomonas aeruginosa.* When the gram-positive organism *Staphylococcus aureus* infects hospitalized individuals, it causes a more serious infection. These staphylococcal infections also are more likely to result in lung necrosis, abscesses, or empyema.

The Legionella species are widely distributed in water environments and are present in cooling systems, condensers, shower heads, and water reservoirs. Infections may occur in outbreaks or sporadically.

Pathogenic microorganisms can reach the lung by inspiration, by aspiration of oropharyngeal secretions, or via the circulation. This last source is usually by systemic infection, sepsis, or contaminated needles of intravenous drug users. The lungs' defense mechanisms, namely, the cough reflex, mucociliary clearance, and phagocytosis by alveolar macrophages, normally prevent infection by these pathogens. The body's immune system and various components of the inflammatory response further aid healthy individuals to prevent disease. In susceptible individuals, the invading pathogen is not contained. Instead, it multiplies and releases damaging toxins and stimulates full-scale inflammatory and immune responses. The immune response and the endotoxins released by some microorganisms damage bronchial mucous membranes and alveolocapillary membranes. Inflammation and edema cause the acinus and terminal bronchioles to fill with infectious debris and exudate; ventilation-perfusion abnormalities follow. If the pneumonia is caused by staphylococcus or gram-negative bacteria, necrosis of lung parenchyma may also occur.

Streptococcus pneumoniae organisms cause most **bacterial infections.** In this bacterial infection, the involved lobe undergoes consolidation or solidification of the tissue as it fills with exudate. A stage of red hepatization follows in which alveoli fill with blood cells, fibrin, edematous fluid, and pneumococci. This gives the lung tissue a red appearance. Next is a stage of gray hepatization in which affected tissues become gray because of fibrin deposition over the pleural surfaces and the presence of fibrin and leukocytes in the consolidated alveoli. Infection is usually limited to one or two lobes; thus the term lobar pneumonia is used.

Viral pneumonia is usually mild and self-limiting, but it can set the stage for a secondary bacterial infection by providing an ideal environment for bacterial growth and by damaging ciliated epithelial cells. Viral pneumonia can be a primary infection or a complication of another viral illness such as chickenpox or measles. Destroyed bronchial epithelium occurs throughout the respiratory tract; thus, a patchy or diffuse distribution is seen radiographically.

Most cases of pneumonia are preceded by an upper respiratory viral infection. Individuals then develop fever, chills, productive or dry cough, malaise, pleural pain, and sometimes dyspnea and hemoptysis. The white blood count is usually elevated, but it may be low if the individual is debilitated. Chest radiographs reveal infiltrates that may involve a single lobe of the lung or may be more diffuse. Purulent sputum is expectorated by individuals with bacterial pneumonia, while viral pneumonia and pneumonia caused by *Mycoplasma pneumoniae* characteristically show scant sputum production.

Antibiotics are used to treat bacterial and mycoplasmal pneumonia. Viral pneumonia is treated with supportive therapy unless secondary bacterial infection is present. Adequate hydration, deep breathing, coughing, chest physical therapy, etc., are important aspects of treatment for all types of pneumonia.

6. Describe the pathogenesis of tuberculosis.
Study text pages 1174-1175.

Tuberculosis is an infection caused by *Mycobacterium tuberculosis*, which is an acid-fast bacillus that usually affects the lungs but may invade other body systems. In the last decade, the number of reported tuberculosis cases has increased. A major reason for this trend is the epidemic of acquired immunodeficiency syndrome (AIDS). Individuals with AIDS are highly susceptible to respiratory infections including tuberculosis. A second important reason is the growing number of drug-resistant strains of tuberculosis bacillus that have developed because a large number of individuals do not consistently take their medications. This allows resistant strains to develop and spread. Emigration of infected individuals from high-prevalence countries, transmission in crowded institutional settings, substance abuse, and lack of access to medical care have also contributed to the growing problem.

Tuberculosis is transmitted from person to person in airborne droplets. Once the bacilli are inspired into the lung, they multiply and cause nonspecific lung inflammation. Some bacilli migrate through the lymphatics and become lodged in the lymph nodes where they encounter lymphocytes and initiate an immune response.

Neutrophils and alveolar macrophages wall off the colonies of bacilli and form a granulomatous lesion called a tubercle. Infected tissues within the tubercle die and form a cheeselike material; this is called **caseation necrosis**. Collagenous scar tissue then grows around the tubercle which prevents further multiplication of bacilli. Once the bacilli are isolated in tubercles and immunity develops, tuberculosis may remain dormant for life. However, if the immune system is impaired or if live bacilli escape into the bronchi, active disease occurs and may spread through the blood and lymphatics to other organs. Endogenous reactivation of dormant bacilli in the elderly may be caused by poor nutritional status, insulin-dependent diabetes, long-term corticosteroid therapy, and other debilitating diseases.

In many infected individuals, tuberculosis is asymptomatic. In others, symptoms develop so gradually that they are not noticed until the disease is well advanced. Common clinical manifestations include fatigue, weight loss, lethargy, loss of appetite, and a low-grade fever that usually occurs in the afternoon. A cough with purulent sputum develops slowly and becomes more frequent after weeks or months. "Night sweats" and general anxiety are often present. Notably, a positive tuberculin skin test indicates that an individual has been infected and has produced antibodies against the bacillus. By itself, the positive skin test does not indicate the presence of active disease. Nodules, calcifications, cavities, and hilar enlargement or enlarged mediastinal lymph nodes are commonly seen in the upper lobes on chest radiographs when active disease is present. The bacillus also can be cultured from the sputum.

Treatment consists of antibiotic therapy to control active or dormant tuberculosis and prevent transmission. Today, with the increased numbers of immunosuppressed and susceptible individuals and drug-resistant bacilli, the recommended treatment for those at high risk is a combination of four drugs: isoniazid, rifampin, pyrazinamide, and ethambutol. Treatment continues until sputum cultures show that the active bacilli have been eliminated. Such therapy may be required for several months.

7. Compare and contrast pulmonary embolism, pulmonary hypertension, and cor pulmonale.
Study text pages 1175-1179; refer to Figures 30-16 and 30-17.

Blood flow through the lungs can be disrupted by a number of disorders that occlude the vessels, increase pulmonary vascular resistance, or destroy the vascular bed. Major disruptive disorders include pulmonary embolism, pulmonary hypertension, and cor pulmonale.

	Embolism	*Hypertension*	*Cor Pulmonale*
Cause	Blood-borne substances from venous stasis, vessel injury or hypercoagulation lodge in a branch of pulmonary artery and obstruct blood flow	Pulmonary arterial pressure is elevated by increased left atrial pressure, pulmonary blood flow or vascular resistance that is secondary to lung disease	Right side heart failure because of primary pulmonary disease and long-standing pulmonary hypertension
Manifestations	Earlier evidence of deep vein thrombosis of legs or pelvis, tachypnea, dyspnea, chest pain, hypotension, shock, possible radiographic wedge shape bordering the pleura	Fatigue, chest discomfort, tachypnea, dyspnea with exercise, a radiograph or electrocardiogram that shows right ventricular hypertrphy	Chest pain, second heart sound or closure of pulmonic valve is accentuated, tricuspid valve murmur, radiograph and electro-cardiogram show right ventricular enlargement
Treatment	Avoid venous stasis, anti-coagulant therapy, fibrinolytic agent if life-threatening	Supplemental oxygen, digitalis, and diuretics are palliative while lung transplantation is therapeutic	Same as pulmonary hypertension

8. Describe the four major histologic types of lung cancer.

Study text pages 1180-1186; refer to Figures 30-20 through 30-22 and Tables 30-4 and 30-5.

Lung cancers or **bronchogenic carcinomas** arise from the epithelium of the respiratory tract. Lung cancer and malignant melanoma are the only major cancers whose incidence is rapidly increasing in the United States. The most common cause of lung cancer is cigarette smoking; heavy smokers have about 25 times greater chance of developing lung cancer than nonsmokers. Cigarette smoke contains several organ-specific carcinogens for organs or tissues other than lung tissue; smoking has been causally related to carcinogenesis of the larynx, oral cavity, esophagus, and urinary bladder.

Genetic predisposition to developing lung cancer also plays a role in lung cancer pathophysiology. DNA mutating agents in cigarettes produce alterations in both oncogenes and tumor-suppressor genes. Individuals with lung cancer demonstrate bronchial epithelial changes progressing from squamous cell alteration or metaplasia to carcinoma in situ. Thickening of the bronchial epithelium, mucous gland hypertrophy, and alveolar cell rupture occur more frequently in smokers than in nonsmokers. Cigarette smokers also have decreased alveolar macrophage function or phagocytosis which may increase the risk for pulmonary infections.

Characteristics of Lung Cancer

Type/ Frequency	Growth Rate	Metastasis	2-Year Prognosis	Manifestations/ Treatment
Adenocarcinoma (35%)	Moderate	Early	< 20%	Pleural effusion; surgical treatment
Squamous cell (30%)	Slow	Late	< 50%	Cough, sputum production, airway obstruction; surgical treatment
Small cell (oat cell) carcinoma (20-25%)	Very rapid	Very early and widespread	< 3-5%	Airway obstruction, excessive ACTH secretion with its signs and symptoms; chemotherapy and radiation to thorax and CNS
Large cell carcinoma (10-15%)	Rapid	Early and widespread	< 12%	Pain, pleural effusion, cough, sputum production, hemoptysis, airway obstruction; surgical treatment

Note: The current accepted system for the staging of lung cancer is the TNM classification. In this system, T denotes the extent of the primary tumor, N indicates the nodal involvement, and M describes the extent of metastasis.

Practice Examination

Match the pulmonary condition with the characteristic.

1. Kussmaul respiration
2. hemoptysis
3. cyanosis
4. Cheyne-Stokes respiration
5. plural space atelectasis
6. bronchiectasis
7. pneumoconiosis
8. flail chest
9. pneumothorax
10. abscess

a. inadequate alveolar ventilation
b. ventilation exceeding metabolic demand
c. coughing blood or bloody secretions
d. abnormal dilation of bronchi
e. fibrous tissue or nodules in lungs
f. fractured ribs or sternum
g. increased ventilatory rate, effortless tidal volume, and no expiratory pause
h. decreased arterial oxygenation
i. alveolar collapse
j. pleural space air
k. pleural space pus
l. apnea, increased ventilations, then apnea again
m. aspiration pneumonia

11. High altitudes may produce hypoxemia by
   a. right-to-left shunts.
   b. hypoventilation.
   c. decreased oxygen inspiration.
   d. diffusion abnormalities.
   e. All of the above are correct.

12. In ARDS, increased alveolocapillary membrane permeability is due to
    a. PAF.
    b. oxygen free radicals.
    c. TNF.
    d. Both a and c are correct.
    e. a, b, and c are correct.

13. Type II pneumocyte damage causes
    a. increased alveolocapillary permeability.
    b. chemotaxis for neutrophils.
    c. exudation of fluid from capillaries into interstitium.
    d. decreased surfactant production.
    e. All of the above are correct.

14. Pulmonary edema may be caused by abnormal
    a. capillary hydrostatic pressure.
    b. capillary oncotic pressure.
    c. capillary permeability.
    d. Both a and c are correct.
    e. a, b, and c are correct.

15. In bronchial asthma,
    a. bronchial muscles contract.
    b. bronchial muscles relax.
    c. mucous secretions decrease.
    d. imbalances within the CNS develop.

16. Intrinsic asthma is precipitated by
    1. IgE.   a. 1
    2. airborne pollens.   b. 2, 3
    3. animal danders.   c. 1, 2, 3
    4. emotional stress.   d. 4

17. In emphysema,
    a. there is increased area for gaseous exchange.
    b. there are prolonged inspirations.
    c. the bronchioles are primarily involved.
    d. there is increased diaphragm movement.
    e. None of the above is correct.

18. Chronic bronchitis
    1. is caused by lack of surfactant.   a. 1, 2, 3, 4
    2. is caused by air pollutants.   b. 1, 3, 4
    3. exhibits a productive cough.   c. 2, 3, 4
    4. causes collapsed alveoli.   d. 2, 3
                                             e. 1

19. Which is inconsistent with pneumonia?
    a. chest pain, cough, and rales
    b. only involves interstitial lung tissue
    c. may be caused by mycoplasmas
    d. can be lobar pneumonia or bronchopneumonia
    e. can be caused by inhaling vomitus

20. Tuberculosis
    1. is caused by an aerobic bacillus.
    2. may affect other organs.
    3. involves a type III hypersensitivity.
    4. antibodies may be detected by a skin test.

    a. 1, 2, 3, 4
    b. 1, 2, 4
    c. 1, 2
    d. 1
    e. 1, 3

21. Pulmonary emboli usually
    1. obstruct blood supply to lung parenchym.
    2. have origins from thrombi in the legs.
    3. occlude pulmonary vein branches.
    4. occlude pulmonary artery branches.

    a. 1
    b. 1, 2, 4
    c. 2, 3
    d. 2, 4

22. Pulmonary hypertension
    a. is seen in elevated left arterial pressure.
    b. involves deep vein thrombosis.
    c. shows right ventricular hypertrophy.
    d. Both a and c are correct.
    e. a, b, and c are correct.

23. Cor pulmonale
    a. occurs in response to long-standing pulmonary hypertension.
    b. is right heart failure.
    c. is manifested by altered tricuspid and pulmonic valve sounds.
    d. Both b and c are correct.
    e. a, b, and c are correct.

24. A lung cancer characterized by many anaplastic figures and the production of hormones is most likely
    a. squamous cell carcinoma.
    b. small cell carcinoma.
    c. large cell carcinoma.
    d. adenocarcinoma.
    e. bronchial adenoma.

25. The metastasis of lung squamous cell carcinoma is
    a. late.
    b. very early and widespread.
    c. early.
    d. early and widespread.
    e. never seen.

Case Study

Mr. S. is a retired 69-year-old county attorney who was on a buying trip with his wife for old, classic cars in the high, mountainous country of Colorado when he became extremely short of breath. His alarmed wife took him to a multispecialty medical clinic for evaluation.

On admission to the clinic, Mr. S. was restless and tachypneic, and breathing through pursed lips. His heart rate was 118 with respirations of 32 and a blood pressure of 144/84. His chest had an increased anteroposterior dimension and his accessory muscles were used for ventilation. While giving his past history, Mr. S. leaned forward with his arms extended and braced on his knees.

His past history revealed a habit of smoking two packages of cigarettes a day for 45 years. During the past few years, Mr. S. had noticed a cough each morning on arising. Recently, while working in his flower garden, he had to stop at times to catch his breath. Even while watching television, he had experienced dyspnea. Also, he indicated a weight loss over the last two months.

A chest radiograph was taken and pulmonary function tests were done. The chest radiograph revealed a flat, low diaphragm with lung hyperinflation but clear fields. Pulmonary function tests showed decreased tidal volume and vital capacity, increased total lung capacity, and prolonged forced expiratory volume.

Which pulmonary disease is exhibited by Mr. S.'s symptoms? Justify your answer.

CHAPTER 31

Alterations of Pulmonary Function in Children

Prerequisite Objectives

a. Identify the major differences between mature and immature pulmonary systems.
   Review text pages 1192-1193; refer to Figure 31-2.

Remember!

- Infants and young children have drastically fewer alveoli than adults, approximately 25 million at birth versus 300 million at eight years of age. These alveoli are much smaller and less complex than those of adults. Due to the relatively small number of alveoli and because the alveoli are functionally immature, infants and young children are at a significant disadvantage when attempting to compensate for processes that interfere with or stress the pulmonary system. The airways of children are shorter and much smaller in lumenal diameter that those of adults. Although the airway grows in length throughout infancy, lumenal diameter does not begin to increase until five years of age. The small-diameter airways produce increased resistance to airflow and are easily obstructed by inflammation, mucus plugging, and bronchospasm. Because of developmental immaturity, the airways and chest wall of the infant are much less rigid than the adult's. During inspiration, the chest wall and airways of the adult resist the negative intrathoracic pressure caused by contraction of the diaphragm and move outward and upward to aid the influx of inspired air. The flexible and compliant infant chest wall may actually flex inward and the airways collapse somewhat during times of respiratory stress, thus limiting respiratory effort. The intercostal muscles of the infant and young child are immature and incapable of the prolonged, heavy effort often required during times of stress. The infant also has a very limited ability to metabolically support such effort. It is possible for the infant and young child to become too fatigued to continue ventilatory effort during times of serious illness because of these limitations. Surfactant production begins at approximately week 24 of gestation and reaches adult levels at term. The premature infant, however, may not have attained adequate surfactant production by birth and will be unable to maintain alveolar surface tension. This leads to severe atelectasis and respiratory distress syndrome of the newborn. By virtue of their immature immune systems and lack of "immune memory," children have many more respiratory infections per year than adults. These infections, coupled with their anatomical respiratory disadvantages, put infants and young children at increased risk for serious respiratory complications due to illness.

b. Describe the structural and physiologic defense mechanisms of the pulmonary system.
   Refer to Table 29-1.

Objectives

After successful study of this chapter, the learner will be able to:

1. Identify two different forms of croup syndrome and differentiate between them by respective etiologies, anatomic involvement, and seriousness.

    Study text pages 1194-1196; refer to Figures 31-3 and 31-4 and Table 31-1.

Croup syndrome is a very generic term that refers to a number of primarily infectious processes of different etiologies affecting the structures of the upper airway. These vary from relatively benign to acutely life-threatening and are usually easily differentiated by matching the symptoms with the probable anatomic site involved.

Epiglottis is an acutely life-threatening emergency. The etiologic agent is usually the bacteria *Hemophilus influenzae* type B. Children aged two to seven years are affected, with the peak incidence at three and one-half years. The affected structures are the epiglottis and the very small glottic space.

Onset is rapid and often without an obvious antecedent illness. Respiratory distress tends to be severe and quickly progresses to respiratory arrest without appropriate intervention. The child will be quite restless and fearful because of air hunger and will generally have severe respiratory stridor and be unable to swallow, causing copious drooling. The child may assume a characteristic "sniffing" position in an instinctive effort to elongate the airway and relieve the obstruction. Symptoms are due to marked edema of the epiglottis secondary to infection. The swollen epiglottis (1) obstructs the esophagus that leads to dysphagia and (2) quickly begins to obstruct the airway, leading to stridor and distress. Total airway obstruction and arrest are imminently probable. The child should be left in whatever position they choose and no procedures should be attempted that might increase agitation. Oxygen may be "blown-by" the face while emergency medical attention is sought. Treatment consists of establishing an emergency airway by endotracheal or surgical means under controlled conditions if possible. Appropriate antibiotics are necessary to treat the underlying infection. No attempt should be made to examine the airway of a child who displays the symptom of epiglottis, as respiratory arrest may result due to laryngospasm.

Laryngotracheobronchitis is most commonly referred to as "croup" or "viral croup" and is generally a more common and benign form of croup syndrome than epiglottis. The etiologic agent is usually parainfluenza virus. The affected age range is usually six months to three years and recurrences are common. Laryngotracheobronchitis often presents in small epidemics during the fall and winter months. Onset is usually gradual.

Classic symptoms are generally preceded by two to three days of "cold" symptoms such as rhinorrhea and low-grade fever that progress to a high-pitched "brassy" or "seal-like" cough, muffled voice, and inspiratory stridor that is variable in intensity but often worse at night. Stridor is caused by turbulent air flow over inflamed vocal cords and trachea; the cough and muffled voice also are caused by laryngeal inflammation. Dysphagia generally is not a clinical manifestation. In some cases, the inflammation may become severe enough to cause respiratory distress marked by stridor, tachypnea, and costal retractions that interfere with oral fluid intake. Affected children often require hospitalization and treatment with intravenous fluid therapy, oxygen supplementation, air humidification or cool mist, and inhaled epinephrine to temporarily decrease airway edema.

2. Identify the most common forms of aspiration syndrome in infants and children and describe the pathophysiology.

    Study text pages 1196-1197.

Foreign body aspiration is common and frequently life-threatening in children. Seriousness depends on the size of the aspirated object, the age of the child and the airway size, and the anatomic area of obstruction. Offending objects are often toys or bits of food. Complete obstruction of the upper airway may lead to acute respiratory arrest. Aspirated foreign objects that reach the lower airways tend to act in a ball-valve manner. As the airways open during aspiration, air tends to pass around the object. When the airways contract elastically during expiration, the object tends to cause total obstruction with resultant air trapping distal to the point of obstruction. Complications include pneumonia, bronchiectasis, and lung abscesses if treatment is delayed.

Foreign substance aspiration, such as chemical or chemical fumes, frequently causes severe airway and lung inflammation. The inflammation may result in chemical pneumonia and respiratory distress. Treatment is usually supportive; prevention is the most effective intervention. Infants may aspirate amniotic fluid which may be contaminated with meconium or bacteria. Meconium, because of its viscosity, may cause ball-valve obstruction and irritation pneumonia. Aspirated bacteria may result in serious bacterial pneumonia. Prevention primarily consists of appropriate suctioning of the infant's upper airway on delivery of the head.

3. Describe the pathophysiologic processes of asthma and relate them to the concept of asthma as a chronic illness of inflammatory nature.

Study text pages 1197-1200; refer to Figure 31-6.

Asthma is a chronic illness of highly variable severity which tends to be punctuated with more or less frequent episodes of acute exacerbation. The pathophysiologic basis of asthma involves hyperresponsive lower airways responding in an exaggerated manner to various triggers. The triggers include allergens, exercise, cold air, viruses and other infectious agents, aerosolized irritants such as pollutants, and cigarette smoke. Responses include spasm of the respiratory smooth muscle that encircles the airways, edema of the airway mucosa, mucus plugging of the airways, and cellular infiltration into the airways. Asthma attacks may have two phases. The early base of the attack is caused by IgE mediation resulting from mast cell degranulation in response to the triggering factor. The late phase follows in six to eight hours and is caused by inflammatory mediators released from cells attracted to the airways. Clinical manifestations may include persistent cough, expiratory wheeze, and signs of respiratory distress. Timing and severity of acute exacerbations are highly variable. The most severe attacks require hospitalization and even mechanical ventilation in severely affected children. Nearly half of affected children seem to outgrow asthma by adolescence. It is not unusual, however, to see classic asthmatic symptoms in an individual who has been symptom-free for years. It is believed that the tendency toward hyperresponsive airways is a lifelong problem.

4. Describe the most common etiologic agents in upper respiratory track infections and pneumonias in infants, children, and adolescents and differentiate them according to general manifestations.

Study text pages 1200-1201; refer to Table 31-2.

Children have approximately six to eight upper respiratory tract infections per year. The majority are viral and are generally well tolerated. **Pneumonia** in the first three months of life is most frequently caused by gram-negative bacteria acquired from the mother during the birth process. Viruses predominate in later infancy and early childhood, particularly respiratory syncytial virus and parainfluenza 3. Most bacterial pneumonias in this age group are due to *S. pneumoniae* followed by *Staphylococcus* and *H. influenzae*. *Mycoplasma pneumoniae* dominates in five- to 10-year-old children and continues into adolescence although the total incidence of pneumonia declines in this age group. The milder viral pneumonias tend to occur in infancy and early childhood and are characterized by an antecedent "cold" followed by cough, fever, tachypnea, and mild systemic symptoms. Respiratory syncytial virus pneumonia can, however, be a rapidly progressive, serious illness with fatal outcome. Bacterial pneumonias tend to have more dramatic systemic features and exhibit high fever, shaking, chills, restlessness, and malaise because they are more lobar in nature and require antibiotic therapy for resolution.

5. Identify the most common etiologic agent in bronchiolitis and describe the pathophysiology and the usual clinical course of the disease.

Study text pages 1202-1203.

The most common cause of **bronchiolitis** is respiratory syncytial virus. Viral infection causes necrosis of the bronchial epithelium and destruction of ciliated epithelial cells. The walls of the bronchi become edematous and plugged with mucus and cellular debris as lymphocytes infiltrate the bronchioles. Cell-mediated hypersensitivity to viral antigens leading to release of lymphokines causes further inflammation and destruction of the bronchiolar epithelium. The usual manifestation is an infant who has been exposed to family members with cold symptoms who develops mild cold symptoms. Over two to three days, these symptoms progress to coughing, expiratory wheeze, and signs of respiratory distress including tachypnea, costal retractions, nasal flaring, and even cyanosis. X-ray may demonstrate hyperinflation of the lungs caused by ball-valve mucus plugs in the bronchioles and flattening of the diaphragm. Infants may have decreased feeding due to respiratory distress. Although most infants improve over three to four days, many require much longer and hospitalization for oxygen therapy and air humidification with cool mist.

6. Describe the pathophysiologic processes involved in respiratory distress syndrome of the newborn.

Study text pages 1203-1205; refer to Figure 31-7.

Respiratory distress syndrome (RDS) of the newborn is a lack of adequate surfactant at birth to reduce alveolar surface tension. Although primarily a disease of preterm infants who have inadequate surfactant production, RDS can appear in term infants, particularly those with diabetic mothers or those who have undergone prenatal or birth insults such as asphyxia or shock. The small, underdeveloped alveoli of preterm infants require very high pressures to inflate. Absence of surfactant compounds this problem and each breath the infant takes requires as much pressure as the first. Widespread atelectasis occurs, causing respiratory distress and increased pulmonary vascular resistance. Increased pulmonary vascular resistance causes shunting of the blood away from the lungs and results in persistent fetal circulation which further compounds the problem of hypoxia and hypercapnia. Hypoxia and hypercapnia trigger vasoconstriction of the pulmonary vascular bed and exacerbate shunting. Capillary permeability increases, resulting in leakage of plasma proteins with clotting and fibrin formation. This process causes the classic **hyaline membrane** seen on histologic examination. Prolonged anaerobic metabolism produces lactic acid and subsequent metabolic acidosis. Treatment is supportive with mechanical ventilation the mainstay. Recently, exogenous surfactant administration has contributed significantly to the treatment of RDS.

Cystic fibrosis is an autosomal recessive, genetically transmitted, multisystem disease in which exocrine or mucus-producing glands secrete abnormally thick mucus that obstructs and eventually damages or destroys the function of affected organs. Thick secretions obstruct the bronchioles in the lung and predispose the child to recurrent or chronic infection. Chronic inflammation leads to destruction of the airway walls and hyperplasia of goblet cells. Bronchiectasis, pneumonia, and widespread pulmonary fibrosis follow. End-stage disease is characterized by cor pulmonale, chronic hypoxia, and pulmonary hypertension. Fortunately, the mean life expectancy is approaching 30 years of age for affected individuals. Treatment includes aggressive chest physiotherapy and the judicious use of antibiotics to control infection. Genetic testing is available to detect carriers. Sweat chloride testing remains the definitive test for the diagnosis of suspected cases.

7. **Describe the pulmonary pathophysiology associated with cystic fibrosis and identify general modes of diagnostic testing and therapy.**
    Study text pages 1206-1207.

Practice Examination

True/False

____ 1. Although the infant has several mechanical disadvantages because of an immature respiratory anatomy, this is well compensated for by the nearly limitless metabolic resources that allow for prolonged, strenuous effort.

____ 2. At birth, the infant has approximately 300 million small, immature alveoli that develop into 25 million fully mature alveoli by approximately eight years of age.

____ 3. Surfactant production begins at birth and accelerates as airway lumenal growth begins at approximately five years of age.

____ 4. Failure to produce surfactant at birth results in severe atelectasis and RDS.

____ 5. Cystic fibrosis is a disease process primarily due to hyperresponsive airways that are sensitive to certain environmental triggers.

____ 6. Bronchiolitis and asthma produce symptoms that are similar.

7. Epiglottis is characterized by
    a. gradual onset.
    b. severe stridor.
    c. drooling.
    d. All of the above are correct.
    e. Both b and c are correct.

8. Laryngotracheobronchitis is characterized by
    a. mild to moderate stridor, often worse at night.
    b. antecedent "cold" symptoms.
    c. a muffled voice.
    d. a "brassy" cough.
    e. All of the above are correct.

9. The most common cause of bronchiolitis is
    a. *H. influenzae*.
    b. exposure to allergens.
    c. parainfluenza virus.
    d. respiratory syncytial virus.

10. Factors related to upper respiratory infections in children include
    a. frequent exposure.
    b. lack of "immune memory."
    c. hyperresponsive airways.
    d. Both a and c are correct.
    e. Both a and b are correct.

11. Amniotic fluid aspiration in newborns is best avoided by
    a. cesarian section delivery.
    b. withholding feedings for two hours after birth.
    c. suctioning the infant's airways on delivery of the head.
    d. thoroughly suctioning the birth canal just prior to delivery.

12. Bronchiolitis peaks at approximately six months of age. This is unfortunate because the
    a. infant's airways are short and narrow at this age.
    b. infant has a relatively compliant chest wall at this age.
    c. infant has a very finite capacity to support prolonged respiratory effort.
    d. All of the above are correct.

13. The following statements about foreign body aspiration are true except
    a. it is a relatively common occurrence in childhood.
    b. the offending objects include food and toys.
    c. it is rarely accompanied by serious complications.
    d. it may cause pneumonias and lung abscess.
    e. Both b and c are correct.

14. Which statement is true concerning cystic fibrosis?
    a. It is a multisystem disease.
    b. Defect results in overproduction of viscous mucus.
    c. It is difficult to detect carriers through genetic testing.
    d. Infectious complications are frequent.
    e. a, b, and d are correct.

15. Which statement is true concerning asthma?
    a. Its triggers include allergy, viruses, and cold air.
    b. Once asymptomatic for a number of years, affected individuals may be assumed to be cured.
    c. It is characterized by hyperresponsive airways.
    d. Both a and c are correct.
    e. a, b, and c are correct.

16. Which statement is true concerning pneumonias?
    a. They are frequently due to viruses.
    b. They are frequently due to bacteria.
    c. Incidence decreases with advancing age toward adolescence.
    d. All of the above are correct.

Match the circumstance or cause with the alteration.

17. chronic condition
18. genetic predisposition
19. may result in persistent fetal circulation
20. may be an outcome of prematurity
21. acute life-threatening infection
22. parainfluenza virus
23. occurs six to eight times per year
24. occurs epidemically in fall and winter
25. inflammatory basis with hyperresponsive airways

a. asthma
b. cystic fibrosis
c. laryngotracheobronchitis
d. upper respiratory tract infections
e. epiglottis
f. respiratory distress syndrome

Case Study

Tyler C. is a two-month-old boy who saw his physician three days ago with a history of mild nasal congestion without fever, cough, vomiting, or other complaints. He was feeding about as well as usual and was felt to have a benign physical examination except for slight rhinorrhea. His parents stated, however, that they were just getting over "terrible winter colds" and hoped they had not given it to Tyler. Tyler was a term baby of an uncomplicated pregnancy and vaginal birth by a 21-year-old mother with no known health problems. He was sent home with his mother at 48 hours of age and has done well.

Tyler is back today because his mother is concerned that he is coughing severely, not feeding well at all, and "breathes funny." He still has no significant fever but is somewhat lethargic with a respiratory rate consistently high at approximately 90/minute with moderate intercostal retractions, nasal flaring, and light expiratory wheeze. A chest x-ray shows no specific areas of consolidation but does show hyperinflation and general "haziness." His oxygen saturation is only 86 percent, which is low, on room air, and he has lost three ounces in weight since last seen. He has not wet a diaper since last evening and has a dry mouth. Tyler is admitted to the hospital for further treatment.

What do Tyler's signs and symptoms suggest and what is pathophysiologically causing his signs? Why is hospitalization necessary?

Structure and Function of the Renal and Urologic Systems

Objectives

After successful study of this chapter, the learner will be able to:

1. **Describe or identify the organs of the urinary system and the gross anatomical features of the kidneys.**
   Review text page 1213; refer to Figures 32-1 and 32-2.

2. **Describe diagrammatically the microscopic structure of the nephron.**
   Review text pages 1213-1217; refer to Figures 32-3 through 32-7.

3. **Identify the determinants of renal blood flow.**
   Review text pages 1219-1221; refer to Figures 32-9 and 32-10.

4. **Describe the process of glomerular filtration.**
   Review text pages 1221-1224; refer to Figure 32-13 and Table 32-1.

5. **Describe the process of tubular reabsorption and tubular secretion.**
   Review text pages 1224-1226; refer to Figure 32-14 and Table 32-2.

6. **Differentiate the substances reabsorbed and secreted by different segments of the nephron tubules.**
   Refer to Figure 32-11.

7. **Describe the purposes of the countercurrent multiplier mechanism.**
   Review text pages 1226-1228; refer to Figure 32-15.

8. **Identify the effects of hormones activated or synthesized by the kidney.**
   Review text pages 1228-1229.

9. **Identify the changes that occur in renal function with advancing age.**
   Review text page 1232.

Practice Examination

1. Which sequence of structures does urine pass through as it leaves the body?
   1. ureter
   2. renal pelvis
   3. urinary bladder
   4. major calyx
   5. urethra
   6. minor calyx

   a. 2, 4, 6, 1, 3, 5
   b. 4, 2, 6, 1, 3, 5
   c. 6, 4, 2, 1, 3, 5
   d. 2, 6, 4, 5, 3, 1
   e. 6, 4, 2, 5, 3, 1

2. The functional unit of the human kidney is the
   a. nephron.
   b. collecting tubule (duct).
   c. major calyx.
   d. minor calyx.
   e. pyramid.

3. One feature of the renal blood circulation that makes it unique is that
   a. blood flows from arterioles into venules.
   b. blood flows from venules into arterioles.
   c. there is a double set of venules.
   d. there are two sets of capillaries.

4. Which has the opposite effect on urine production from the others?
   a. decreased solutes in blood
   b. decreased blood pressure
   c. increased ambient temperature
   d. dehydration
   e. reducing water consumption

5. The maintenance of a relatively high blood pressure in the glomerulus of the kidney is because
   a. the afferent arteriole arises from the arcuate artery.
   b. the efferent arteriole is larger than the interlobular artery.
   c. the glomerulus is constricted.
   d. the afferent arteriole is larger than the efferent arteriole.
   e. ADH from the anterior pituitary causes vasoconstriction of the renal arteries.

6. If the following hypothetical conditions exist in the nephron, what would be the net (effective) filtration pressure?

   glomerular blood hydrostatic = 80 mm Hg
   glomerular blood osmotic = 20 mm Hg
   capsular hydrostatic = 30 mm Hg

   a. 40 mm Hg
   b. 30 mm Hg
   c. 20 mm Hg
   d. 10 mm Hg

7. The capillaries of the glomerulus differ from other capillary networks in the body because they
   a. have a larger area of anastomosis.
   b. branch from and drain into arterioles.
   c. lack endothelium.
   d. force filtrate from the blood.

8. Which is not a function of the kidney?
   a. water volume control
   b. blood pressure control
   c. urine storage
   d. converts vitamin D to an active form

9. Potassium is secreted and reabsorbed respectively by the
   1. Bowman's capsule.
   2. proximal convoluted tubule.
   3. loop of Henle.
   4. distal convoluted tubule.
   5. collecting ducts.

   a. 1, 3
   b. 2, 4
   c. 3, 5
   d. 4, 2
   e. 5, 3

10. The primary receptors sensitive to the oncotic pressure of blood are found in the
    a. kidney's cortex.
    b. the kidney's medulla.
    c. hypothalamus.
    d. juxtaglomerular apparatus.

11. Water reabsorbed from the glomerular filtrate initially enters the
    a. afferent arterioles.
    b. efferent arterioles.
    c. Bowman's capsule.
    d. glomerulus.
    e. vasa recta.

12. Plasma contains a much greater concentration of _____ than the glomerular filtrate.
    a. sodium
    b. protein
    c. urea
    d. creatinine

13. An increase in water permeability of the distal convoluted tubules and collecting duct is due to
    a. a decrease in the production of ADH (anti-diuretic hormone).
    b. an increase in production of ADH.
    c. a decrease in blood plasma osmolality.
    d. an increase in water content within tubular cells.
    e. None of the above is correct.

14. The descending loop of the nephron allows
    a. sodium secretion.
    b. potassium secretion.
    c. hydrogen ion secretion.
    d. water reabsorption.

15. Which most accurately describes the pressures affecting net glomerular filtration?
    a. Blood osmotic opposes capsular hydrostatic and blood hydrostatic.
    b. Blood hydrostatic opposes capsular hydrostatic and blood oncotic.
    c. Capsular hydrostatic opposes blood osmotic and blood hydrostatic.
    d. None of the above is correct.

16. Tubular secretion is accomplished in
    a. the glomerulus.
    b. the urethra.
    c. the renal pelvis.
    d. the distal convoluted tubule.
    e. None of the above is correct.

17. Tubular reabsorption and tubular secretion differ in that
    a. secretion adds material to the filtrate; reabsorption removes materials from the filtrate.
    b. secretion is a passive process; reabsorption is an active transport process.
    c. reabsorption tends to increase urine volume; secretion tends to decrease urine volume.
    d. secretion adds materials to the blood; reabsorption removes materials from the blood.

18. The kidneys
    1. conserve H^+.
    2. conserve NH^+_4.
    3. eliminate H^+.
    4. eliminate NH^+_4.
    5. conserve HCO_3^-

    a. 2, 4
    b. 1, 3, 4
    c. 1, 3, 5
    d. 3, 4
    e. 3, 4, 5

19. If a small person excretes about 1 liter of urine during a 24-hour period, estimate the total amount of glomerular filtrate formed.
    a. 4 liters
    b. 10 liters
    c. 18 liters
    d. 100 liters

20. Which should not appear in the glomerular filtrate (in any significant quantity) just after the process of glomerular filtration has been accomplished?
    a. protein
    b. urea
    c. glucose
    d. Both a and b are correct.

21. Loop of Henle is to vasa recta as convoluted tubules are to the
    a. afferent arterioles.
    b. peritubular capillaries.
    c. efferent arterioles.
    d. renal arteries.

22. The two "currents" used in the counter current multiplier mechanism are the
    a. afferent and efferent arterioles.
    b. glomerulus and glomerular (Bowman's) capsule.
    c. ascending and descending limbs.
    d. proximal and distal tubules.
    e. All of the above are correct.

23. The counter current multiplier
    a. prevents water reabsorption from the collecting duct.
    b. concentrates sodium in the renal cortex.
    c. facilitates osmosis.
    d. concentrates chloride in the renal cortex.
    e. None of the above is correct.

24. As ambient temperature increases, what usually happens to the volume of urine production?
    a. no effect at all
    b. either more or less depending on other factors
    c. more urine output
    d. less urine output

25. A waste product of protein metabolism is
    a. pepsinogen.
    b. trypsin.
    c. amino acid.
    d. urea.
    e. urine.

CHAPTER 33

Alterations of Renal and Urinary Tract Function

Prerequisite Objectives

a. Define the renal processes of filtration, reabsorption, and secretion.
   Refer to Figure 32-12.

> **Remember!**
>
> - Glomerular filtration is the first step in urine formation in which permeable substances from the blood are filtered at the endothelial-capsular membrane and the filtrate enters the proximal convoluted tubule.
>
> - Tubular reabsorption retains substances needed by the body including water, glucose, sodium, potassium, and bicarbonate. This process removes materials from the filtrate and returns them to the blood.
>
> - Tubular secretion excretes chemicals not needed by the body including hydrogen and some amino acids, urea, creatinine, and some drugs. Secretion adds material to the filtrate from the blood.
>
> - In electrolyte movement between body fluids and cells, electrolyte neutrality must be maintained in both extracellular and intracellular compartments. It is necessary that the number of cations equal the number of anions present. This principle is particularly important in renal function.

b. Identify the forces and factors determining net filtration pressure; explain cause and effect of decreased filtration pressure.
   Review text pages 1219-1221.

> **Remember!**
>
> - Net filtration pressure is equal to glomerular blood hydrostatic pressure minus capsular hydrostatic pressure plus blood oncotic pressure. Stated mathematically, the formula is NFP = GBHP - (CHP + BOP). The pressure promoting filtration into Bowman's space is 47 mm Hg due to GBHP while the pressure resisting flow to Bowman's space is 35 mm Hg due to 10 mm Hg of pressure from Bowman's capsule HP and 25 mm Hg from BOP. This provides a small net
>
> *(Continued)*

Remember! *(cont'd)*

filtration pressure of 12 mm Hg. This net filtration pressure can be reduced by renal vasoconstriction, hypotension, hypovolemia, or low cardiac output. Any of these circumstances will reduce GFR. The GFR is directly related to renal blood flow (RBF) which is regulated by intrinsic neural and hormonal autoregulation. The blood flow is determined by arteriovenous pressure differences across the vascular bed divided by the vascular resistance or, stated mathematically, RBF = PA-PV/R. As pressure increases and resistance decreases, renal blood flow increases. Sympathetic nerve activity stimulates renal arteriolar vasoconstriction and decreases both RBF and GFR.

Effects of Renin-Angiotensin System

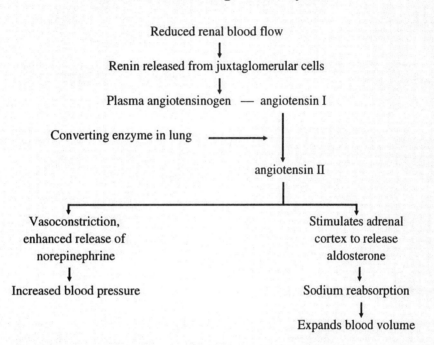

Reduced renal blood flow
↓
Renin released from juxtaglomerular cells
↓
Plasma angiotensinogen — angiotensin I

Converting enzyme in lung ⟶

angiotensin II

Vasoconstriction, enhanced release of norepinephrine
↓
Increased blood pressure

Stimulates adrenal cortex to release aldosterone
↓
Sodium reabsorption
↓
Expands blood volume

Note: The increase in circulating blood volume increases venous return and arterial pressure. The renin-angiotensin system impacts both the renal and cardiovascular systems.

c.   Explain the basis of serum and urinalysis examinations to evaluate renal function.
     Review text pages 1230-1232.

Remember!

Laboratory Tests for Kidney Function:

- **Blood urea nitrogen** (BUN) measures the concentration of urea in the blood. Urea is formed from protein metabolism and is elevated in reduced glomerular filtration. Normal BUN is 10-20 mg/dl. The BUN rises in states of dehydration and acute and chronic renal failure as passage of fluid through the tubules is slowed.

(Continued)

255

- The **serum creatinine level** should have a stable value because creatinine is a byproduct of muscle metabolism and its levels of production are constant and are proportional to muscle mass. Normally, it is not reabsorbed. If normal serum levels of 0.7 to 1.2 mg/dl exist, it indicates normal renal function. When creatinine rises and accumulates in the plasma, it represents decreasing GFR. If doubled, renal function is probably half of normal. If three times, about 75 percent of renal function is lost.

- **Creatinine clearance** is the amount of blood theoretically "cleared" of creatinine by the kidney in one minute of filtration; 90-130 ml/min is normal. Creatinine clearance provides a good measure of renal blood flow and GFR as serum levels are related to a 24-hour urine volume. Inulin, a substance with a stable plasma concentration, can be used to assess clearance. The amount of inulin filtered is equal to the volume of plasma filtered multiplied by the plasma concentration of inulin.

  Normally in 24 hours, the following may be observed as substances are filtered, reabsorbed, and secreted:

	Filtrate (enters glomerular capsule/day)	Reabsorbed (returned to blood/day)	Urine (excreted/day)
Glucose	180g	180g	0
Urea	53g	28g	25g
Creatinine	1.6g	0	1.6g

- The **urinalysis** is an essential part of the examination of all patients who may have renal disease since materials in the urine can be diagnostic for many disorders. It is normal to have inorganic material such as Na^+, Cl^-, Mg^{++}, SO_4^{--}, PO_4^{---}, NH_4^+ and organic materials such as urea, creatinine, and uric acid in the urine. It is abnormal to find RBCs, more than a few WBCs, bacteria, protein, glucose, or ketones in the urine.

Objectives

After successful study of this chapter, the learner will be able to:

1. Describe the characteristics of a patient suffering an acute renal calculi episode or ureteral stones.
   Study text pages 1237-1238; refer to Figures 33-1 and 33-2.

Calcium is a common constituent of renal stones; about 80 percent of **renal calculi** are composed of calcium oxalate, calcium phosphate, or a combination of both. Another stone, the struvite stone, which is composed of magnesium ammonium phosphate, is caused by the action of some urea-splitting bacteria. These stones, unlike the others, are seen more often in women and account for 10 to 15 percent of all stones. Uric acid stones, about 5 percent of stones, may be seen with gout. Rarely, cystine stones are seen in individuals with a genetic defect in transporting cystine.

A colicky pain occurs as the rhythmic contractions of the ureter attempt to dislodge and advance the sharp-edged stone. The accumulation of urine behind the stone causes distention and spasm of the ureter. The pain may be in the flank or between the last rib and the lumbar vertebrae, or it may radiate into the groin depending on the stone's location.

Treatment involves dilution of stone-forming substances by a high fluid intake, extraction of small stones by instrumentation, fragmentation of stones by ultrasonic lithotripsy, and laser treatment. Some smaller stones may pass spontaneously.

2. Characterize neurogenic bladder.
Study text pages 1238-1239; refer to Table 33-1.

Neurogenic bladder is a functional urinary tract obstruction caused by an interruption of the nerve supply to the bladder. The neurologic disruption can occur in the central nervous system or at the level of the spinal cord. Resulting bladder paralysis interferes with the normal flow of urine. Upper motor neuron lesions occur in the cortex or below the cortex but above the sacral level of the spinal cord and cause loss of voluntary control of voiding. Lower motor neuron lesions occur at the sacral level of the spinal cord and cause loss of both voluntary and involuntary control of urination.

3. Explain the development of acute urinary tract infections, the predisposing risk factors, and the most likely pathogens responsible for the infection.
Study text page 1242.

In these infections, predisposing factors are very important. Factors include fecal contamination of the urethra particularly in the female, sexual activity, catheterization or instrumentation of the urinary tract, urinary obstruction so the flushing effects of urination are reduced, and diaphragm spermatocidal usage.

The most common route in the development of acute urinary tract infection is by an ascending infection. Common pathogens in these infections are the gram-negative rods, namely *E. coli, Klebsiella, Proteus, and Pseudomonas*. Other possible infectious agents are gram-positive cocci, mycobacteria, and fungi.

4. Compare and contrast the signs, symptoms, and etiology of cystitis and pyelonephritis.
Study text pages 1242-1244; refer to Figure 33-5 and Table 33-4.

Cystitis and Pyelonephritis

	Cystitis (bladder) *Lower Tract Infection*	*Pyelonephritis (kidney tubules, pelvis, and interstitium)* *Upper Tract Infection*
Signs/Symptoms	Low abdominal, back pain, painful, burning urination, frequent voiding/urgency, hematuria, cloudy urine	Fever, chills, backache, abdominal pain, nausea, vomiting, urinary urgency and frequency, oliguria
Etiology	Urinary obstruction, prostatitis, ascending infection with gm negative rods ("honeymoon cystitis"), irritable bladder from sphincter dysfunction, interstitial cytosis caused by an inflammatory autoimmune response	Inflammation or scarring of the interstitial tissue and tubules, causative organism is usually an ascending gm negative rod but can be fungi or viruses; a risk factor is any urinary obstruction or condition that causes urine reflux or residual urine since bacteria are trapped, are able to ascend, or are not flushed

5. Describe the types of glomerulonephritis, its features, manifestations, and treatment.

Study text pages 1244-1251; refer to Figures 33-6 through 33-9 and Tables 33-5 through 33-7.

Common Types of Glomerulonephritis

Poststreptococcal Group A - beta hemolytic streptococci	Diffuse, subepithelial deposits of IgG and complement complexes, phagocytic infiltration, proliferation of mesangial and epithelial cells, occlusion of glomerular capillary blood flow, decreased glomerular filtration
Rapidly progressive or crescentic Nonspecific response to glomerular injury	Diffuse, accumulation of fibrin or macrophages or epithelial cell proliferation into Bowman's space form crescents and occlude glomerular filtration, antiglomerular basement membrane antibodies lead to necrotizing and proliferative tissue and renal failure
Membranoproliferative Usually idiopathic, associated with activation of complement pathways	Diffuse, mesangial cell proliferation, thickened basement membrane, subendothelial deposits of immune complex occlude glomerular capillary blood flow and decrease glomerular filtration
IgA Nephropathy Usually idiopathic	Focal, some diffuse lesions, mesangial cell proliferation with IgA deposits, release of inflammatory mediators with crescent formation, sclerosis, interstitial fibrosis, decreased GFR
Minimal change disease or lipoid nephrosis Usually idiopathic	Diffuse fusion of epithelial processes, loss of negative charge in basement membrane and increased permeability lead to severe proteinuria and nephrotic syndrome
Focal glomerulosclerosis Usually idiopathic	Similar pathology to minimal change disease with focal glomerulosclerosis from hyaline deposits in the glomerular membrane, proteinuria and nephrotic syndrome
Membranous nephropathy Usually idiopathic, can be associated with systemic disease	Diffuse thickening of glomerular basement membrane and capillary wall from deposits of antibody and complement, increased permeability with proteinuria and nephrotic syndrome

Glomerular damage generally occurs from activation of biochemical mediators of inflammation, namely complement, leukocytes, and fibrin. Damage begins after the antibody or antigen-antibody complexes have localized in the glomerular capillary wall. Complement is deposited with the antibodies. Complement activation attracts neutrophils and monocytes. The neutrophils and monocytes further the inflammatory reaction by releasing lysosomal enzymes which damage glomerular walls and increase glomerular capillary wall permeability. Membrane damage can lead to platelet aggregation and degranulation wherein platelets release vaso-active amines such as serotonin or histamine. Changes in membrane permeability permit the passage of protein molecules and red blood cells into the urine causing proteinuria and hematuria.

The coagulation system also may be activated and lead to fibrin deposition in Bowman's space. Membrane proliferation deposits in the membrane, mesangial proliferation, and swelling will reduce renal blood flow and depress glomerular filtration. Depending on the cause, extent, and degree of damage to the glomerulus, increased or decreased filtration results. Mild proteinuria and hematuria occur during the early years of the disease. Blood pressure may be normal. After 10 or 20 years, renal insufficiency will develop followed by nephrotic syndrome and an accelerated progression to end-stage renal failure.

The diagnosis of glomerular disease is confirmed by an urinalysis that shows proteinuria, red blood cells, white blood cells, and casts. In acute poststreptococcal glomerulonephritis, antistreptolysin-O (ASO) and antistreptokinase (ASK) are elevated and serum complement is decreased. Creatinine clearance evaluates the extent of glomerular damage.

The basic principles for treating glomerulonephritis are related to treating the primary disease, preventing or minimizing immune responses, and correcting accompanying problems such as edema, hypertension, and hyperlipidemia. Antibiotic therapy is essential for management of underlying infections. Dialysis or kidney transplantation ultimately may be necessary.

6. Identify and explain key features of nephrotic syndrome.
Study text pages 1251-1253; refer to Table 33-8.

In **nephrotic syndrome,** there is increased glomerular permeability and protein leakage. It is not a disease but a symptom complex that is the consequence of a variety of long-standing glomerular lesions. No immune complexes are found in nephrotic syndrome.

The key features of nephrotic syndrome include proteinuria, edema, hypoalbuminemia, hyperlipidemia, and lipiduria. Proteinuria occurs with protein leakage from the serum into the urine; this process reduces blood oncotic pressure. Thus, water leaves the capillaries more easily and tissue edema follows. The water is forced through the capillary walls by increased hydrostatic pressure as water moves from high concentration to low concentration and to dilute the interstitial solute. The edema is soft, pitting, and generalized. Hypoalbuminemia develops as albumin leaks through the capillaries and depletes its serum level. Hyperlipidemia occurs as the liver responds to the hypoalbuminemia by synthesizing replacement albumin. While synthesizing albumin, the liver also synthesizes lipoproteins in large amounts; therefore, hyperlipidemia develops. As tubular cells containing fat are sloughed into the urine, lipiduria can be seen. Also, free fat from the hyperlipidemia leaks across the glomerulus. Loss of protein immunoglobulins increases susceptibility to infection in nephrotic syndrome.

7. Define and identify the common etiologies for prerenal, intrarenal, and postrenal disease.
Study text pages 1253-1257; refer to Figure 33-10 and Tables 33-9 and 33-10.

Acute renal failure is the rapid deterioration of renal function with accompanying elevation of BUN and plasma creatinine; oliguria also develops. The etiology may be either prerenal because of renal hypoperfusion, intrarenal from renal functional impairment, or postrenal following obstruction of urinary flow.

Causes of Acute Renal Failure

Prerenal	Intrarenal	Postrenal
Hypovolemia	Prolonged renal ischemia	Urethral obstructions
Dehydration	Nephrotoxins	Edema, tumors,
Gastrointestinal	Glomerulonephritis	stones, clots
fluid loss	Intratubular obstructions	Bladder outlet obstruction
Hemorrhage	or necrosis	Prostatic hypoplasia,
		urethral structures
Hypotension		
Septic shock		
Shock		
Cardiac failure		
Pulmonary embolism		
Interruption of renal		
artery flow		

8. State the outcome of chronic renal failure.
    Study text pages 1257-1261; refer to Figure 33-11 and Table 33-11.

    Chronic renal failure symptoms and signs usually do not develop until GFR declines to 25 percent of normal. The chronic alteration is primarily because of loss of nephron mass. The clinical manifestations of chronic renal failure are described as **uremia**. The uremic state is characterized by a decline in renal function and the accumulation of toxins in the blood. If the lesions are tubular, electrolyte imbalances, volume depletions, and metabolic acidosis occur. In glomerular lesions, hematuria and nephrotic syndrome develop.

9. Identify the systemic manifestations of uremia.
    Refer to Table 33-12.

    Uremia is a toxic condition associated with widespread effects on all body systems.

Uremia

Musculoskeletal	*Cardiopulmonary*	*Neurologic*	*Hematologic*
Bone demineralization	Hypertension	Fatigue	Anemia
Soft tissue calcification	Pericarditis	Attention deficit	Bleeding
	Pulmonary edema	Irritability	Infection
	Pleuritis	Retinopathy	Suppressed immunity
		Depression	
		Stupor	
		Coma	

Metabolic	*Gastrointestinal*	*Integumentary*	*Reproductive*
Acidosis	Diarrhea	Pruritus	Infertility
Hyperuricemia	Nausea	Pigmentation	Decreased libido
Hyperglycemia	Vomiting	Decreased perspiration	Impotence
Hypothyroidism	Anorexia		Amenorrhea
Hyperparathyroidism	Urinous breath		

Note: If chronic renal failure cannot be managed with diet, diuretics, and fluid restriction, dialysis or transplantation becomes necessary.

Practice Examination

1. Renal function tests include
    a. the urinalysis.
    b. BUN and serum creatinine.
    c. SGOT/SGPT.
    d. Both a and b are correct.
    e. a, b, c are correct.

2. Which of the following substances is an abnormal constituent of urine?
    a. urea
    b. glucose
    c. sodium chloride
    d. creatinine

3. The presence of albumin in the urine would indicate probable damage to
   a. glomeruli.
   b. renal columns.
   c. collecting tubules.
   d. pyramids.
   e. None of the above is correct.

4. Which of the following is not true concerning urinary tract infections?
   a. Once cystitis develops, pyelonephritis will certainly occur.
   b. They are usually due to coliforms, especially *E. coli.*
   c. Organisms probably entered the bladder by way of the urethra.
   d. The patient may be asymptomatic.

5. Renal calculi may be composed of
   a. calcium oxalate.
   b. uric acid.
   c. cholesterol.
   d. All of the above are correct.
   e. Both a and b are correct.

6. Which of the following is characteristic of ureteral stones?
   a. severe pain in back
   b. severe pain in abdomen
   c. nausea and vomiting
   d. All of the above are correct.
   e. Both a and c are correct.

7. Predisposing factors for acute urinary tract infections are
   1. congenital deformities of urinary tract.   a. 1
   2. the sex of the patient.   b. 1, 2, 3
   3. decreased urine flow.   c. 2, 3, 4
   4. increased urine flow.   d. 1, 4, 5
   5. increased fluid intake.   e. 1, 2, 3, 4, 5

8. A common cause of both pyelonephritis and cystitis is
   a. urinary calculi.
   b. invading microorganisms, such as *E coli.*
   c. allergy reactions.
   d. heavy metals.

9. Uremia exhibits
   a. polycythemia.
   b. retention of metabolic acids.
   c. low plasma calcium levels.
   d. increased erythropoiesis.
   e. Both a and d are correct.

10. Pyelonephritis
    1. is an inflammation and infection of the urinary bladder.   a. 1, 2, 3
    2. is characterized by fever, chills, and flank pain.   b. 1, 2, 3, 4
    3. is characterized by pyuria, bacteriuria, and hematuria.   c. 2, 3, 4
    4. is more common in young women than in young men.   d. 2, 3, 4

11. Which renal condition usually has a history of recent infection with beta-hemolytic streptococci?
    a. pyelonephritis
    b. chronic renal failure
    c. nephrosis
    d. glomerulonephritis
    e. calculi

12. Which of the following is not true concerning glomerulonephritis?
    a. Significant damage to kidneys occurs during the body's response to an infection.
    b. Fever and flank pain occur.
    c. It is Type III hypersensitivity.
    d. It is characterized by hematuria, proteinuria and the presence of casts.
    e. Approximately 90 percent of individuals develop chronic disease.

13. Nephrotic syndrome is associated with _____ to plasma _____.
    a. increased glomerular permeability / urea
    b. decreased glomerular permeability / proteins
    c. decreased glomerular permeability / tubular filtrate
    d. increased glomerular permeability / proteins

14. Causes of acute renal failure include
    a. cholecystitis.
    b. stones and strictures in kidneys or ureters.
    c. heart failure leading to poor renal perfusion.
    d. Both b and c are correct.
    e. a, b, and c are correct.

15. Which of the following describe a patient in acute renal failure?
    1. elevated serum creatinine
    2. leukocytosis
    3. low BUN
    4. fever
    5. oliguria

    a. 1, 2, 3, 4, 5
    b. 1, 3, 5
    c. 2, 4
    d. 1, 2, 3, 5
    e. 1, 5

16. Which of the following is not true of chronic renal failure?
    a. hyperkalemia
    b. anuria
    c. anemia
    d. pruritus
    e. acidosis

17. Chronic renal failure
    a. may result from hypertension.
    b. is usually the result of chronic inflammation of the kidney.
    c. may be treated with dialysis or transplants.
    d. All of the above are correct.
    e. Both a and c are correct.

18. An individual has an elevated blood level of urea and creatinine because of complete calculi blockage of one ureter. This is referred to as
    a. prerenal disease.
    b. intrarenal disease.
    c. postrenal disease.
    d. preeclampsia.
    e. hypercalcemia.

19. Nephrotoxins such as the antibiotics may be responsible for
    a. acute tubular necrosis.
    b. acute glomerulonephritis.
    c. pyelonephritis.
    d. cystitis.

20. Uremia, as seen in chronic renal failure, would include
    a. metabolic acidosis.
    b. elevated BUN and creatinine.
    c. cardiovascular disturbances.
    d. All of the above are correct.

21. The earliest symptom of chronic renal failure is
    a. pruritus.
    b. oliguria.
    c. polyuria.
    d. decreased BUN.

22. In chronic renal failure, tubulointerstitial disease leads to
    a. sodium retention.
    b. sodium wasting.
    c. no significant changes in sodium levels.
    d. increased phosphate excretion.

Match the condition with the etiology.

23. Goodpasture syndrome
24. hypovolemia
25. uremia

a. prerenal failure
b. postrenal failure
c. chronic glomerulonephritis
d. rapidly progressive glomerulonephritis
e. pruritus

Case Study

Mr. and Mrs. C. returned from a weekend of downhill skiing to find their 9-year-old-son, Eddie, with bloody urine. About six weeks earlier they had spent a week skiing during which Eddie had a severe sore throat that was not treated since his teenage sitter did not take him to a physician.

Eddie was taken to his pediatrician where it was established that he had been lethargic and without appetite for the past ten days and had complained of back pain. His physical examination showed a temperature of 101° F and a blood pressure of 140/102. The remainder of the physical was noncontributory. Eddie's urinalysis showed blood, protein, and RBC casts with an elevated specific gravity. BUN, serum creatinine, and ASO liter levels were elevated.

What do you think is the likely cause of Eddie's symptoms and signs? What do you think the pediatrician will do?

CHAPTER 34

Alterations of Renal and Urinary Tract Function in Children

Prerequisite Objectives

a. Briefly describe the embryologic development of the renal system and urinary tract and urine formation and excretion in children.
   Review text pages 1265-1266; refer to Figure 34-1 and Table 34-1.

Remember!

- The kidneys develop from three distinct tissues: the pronephros, mesonephros, and the metanephros. The tissue is present by the third week of gestation and excretory function is evident by six weeks. Actual urine formation occurs by three months' gestation, and the collecting system develops from the metanephric duct and is in place by the fifth month. After the primitive glomeruli and uriniferous tubules develop from the metanephrogenic tissue on the top of the collecting ducts, they continue to develop into the tenth month. The other structures of the urinary tract form as the kidneys mature. The cloaca becomes the urogenital sinus and follows a differentiation process that develops into the bladder and the urethra. If at any point during this process an injury or insult occurs to the embryo, congenital anomalies may result that will have a major impact on the structure and function of the system. All the nephrons are present at birth, and their number does not increase as the kidney grows and matures. Maturation of the tubular system increases the size and weight of the kidney tenfold from birth. Urine formation and excretion begin by the third month of gestation and contribute to the amniotic fluid. Immediately at birth, the renal blood flow and glomerular filtration rate (GFR) increase due to a decrease in vascular resistance and required excretory functions no longer performed by the placenta. The resistance progressively declines during the first year of development and an increasing fraction of the cardiac output goes to the kidney. The GFR continues to increase but remains at 30 to 50 percent of adult levels until the end of the first year.

---

b. Describe fluid and electrolyte balance in children; explain the implications of imbalances of either.
   Review text pages 1266-1267.

Remember!

- Infants and young children have a larger ratio of body water to body weight than adults; a large proportion of this water is in the extracellular compartment. Children exchange half of their extracellular water each day. Factors that influence water movement are those that affect osmolality. When children become ill, they tend to retain fluid due to the effects of antidiuretic hormone

(Continued)

and increased levels of aldosterone in response to "stress." Both factors decrease urine volume and increase urine concentration. However, the infant has limited ability to concentrate urine because of decreased renal blood flow, high renal vascular resistance, shorter tubular length, and a limited amount of urea available in the loop of Henle. There also is a lower threshold for bicarbonate reabsorption and limited acid excretion. This increases the child's risk for developing metabolic acidosis. Fluid and electrolyte balance is very sensitive to the slightest changes in any of these factors. Imbalance may occur rapidly and can precipitate life-threatening crises.

Objectives

After successful study of this chapter, the learner will be able to:

1. Describe the common congenital anomalies that occur within the renal and urologic system.

> Study text pages 1267-1269; refer to Figures 34-2 through 34-4.

Structural defects range from mild to severe and from simple to complex. The extent of the defect is directly related to the injury, insult, or interruption occurring during embryologic development. **Hypospadias**, with or without chordee and its band of fibrous tissue that deviates the penis ventrally, and **epispadias** are defects in the placement of the urethral meatus. Hypospadias is the more common penile defect, with an incidence of one in 300 infant boys, and is usually easily corrected with surgery. Epispadias is a more complex problem but has a lower incidence rate, approximately one in 200,000 boys and one in 400,000 girls. This can also be surgically corrected but requires a more involved intervention.

Exstrophy of the bladder is a defect wherein the bladder and associated urinary tract structures are exposed to the surface of the body. This defect involves the abdominal wall and the pubic bone. Incidence is one in 40,000 of which two-thirds are boys. This defect allows urine to leak from the ureters into the abdominal wall leading to excoriation of the skin and the persistent odor of urine. The exposed mucosa becomes edematous, bleeds easily, and is painful. Surgical repair requires several stages with the first during the first few days of life. Neoplastic changes have been associated with exstrophy of the bladder.

Structural changes of the kidney may be categorized as those that affect renal function and those that do not; they may occur unilaterally or bilaterally. **Unilateral agenesis** occurs in approximately one in 1000 births and has little or no effect on function if one of the kidneys is normal. **Bilateral agenesis**, or Potter syndrome, occurs in approx-

imately one in 3000 births, is usually associated with other anomalies, and has a high mortality rate. **Hypoplastic kidney** may be small but functionally normal or underdeveloped and functionally abnormal. The bilateral form is a common cause of chronic renal failure. **Dysplastic kidney** is associated with obstructions of the renal collecting system. **Ectopic kidney** is usually functionally normal but lies in the pelvic region rather than in the abdomen. **Horseshoe kidney**, or fused kidney, is associated with hydronephrosis, infection, and stone formation.

2. Describe the pathophysiology and clinical manifestations of hemolytic uremic syndrome and its treatment.

> Study text page 1272.

Hemolytic uremic syndrome is believed to be associated with a viral or bacterial illness because it is usually preceded one or two weeks by an upper respiratory or gastrointestinal infection. The result of this illness may include the development of a hemolytic anemia with thrombocytopenia and acute renal failure. A noxious stimulus that could be an antecedent infection causes endothelial injury to the glomerular arterioles. This event triggers the inflammatory cascade resulting in platelet aggregation and fibrin clot formation that narrows the arterioles. Anemia results when erythrocytes and platelets are damaged while passing through narrowed and inflamed glomerular arterioles and sequestered by the spleen. This same thrombocyte and fibrin clot mechanism activates the fibrinolytic cascade that prompts the release of damaged platelets from the arterioles. These damaged platelets are also sequestered by the spleen. Thrombocytosis eventually results. Classic symptoms of hemolytic uremic syndrome are pallor, bruising, and oliguria that may be accompanied by fever, vomiting, bloody diarrhea, abdominal pain, and jaundice. Central nervous system involvement may be a feature of severe disease. Treatment is supportive and includes transfusions of red blood cells and platelets to treat the anemia and thrombocytopenia. Either hemodialysis or peritoneal dialysis may be required to regulate fluids and electrolytes until renal function returns to normal.

3. Identify the structural cause of vesicoureteral reflux and explain the potential effects on renal function.

Study text pages 1272-1274; refer to Figures 34-6 and 34-7.

Primary vesicoureteral reflux is caused by the congenital malpositioning of a ureter or ureters into the bladder that allows urine to retrograde up the ureters. If the urine contains microorganisms and can reach the renal parenchyma, chronic infection and scarring may result. This reflux of urine returns to the bladder after the child voids; the incomplete emptying of the bladder predisposes the child to infection. This condition is classified by a grading system with grade I the most mild and grade V the most severe.

Secondary vesicoureteral reflux occurs because an infection causes mucosal edema and interferes with the antireflux mechanisms of the urinary tract. Antireflux mechanisms that are somewhat immature at birth become efficient as the urinary tract matures. Symptoms associated with vesicoureteral reflux include fever, recurrent urinary tract infections, and poor feeding. Diagnosis is confirmed by a radiologic procedure that allows visualization of reflux during voiding. Treatment goals are to prevent infection and to protect and preserve renal function. Recurrent infection is an indication for surgical repair.

4. Characterize Wilms tumor.

Study text pages 1274-1275; refer to Tables 34-4 and 34-5.

Wilms tumor, or nephroblastoma, is an embryonic tumor with cellular components that are stromal, epithelial, and blastermal. The peak age of diagnosis is two to three years of age with an incidence of approximately 400 cases diagnosed yearly in the United States. Wilms tumor may occur as a sporadic phenomenon or it may be inherited. The tumor is smooth, firm, and usually encapsulated and separated from the renal parenchyma. The inherited form is an autosomal dominant disorder but is rare. The occurrence has been found to be caused by the deletion or inactivation of genes on the short arm of chromosome 11. This finding tends to support the theory of tumor-suppressor genes. Other congenital anomalies have been associated with Wilms tumor in 18 percent of children. These children may be asymptomatic or may present with vague abdominal pain, hematuria, fever, or hypertension. Diagnosis is made by locating the tumor and assessing its site by radiologic procedures such as ultrasound, computerized tomography (CT scan), or magnetic resonance imaging (MRI). Treatment is surgical excision with a heminephrectomy or total nephrectomy. Depending on the stage of the tumor, chemotherapy or radiation therapy or both may be required. Prognosis is affected by tumor weight and histologic category, the age of the child, and the extent of lymph node involvement. The survival rate of Wilms tumor is approximately 90 percent for those with a histologically favorable tumor and lack of metastatic disease.

5. Define primary and secondary enuresis; discuss their likely causes and common approaches to management.

Study text pages 1276-1277; refer to Table 34-6.

Enuresis can be classified in two categories: **primary enuresis** occurs when a child has never obtained continence and **secondary enuresis** occurs when a child has had and then lost bladder control. Secondary enuresis is also termed acquired enuresis. Statistics are not helpful in determining the incidence of this problem because it is a subject that is not usually reported or discussed. The origin may be neurologic, anatomical, or functional. Psychological problems have been related to enuresis in some cases and must be considered a legitimate cause in the absence of organic findings. All efforts are initially focused on identifying an organic, underlying problem including urinary tract infection, a congenital defect of the urinary tract, or neurologic dysfunction. The child who exhibits smaller functional bladder capacity or experiences episodes of enuresis during "deep sleep" will most likely "outgrow" the problem. Management depends on cause and may include a combination of interventions such as medication, limited fluid intake, behavior modification, alarms, or periodic awakenings during sleep. Psychological counseling may also benefit the child and family.

Practice Examination

True/False

_____ 1. The bladder is a pelvic organ during infancy.

_____ 2. Vesicoureteral reflux is caused by a congenitally malpositioned insertion of the ureter or ureters into the bladder.

_____ 3. Children are at no greater risk for fluid and electrolyte imbalances than adults.

_____ 4. Grade V vesicoureteral reflux can be medically managed.

_____ 5. Wilms tumor is an embryonic tumor of the kidney.

_____ 6. Secondary enuresis occurs when the child has never been continent.

7. At what time during embryologic development does urine form and excretion begin?
   a. six weeks
   b. six months
   c. three months
   d. None of the above is correct.

8. Which of the following represents the final stage in the embryonic development of the kidney?
   a. metanephros
   b. mesonephros
   c. pronephros
   d. endonephros

9. Infants cannot concentrate urine because of
   a. decreased urea in the loop of Henle.
   b. decreased tubular weight.
   c. decreased blood flow to the kidneys.
   d. Both a and c are correct.
   e. a, b, and c are correct.

10. Vesicoureteral reflux causes urine to _____ up the ureters and places the young child at risk for _____.
   a. retrograde / glomerulonephritis
   b. regrade / nephrotic syndrome
   c. retrograde / pyelonephritis
   d. regrade / cystitis

11. Which of these manifestations may be associated with vesicoureteral reflux?
   a. recurrent urinary tract infections
   b. poor growth
   c. irritability
   d. Both a and b are correct.
   e. a, b, and c are correct.

12. Children are at risk of acidosis and dehydration during
   a. restricted fluid intake.
   b. vomiting and/or diarrhea.
   c. improper nutrition.
   d. All of the above are correct.

13. Organic causes of enuresis may include
   a. congenital abnormalities of the urinary tract.
   b. a neurologic origin.
   c. diabetes insipidus.
   d. All of the above are correct.

267

14. Children may "outgrow" enuresis if there is
   a. small bladder size.
   b. general developmental delay.
   c. "deep sleep" enuresis.
   d. All of the above are correct.

15. Which clinical manifestations suggest hemolytic uremic syndrome?
   a. oliguria
   b. pallor and bruising
   c. fever, vomiting, and diarrhea
   d. All of the above are correct.
   e. Both a and b are correct.

16. Identify the sequence of events in hemolytic uremic syndrome that cause anemia.
   1. The damaged cells are removed from the circulation by the spleen.   a. 1, 3, 4
   2. The endothelial lining of the glomerular arterioles becomes swollen.   b. 2, 4, 1
   3. Narrowed vessels damage erythrocytes.   c. 3, 1, 2
   4. Fibrin split-products appear in the urine and serum.   d. 2, 3, 1

17. Which of these factors influences the prognosis of a child with Wilms tumor?
   a. the child's weight
   b. histologic category of the tumor
   c. lymph node invasion
   d. tumor weight
   e. b, c, and d are correct.

18. What symptoms may a child with Wilms tumor develop?
   a. fever
   b. hypertension
   c. hematuria
   d. Both b and c are correct.
   e. a, b, and c are correct.

Match the description with the structural abnormality.

19. small normally developed kidney
20. usually normal kidneys remain in the pelvis
21. urethral opening on the dorsal surface of the penis, a cleft along the ventral urethra in girls
22. results from abnormal differentiation of renal tissue
23. exposed bladder mucosa through a fissure in the abdominal wall
24. urethral meatus opening on the ventral side of the penis
25. absence of the kidneys

a. hypospadias
b. epispadias
c. bladder exstrophy
d. hypoplastic kidney
e. renal dysplasia
f. ectopic kidney
g. renal aplasia

Case Study

A three-year-old girl is brought to the emergency room of a local hospital because she has bloody stools. The parents complain that "her eyes are puffy and she looks very pale." Her parents reveal a history of gastrointestinal illness two weeks ago after a weekend of camping. The girl has been well since the GI illness until yesterday when the bloody stools began. At that time, they noticed how pale she was and believe she has not voided at all today. Her assessment reveals pallor, bruising, and petechiae. She has general edema. A urine collection bag was placed on the child; however, she never voided while in the emergency room. A complete blood count revealed low Hgb, Hct, and platelets. Serum levels showed Na^+ and K^+ all elevated and albumin and protein low; pH was 7.30.

From the laboratory values, what diagnosis is likely? What treatment will she require?

Structure and Function of the Digestive System

Objectives

After successful study of this chapter, the learner will be able to:

1. **List sequentially the parts of the alimentary canal from mouth to anus.**
   Refer to Figure 35-1.

2. **Describe the structural layers of the gastrointestinal tract.**
   Review text page 1284; refer to Figure 35-2.

3. **Describe the mouth and esophagus noting specific structural functions.**
   Review text pages 1283-1286; refer to Figures 35-3, 35-4, and 35-11.

4. **Describe the stomach noting specific structural function.**
   Review text pages 1286-1291; refer to Figures 35-5 through 35-9 and 35-11 and Table 35-1.

5. **Describe the small intestine noting specific function and secretions.**
   Review text pages 1291-1300; refer to Figures 35-10 through 35-15 and Table 35-2.

6. **Describe the structure and function of the large intestine and identify normal intestinal flora and their activities.**
   Review text pages 1300-1303.

7. **Describe the structure and function of the liver and gall bladder.**
   Review text pages 1303-1308; refer to Figures 35-17 through 35-22.

8. **Explain the relationship between cell types and function of the pancreas.**
   Review text pages 1308-1310; refer to Figure 35-22.

9. **Describe the alterations in the digestive system associated with normal aging.**
   Review text page 1315.

Practice Examination

1. The muscularis of the gastrointestinal tract is
   a. skeletal muscle throughout the tract, particularly in the esophagus and large intestine.
   b. the layer which contains the blood capillaries for the entire wall of the tract.
   c. composed principally of keratinized epithelium.
   d. composed of circular fibers and longitudinal fibers.

2. The digestive functions performed by the saliva and salivary amylase respectively are
   a. moistening and protein digestion.
   b. deglutition and fat digestion.
   c. peristalsis and polysaccharide digestion.
   d. lubrication and carbohydrate digestion.

3. The nervous pathway involved in salivary secretion requires stimulation of
   a. receptors in the taste buds, impulses to the motor cortex, and somatic motor impulses to salivary glands.
   b. receptors in the mouth, sensory impulses to a center in the brain stem, and parasympathetic impulses to salivary glands.
   c. taste receptors, sensory impulses to centers in the brain stem, and somatic motor impulses to salivary glands.
   d. pressoreceptors in blood vessels, motor impulses, and autonomic impulses to salivary glands.

4. Food would pass rapidly from the stomach into the duodenum if it were not for the
   a. fundus.
   b. epiglottis.
   c. rugae.
   d. cardiac sphincter.
   e. pyloric sphincter.

5. The secretion of gastric juice
   a. occurs only when the stomach comes in contact with swallowed food.
   b. is entirely under the control of the hormone gastrin.
   c. is entirely under the control of the hormone enterogastrone.
   d. is stimulated by the presence of saliva in the stomach.
   e. occurs in three phases: cephalic, gastric, and intestinal.

6. During nervous control of gastric secretion, the gastric glands secrete before food enters the stomach. This stimulus to the glands comes from
   a. gastrin.
   b. impulses over somatic nerves from the hypothalamus.
   c. motor impulses from the cerebral cortex and cerebellum.
   d. parasympathetic impulses over the vagus nerve.

7. Pepsinogen
   a. must be activated by HC1.
   b. is secreted by the chief cells.
   c. is important in breakdown of proteins.
   d. All of the above are correct.

8. Beginning at the lumen of the tube, the sequence of layers of the gastrointestinal tract is
   a. mucosa, submucosa, muscularis, serosa.
   b. submucosa, mucosa, serous membrane, muscularis.
   c. submucosa, mucosa, muscularis, skeletal muscle.
   d. serous membranes, muscularis, mucosa, submucosa.

9. Normally, when chyme leaves the stomach,
    a. the nutrients are ready for absorption into the blood.
    b. the amount of inorganic salts have been increased by the action of hydrochloric acid.
    c. its pH is neutral.
    d. the proteins have been partly digested.
    e. All of the above are correct.

10. Which layer of the small intestine includes microvilli?
    a. submucosa
    b. mucosa
    c. muscularis
    d. serosa

11. Which is not an example of mechanical digestion?
    a. chewing
    b. churning and mixing of food in the stomach
    c. peristalsis and mastication
    d. conversion of protein molecules into amino acids

12. Pancreatic juice is to trypsin as gastric juice is to
    a. salivary amylase.
    b. pepsin.
    c. mucin.
    d. intrinsic factor.

13. Which part of the small intestine is most distal from the pylorus?
    a. jejunum
    b. pyloric sphincter
    c. duodenum
    d. cardiac sphincter
    e. common bile duct

14. The pancreas
    a. lies mostly on the left side of the abdominal cavity, anterior to the stomach and the spleen.
    b. secretes all of its products directly into the blood stream.
    c. is a slender, flattened gland with its duct ultimately opening into the duodenum.
    d. contains cells with endocrine function for the determination of secondary sex characteristics.
    e. is classified as a digestive exocrine gland, not having endocrine functions.

15. The chief role played by the pancreas in digestion is to
    a. secrete insulin and glucagon.
    b. churn the food and bring it into contact with digestive enzymes.
    c. secrete enzymes which digest food in the small intestine.
    d. assist in absorbing the digested foods.

16. Among the structural features of the small intestine are villi, microvilli, and circular folds. Their function is to
    a. liberate hormones.
    b. promote peristalsis.
    c. liberate digestive enzymes.
    d. increase the surface area for absorption.

17. The fate of carbohydrates in the small intestine is
    a. digestion by amylase, sucrase, maltase, and lactase to monosaccharide.
    b. conversion to simple sugars by the activity of trypsin and lipase.
    c. hydrolysis to amino acids by the activity of amylase, sucrase, maltase, and lactase.
    d. conversion to glycerol and fatty acids by the activity of lipase and amylase.

18. The immediate fate of the end products of digestion may be summarized as
    a. most fatty acids are absorbed into the blood; glucose and amino acids are absorbed into the lymphatic system.
    b. amino acids and monosaccharides are absorbed into blood capillaries; most fatty acids are absorbed into lymph.
    c. amino acids and fatty acids are absorbed into the lymph capillaries; glycerol and glucose are absorbed into the blood capillaries.
    d. fatty acids are absorbed into blood capillaries; glycerol, glucose, and amino acids are absorbed into lymph.

19. A lobule of the liver contains a centrally located
    a. vein with radiating hepatocytes and sinusoids.
    b. arteriole with radiating capillaries and Kupffer cells.
    c. hepatic sinus with radiating sinusoids.
    d. hepatic duct with radiating Kupffer cells and cords of hepatic cells.

20. An obstruction of the common bile duct would cause blockage of bile coming from
    a. the gall bladder.
    b. the liver but not from the gall bladder.
    c. both the liver and the gall bladder.
    d. the pancreatic duct but not from the gall bladder.

21. The human adult liver does not
    a. store glycogen.
    b. produce erythrocytes.
    c. convert ammonia to urea.
    d. produce blood coagulation proteins.

22. The chyme which enters the large intestine is converted to feces by activity of
    a. specific mucosal enzymes.
    b. gastric and duodenal hormones.
    c. bacteria, water reabsorption.
    d. the microvilli, villi, and circular muscles.

Match the substance with its function.

23. mucus
24. intrinsic factor
25. cholecystokinin

    a. stimulates gall bladder to eject bile
    b. activates pepsinogen
    c. required for vitamin B_{12} absorption
    d. increases gastrointestinal mobility
    e. protects gastric mucosa from digestion
    f. stimulates liver to secrete bile

CHAPTER 36

Alterations of Digestive Function

Prerequisite Objectives

a. Describe the structure and function of the gastrointestinal tract and accessory organs of digestion. Refer to Figure 35-1.

Remember!

- The gastrointestinal system includes the oral structures (mouth, salivary glands, pharynx), the alimentary tract (esophagus, stomach, small intestine, large intestine, appendix, anus), and the accessory organs of digestion (liver, gallbladder, bile ducts, pancreas). The function of the alimentary tract is to digest masticated food, to absorb digestive products, and to excrete the digestive residue and certain waste products excreted by the liver through the bile duct.

- The esophagus is a straight tube that carries food from the pharynx to the stomach. The stomach is a distensible organ. The stomach's mucosal cells secrete hydrochloric acid and proteolytic enzymes which aid in digestion. The mucosa of the lower part of the stomach is lined by mucous cells. The distal end of the stomach is called the pylorus. The small intestine is divided into the duodenum, jejunum, and ileum. The large intestine or colon consists of the cecum, ascending colon, transverse colon, descending colon, sigmoid colon, and rectum. The vermiform appendix is a nonfunctional vestigial structure attached to cecum. The colon is a storage reservoir for undigested food and a site for water absorption.

- The alimentary tract has four layers: mucosa, submucosa, muscularis, and serosa. The mucosal layer consists of epithelial cells lining the lumen's surface, supporting connective tissue called the lamina propria, and a unique thin, muscular layer called the muscularis mucosae. The structure of inner mucosal layer varies to provide specialized function at each part of the tract. The esophagus is lined by stratified squamous epithelium which enables rapid gliding of masticated food from the mouth to the stomach. The stomach has a thick glandular mucosa which provides mucus, acid, and proteolytic enzymes to help digest food. The small intestinal mucosa has a villous structure to provide a large surface of cells for active absorption. The large intestinal mucosa is lined by abundant mucus-secreting cells which facilitate storage and evacuation of the residue. Beneath the mucosa is the submucosa which gives structural support to the tract because of its abundant collagenous tissue. The muscle layer contracts rhythmically to move materials through the alimentary tract. The serosal layer is a thin, smooth membrane present on the outer surface of the alimentary tract. It keeps the tortuous loops of bowel from becoming tangled and is continuous with the mesentery. The mesentery is a connective tissue attachment of the bowel to the abdominal wall; it contains blood vessels, lymphatics, and nerves.

(Continued)

Remember! *(cont'd)*

- A wave of muscle contraction carries a bolus of swallowed food down the esophagus where a sphincter at the lower end of the esophagus prevents regurgitation. Contractions in the stomach mix the food and push the partially digested contents into the duodenum. The muscle of the pylorus only partially closes the outlet to the stomach so intestinal contents can regurgitate into the stomach if the small intestine is not emptying properly. Normally, movement of lumenal contents in the small intestine is more rapid in the upper small intestine and slows as chyme moves distally. Contents pass from the ileum into the colon where reverse proximal movement is partially prevented by the ileocecal valve. Water is absorbed in the colon and the contents become solid; the solid residue is moved to the left side of the colon and rectum. When the rectum becomes distended, an urge for defecation develops.

- The liver and the pancreas are glandular organs with excretory ducts emptying into the duodenum at a site called the ampulla of Vater. The excretory ducts of the liver are called bile ducts. The gallbladder is a storage reservoir connected to the bile ducts by the cystic duct.

- Most of the blood from the abdominal organs is carried to the liver via the portal veins. Therefore, blood is filtered by the glandular cells of the liver before it returns to the heart via the hepatic vein and vena cava. Because portal blood has little oxygen left after passing through the abdominal organs, the liver has the hepatic artery to provide oxygenated blood. The bulk of the liver is composed of hepatocytes which are aligned in cords with sinusoids between the cords to diffuse the blood from the portal areas to the central vein. Between adjacent hepatocytes are tiny canaliculi that carry bile produced by the hepatocytes to the portal area where they empty into epithelial-lined bile ducts. In the sinusoids, waste products and nutrients are removed and metabolized by the hepatocytes. The metabolites may be returned to the blood, stored in the hepatocytes, or excreted into bile canaliculi. The liver also contains many mononuclear cells or Kupffer cells that line the sinusoids. They phagocytize particulate material from the blood. Metabolically, the liver (1) produces bile salts, (2) excretes bilirubin, (3) metabolizes nitrogenous substances, (4) produces serum proteins, and (5) detoxifies drugs and poisons.

- The gallbladder is a distension of the common bile duct that becomes a storage reservoir for bile. The gallbladder empties its contents into the duodenum after meals when bile salts are needed for fat absorption. This reservoir function is not essential, as the gallbladder can be removed without loss of digestive function.

- The pancreas is a long, narrow glandular organ lying horizontally and retroperitoneally in the midabdomen region. The pancreatic duct runs the length of the pancreas and empties into the duodenum after joining the bile duct. The bulk of the pancreas is made up of glands that secrete digestive enzymes into the pancreatic duct. When activated by intestinal juices, these enzymes digest carbohydrate, fat, and protein. Pancreatic enzymes are essential for life. Scattered among the pancreatic glands are clusters of endocrine cells known as the islets of Langerhans, which produce insulin and other hormones.

- The digestive process begins in the mouth, where carbohydrate-splitting enzymes or amylases from the salivary glands mix with food during mastication. In the stomach, proteolytic pepsin and hydrochloric acid are added to speed the digestive process. The greatest volume of digestive enzymes originates from the pancreas and is added to the digesting mixture of food in the duodenum. These include amylases, proteolytic trypsin, and fat-splitting enzymes or lipases. In addition, bile salts secreted by the liver and stored in the gallbladder are added to emulsify lipids into small water-soluble micelles. The final phase of the digestive process occurs at the surface of small intestinal epithelial cells. Here, carbohydrate-splitting disaccharidases and protein-splitting dipeptidases continue the process. Complex endocrine and nervous mechanisms coordinate the timing of the secretion of digestive enzymes, hydrochloric acid, and bile salts. The sight of food may cause salivation and gastric secretions because of nervous stimulation. Distention of the stomach causes release of gastrin which stimulates acid production and gastric emptying. Movement of food into the duodenum causes the pancreas to secrete more fluid and enzymes and the gallbladder to release bile. The products of both enter the duodenum.

b. Describe tests used to evaluate the structure and function of the digestive system
   Refer to Tables 35-4 through 35-8.

Remember!

- The structure and function of the gastrointestinal tract can be assessed by x-ray films using contrast media such as barium- or iodine-containing compounds to outline the gastrointestinal lumen, biliary tree and pancreatic ducts, fistulas, and arteriovenous systems. CT scanning is used for diagnosis of pancreatic or hepatic tumors or cysts. Ultrasonic scanning can detect liver-related jaundice and intra-abdominal masses. Fiberoptic endoscopy with flexible endoscopes permits direct visualization of the upper and lower gastrointestinal tract; a biopsy channel in the endoscope allows tissue sampling. Suction can be used to remove gastrointestinal secretions or blood to assess infection, malabsorption syndromes, ulcerative lesions, and tumor growth.

- Imaging techniques similar to those used for the gastrointestinal tract also are useful to evaluate liver structure and function. Serum enzymes are elevated in many liver diseases; aminotransferase and lactate dehydrogenate are released into the circulation when there is damage to hepatocytes. Obstruction of bile canaliculi or ducts causes regurgitation of bile back into the hepatic sinusoids and into the circulation, which elevates bilirubin levels. Blood coagulation times are often prolonged with both hepatitis and chronic liver disease. Serum albumin and globulins may be lowered because of hepatocyte damage. Liver biopsies may be performed to evaluate the extent of liver involvement or degeneration in either cirrhosis or hepatitis.

- Evaluation of structural alterations in the gallbladder uses imaging techniques. Both conjugated and total serum bilirubin values are elevated, urine urobilinogen is increased, stools are clay-colored, and jaundice develops if bile flow to the gastrointestinal tract is obstructed. During inflammation of the gallbladder, the white cell count is elevated. Inflammation or obstruction of the pancreas results in an increase in serum amylase levels. Increased stool fat indicates pancreatic insufficiency because of decreased lipase secretion.

Objectives

After successful study of this chapter, the learner will be able to:

1. Describe the common terms used in identifying the signs and symptoms of gastrointestinal dysfunction.
   Study text pages 1321-1326; refer to Figure 36-1 and Table 36-1.

Anorexia is the absence of a desire to eat despite physiologic stimuli that would normally produce hunger. Anorexia is a nonspecific symptom often associated with nausea, abdominal pain, and diarrhea. Disorders of other systems besides the digestive system are accompanied by anorexia. These include cancer, heart disease, and renal disease.

Vomiting is the forceful emptying of stomach and intestinal contents or chyme through the mouth. The vomiting reflex is stimulated by presence of ipecac or copper salts in the duodenum, severe pain, or distention of the stomach or duodenum. Torsion or trauma affecting the ovaries, testes, uterus, bladder, or kidney also elicit vomiting.

Nausea and retching usually precede vomiting. **Nausea** is a subjective experience associated with many different conditions. **Retching** is a strong involuntary effort to vomit. In retching, the lower esophageal sphincter and body of the stomach relax but the duodenum and antrum of the stomach go into spasm. The reverse peristalsis forces chyme from the stomach and duodenum up into the esophagus. Since the upper esophageal sphincter is closed, chyme does not enter the mouth. As the abdominal muscles relax, the contents of the esophagus drop back into the stomach. This process may be repeated several time before vomiting occurs.

Vomiting occurs when the stomach is full of gastric contents and the diaphragm is forced high into the thoracic cavity by strong abdominal muscle contractions. The higher intrathoracic pressure forces the upper esophageal sphincter to open and chyme is discharged from the mouth. Spontaneous vomiting not preceded by nausea or retching is called projectile vomiting. This vomiting is caused by direct stimulation of the vomiting center because of neurologic lesions involving the brain stem. The metabolic consequences of vomiting are fluid, electrolyte, and acid-base disturbances.

Constipation is difficult or infrequent defecation involving decreased numbers of bowel movements per week, hard stools, and difficult evacuation. Constipation is frequently caused by unhealthy dietary and bowel habits combined with inadequate exercise. It also can occur as a result of intestinal immobility or obstruction disorders. Constipation resulting from lifestyle or bowel habits usually has a long duration. Dysfunctional constipation is more likely to be sudden and can accompany the development of organic lesions.

Diarrhea is increased frequency of defecation accompanied by changes in fecal fluidity and volume. In osmotic diarrhea, the presence of nonabsorbable substances in the intestine causes water to be drawn into the lumen by osmosis. The excess water and the nonabsorbable substances increase stool weight and volume. This causes **large-volume diarrhea**. Secretory diarrhea is a form of large-volume diarrhea caused by excessive mucosal secretion of fluid and electrolytes. Excessive intestinal secretion is mostly caused by bacterial enterotoxins released by cholera or strains of *Escherichia coli*. Gastrinoma or thyroid carcinoma produce hormones that may stimulate intestinal secretion. A lesion that impairs autonomic control of motility such as diabetic neuropathy can cause large-volume diarrhea. Excessive motility decreases transit time, mucosal surface contact, and opportunities for fluid absorption. Motility diarrhea can be caused by resection of the small intestine, surgical bypass of an area of the intestine, or fistula formation between loops of the intestine.

Small-volume diarrhea is usually caused by inflammatory disorders of the intestine or by fecal impaction from severe constipation. In the latter case, the diarrhea consists of mucus and fluid produced by the colon to lubricate the impacted feces and move it toward the anal canal.

Abdominal pain is observed in a number of gastrointestinal diseases. Abdominal organs are sensitive to stretching and distention which can activate nerve endings in both hollow and solid structures. Histamine, bradykinin, and serotonin, when released during inflammation, stimulate organic nerve endings and produce abdominal pain. The edema and vascular congestion that accompany inflammation also cause painful stretching. Any obstruction of blood flow because of distention of bowel obstruction or mesenteric vessel thrombosis produces ischemic pain. **Parietal pain** arises from the parietal peritoneum and is more localized and intense than **visceral pain**, which arises from the organs themselves. **Referred pain** is visceral pain felt at some distance from a diseased or affected organ. Referred pain is usually well localized and is felt in the skin or deeper tissues which share a central, common afferent pathway with the affected organ.

Numerous disorders cause gastrointestinal tract bleeding. Acute **gastrointestinal bleeding** is usually characterized by **hematemesis** or the presence of blood in the vomitus, **hematochezia** or frank bleeding from the rectum, or **melena**, which is dark, tarry stools. **Occult bleeding** is slow, chronic blood loss that results in iron-deficiency anemia as iron stores in the bone marrow are slowly depleted.

2. Compare and contrast the various disorders of digestive motility.
Study text pages 1326-1332; refer to Figures 36-2 through 36-4 and Tables 36-2 and 36-3.

Motility Disorders

	Causes	*Manifestations*
Dysphagia (swallowing difficulty)	Esophageal obstruction Tumors, strictures, or diverticula Impaired esophageal motility Neural dysfunction, muscular disease, CVA Achalasia (decreased ganglion cells in myenteric plexus, muscle cell atrophy)	Distention and spasm of esophagus after swallowing, regurgitation of undigested food

(Continued)

Motility Disorders *(cont'd)*

	Causes	Manifestations
Gastroesophageal reflux (chyme reflux into esophagus)	Increased abdominal pressure, ulcers, pyloric edema and strictures, hiatal hernia	Regurgitation of chyme within one hour of eating
Hiatal hernia (protrusion of upper stomach through diaphragm into thorax)	Congenitally short esophagus, trauma, weak diaphragmatic muscles at gastroesophageal junction, increased abdominal pressure	Gastroesophageal reflux, dysphasia, epigastric pain
Pyloric obstruction (narrow pylorus)	Peptic ulcer or carcinoma near pylorus	Epigastric fullness, nausea and pain, vomitus without bile
Intestinal obstruction (impaired chyme flow through intestinal lumen)	Hernia, telescoping of one part of intestine into another, twisting, inflamed diverticula, tumor growth, loss of peristaltic activity	Colicky pain to severe and constant pain, vomiting, diarrhea, constipation, dehydration and hypokalemia and acidosis with their complications

3. Describe the pathogenesis of acute and chronic gastritis.

Study text pages 1332-1333.

Gastritis is an inflammatory disorder of the gastric mucosa that may be acute or chronic and affects the fundus or antrum or both. Aspirin and other anti-inflammatory drugs are known to cause **acute gastritis** which erodes the epithelium, probably because they inhibit prostaglandins that normally stimulate the secretion of protective mucus. Alcohol, histamine, digitalis, and metabolic disorders such as uremia are contributing factors for gastritis. The clinical manifestations of acute gastritis can include vague abdominal discomfort, epigastric tenderness, and bleeding. Healing usually occurs spontaneously within a few days. Discontinuing injurious drugs, using antacids, or decreasing acid secretion with drugs facilitates healing.

Chronic gastritis is a progressive disease that tends to occur in elderly individuals. This gastritis causes thinning and degeneration of the stomach wall.

Chronic fundal gastritis is the most severe type, as the gastric mucosa degenerates extensively. The loss of chief cells and parietal cells diminishes secretion of pepsinogen, hydrochloric acid, and intrinsic factor. Pernicious anemia develops because intrinsic factor is unavailable to facilitate vitamin B_{12} absorption. Chronic fundal gastritis becomes a risk factor for gastric carcinoma, particularly in individuals who develop pernicious anemia. A sig-nificant number of individuals with chronic fundal gastritis have antibodies to parietal cells, intrinsic factor, and gastric cells in their sera thus suggesting an autoimmune mechanism in the pathogenesis of the disease.

Chronic antral gastritis is more frequent than fundal gastritis. It is not associated with decreased hydrochloric acid secretion, pernicious anemia, or the presence of parietal cell antibodies. *Helicobacteria pylori* is a major etiologic factor associated with the inflammation seen in chronic gastritis. The longstanding inflammatory process and gastric atrophy may develop without a history of abdominal distress. Individuals may report vague symptoms including anorexia, fullness, nausea, vomiting, and epigastric pain. Gastric bleeding may be the only clinical manifestation of gastritis.

4. Compare duodenal, gastric, and stress ulcers; identify the complications of surgical management of ulcers.

Study text pages 1333-1339; refer to Figures 36-5 through 36-7 and Tables 36-4 and 36-5.

A **peptic ulcer** is a break or ulceration in the protective mucosal lining of the lower esophagus, stomach, or duodenum. Such breaks expose submucosal areas to gastric secretions and autodigestion. Normally, the gastric and duodenal mucosa are protected from acid and pepsin by mucous and bicarbonate that are secreted by surface epithelial cells. Also, cellular tight junctions prevent back-diffusion of acid.

Risk factors for peptic ulcer disease are smoking and habitual use of NSAIDs or alcohol. Some chronic diseases such as emphysema, rheumatoid arthritis, and cirrhosis are associated with the devel opment of peptic ulcers. Infection of the gastric and duodenal mucosa with *H. pylori* may cause peptic ulcers. Studies of life stress and ulcer disease are inconclusive regarding causation of peptic ulcers.

Features of Ulcers

	Duodenal	*Gastric*	*Stress*
Age incidence	25-50 years	50-70 years	Related to severe stress, trauma, sepsis, head injuries
Sex prevalence	Men	No sex difference	No sex difference
Stress factors	Average	Increased	Increased
Acid production	Increased	Normal to low	Increased
Ulcerogenic drugs	Increased use of alcohol and tobacco	Moderate use of alcohol and tobacco	Increased use of alcohol and aspirin
Associated gastritis	Seldom	Common	Acute, common
Helicobacteria pylori	Often present	May be present	
Pain	Pain-food-relief, common nocturnal pain, remission and exacerbations	Pain-food-relief, uncommon nocturnal pain, chronic, no remission and exacerbations	Asympathetic until hemorrhage or perforation
Hemorrhage	Common	Less Common	Very common (most frequent complication)
Malignancy	Almost never	Possible	

Note: Medical treatment is directed toward inhibiting or buffering acid secretions to relieve symptoms and promote healing. Antiacids, dietary management, anticholinergic histamine blockers, and physical and emotional rest are used to accomplish relief and promote healing.

Postgastrectomy syndromes are a group of signs and symptoms that occur after gastric resection. They are caused by alterations in motor and control functions of the stomach and upper small intestine. **Dumping syndrome** is the rapid emptying of hypertonic chyme from the surgically reduced and smaller stomach into the small intestine 10 to 20 minutes after eating. Rapid gastric emptying and creation of a high osmotic gradient within the small intestine cause a sudden shift of fluid from the vascular compartment to the intestinal lumen. Plasma volume decreases may cause increased pulse rate, hypotension, weakness, pallor, sweating, and dizziness. Rapid distention of the intestine produces a feeling of epigastric fullness, cramping, nausea, vomiting, and diarrhea. After a high-carbohydrate meal, hypoglycemia can develop because of an increase in insulin secretion stimulated by the hyperglycemia that follows eating. The symptoms include weakness, diaphoresis, and confusion.

Alkaline reflux gastritis is stomach inflammation caused by reflux of bile and alkaline pancreatic secretions that contain proteolytic enzymes which disrupt the mucosal barrier. Clinical manifestations include nausea, vomiting in which the vomitus contains bile, and sustained epigastric pain that worsens after eating and is not relieved by antacids.

Afferent loop obstruction is a problem caused by volvulus, hernia, adhesion, or stenosis in the duodenal stump on the proximal side of the surgery. Partial obstruction causes bile and pancreatic secretions to accumulate, distend the loop, and delay emptying. The symptoms of afferent loop obstruction include intermittent severe pain and epigastric fullness after eating.

Diarrhea is one of the most common long-term alterations caused by gastric surgery. Postgastrectomy diarrhea appears to be related to rapid gastric emptying of large amounts of high carbohydrate liquids that increase the osmotic gradient and attract water into the intestinal lumen.

Many individuals cannot tolerate carbohydrates or a normal-sized meal. **Weight loss** frequently follows gastric resection.

Anemia after gastrectomy results from iron, vitamin B_{12}, or folate deficiency. Iron malabsorption may be caused by decreased acid secretion which makes it more difficult to absorb iron. The duodenum may no longer be available to absorb iron after gastrectomy. Vitamin B_{12} deficiency may occur because of fewer parietal cells to secrete intrinsic factor that facilitates absorption of vitamin B_{12}.

5. Define malabsorption syndrome and maldigestion; characterize pancreatic insufficiency and lactose and bile salt deficiency.
Study text pages 1339-1340.

Malabsorption syndromes interfere with nutrient absorption in the small intestine; the intestinal mucosa fails to absorb or transport the digested nutrients into the blood. **Malabsorption** is the result of mucosal disruption caused by gastric or intestinal resection, vascular disorders, or intestinal disease. **Maldigestion** is failed or faulty digestion because of deficiencies of chemical enzymes.

Pancreatic insufficiency occurs because of deficient production of lipase, amylase, trypsin, or chymotrypsin by the pancreas. Causes of pancreatic insufficiency include chronic pancreatitis, pancreatic carcinoma, pancreatic resection, and cystic fibrosis. Fat maldigestion is the chief problem since salivary amylase and enzymes secreted by the intestinal brush border assist in carbohydrate and protein digestion but do not digest fats. A large amount of fat in the stool is the most common sign of pancreatic insufficiency.

Lactase deficiency inhibits the breakdown of lactose or milk sugar into monosaccharides and therefore prevents lactose digestion and absorption across the intestinal wall. Lactase deficiency is most common in blacks. The undigested lactose remains in the intestine where bacterial fermentation causes gases to form. The osmotic gradient in the intestine also increases which causes irritation and osmotic diarrhea.

Conjugated bile acids or bile salts are necessary for the digestion and absorption of fats. When bile from the liver enters the duodenum, the bile salts aggregate with fatty acids and monoglycerides to form micelles. Micelle formation solubilizes fat molecules and allows them to pass through the unstirred layer at the brush border. Advance liver disease which causes **bile salt deficiency**, obstruction of the common bile duct, intestinal immotility, and diseases of the ileum leads to poor intestinal absorption of fat and fat-soluble vitamins A, D, E, and K. Increased fat in the stool leads to diarrhea and decreased plasma proteins. The loss of fat-soluble vitamins causes night blindness, bone demineralization, and bleeding abnormalities.

6. Characterize the disorders of overnutrition and undernutrition.
Study text pages 1344-1346.

Overnutrition or excessive caloric intake leads to **obesity** or excessive body fat which is associated with three leading causes of death: cardiovascular disease, cancer, and diabetes mellitus. Obesity also is a risk factor for breast, cervical, endometrial, and liver cancer in women. Obese men are at greater risk for prostatic, colon, and rectal cancer than non-obese men. Obesity is classified by cause as either exogenous, resulting from an excess of ingested calories, or endogenous, resulting from inherent metabolic problems. Physiologically, obesity can be (1) hyperplastic; that is, caused by a greater-than-normal number of fat cells; or (2) hypertrophic; that is, caused by a greater-than-normal size of fat cells. In children, the adipose tissue is dispersed over the entire body and is both hyperplastic and hypertrophic with few metabolic abnormalities. Adult-onset obesity is hypertrophic, with the adipose tissue centrally located and metabolic abnormalities are more common. Genotype is an important predisposing factor.

A number of theories have been postulated to explain the physiology of obesity. In the lipoprotein-lipase (LPL) theory, lipase hydrolyzes triglycerides into glycerol and free fatty acids which then enter the fat cells and are converted back into triglycerides; LPL promotes fat storage.

The lipostatic theory states that every individual has a biologic "set point" that maintains body weight. The set point is controlled by the ventromedial hypothalamus that regulates an individual's appetite. Obese individuals are believed to have a higher set point.

Another theory of obesity is based on the thermogenesis of brown adipose tissue that is responsible for heat production. Subcutaneous brown fat cells release excess energy through heat production instead of converting the energy to fat stores; obese people are believed to have very few brown fat cells compared with the average individual.

The sodium-potassium-adenosine triphosphatase (ATPase) pump transports sodium out of the cell and potassium into the cell and splits adenosine triphosphate thus releasing energy. Obese people have an average of 22 percent fewer ATPase pumps than non-obese individuals, which could lead to less energy release and obesity.

Obesity probably has psychologic as well as physiologic causes. One theory proposes that obese people are directed more by the sight, smell, and taste of food than by hunger and satiety. Another psychologic theory is that eating creates the desire to eat more. Some obese individuals eat more food after a snack than non-obese individuals, who reduce food intake after a snack.

Type II or non-insulin-dependent type of diabetes mellitus is often associated with obesity. The decrease of insulin receptor sites decreases the amount of glucose that can enter the cells; high blood levels of glucose follow. The excess glucose is stored as glycogen in the liver or as triglycerides in adipose cells thus enhancing hypertrophy and hyperplasia of fat cells.

Treatment for obesity caused by excessive nutrient intake is a regimen of reduced nutrient intake and increased energy expenditure. Individuals with adult-onset obesity can reduce the size of the adipose cells and achieve a standard weight. Those with child-onset obesity may never achieve standard weight. Additional treatments such as psychotherapy, behavioral modification, medications, and surgery may be needed.

Many young adults and adolescents in the United States are affected by two complex and related eating disorders, anorexia nervosa and bulimia. **Anorexia nervosa** is characterized by refusal to eat because of distorted body image perceptions that one is too fat. As the disease progresses, muscle and fat depletion give the individual a skeleton- like appearance. The loss of 25 to 30 percent of ideal body weight can eventually lead to death caused by starvation-induced cardiac failure. Treatment objectives for anorexia nervosa include reversing the compromised physical state, promoting insights and knowledge about the disorder, and modifying food habits.

Bulimia is characterized by binging or the consumption of normal to large amounts of food followed by self-induced vomiting or purging of the intestines with laxatives. Although individuals with bulimia are afraid of gaining weight, their weight usually remains within normal range. Because of negative connotations associated with vomiting and purging, individuals who have bulimia often binge and purge secretly. Bulimics may binge and purge as often as 20 times a day. Continual vomiting of acidic chyme can cause pitted teeth, pharyngeal and esophageal inflammation, and tracheoesophageal fistulas. Overuse of laxatives can cause rectal bleeding.

Starvation can be either short-term or long-term. Therapeutic short-term starvation is part of many weight-reduction programs, while therapeutic long-term starvation is used in medically controlled environments to facilitate rapid weight loss in morbidly obese individuals. Pathologic long-term starvation can be caused by poverty or chronic diseases such as cardiovascular, pulmonary, hepatic, and digestive disorders, malabsorption syndromes, and cancer.

Short-term starvation consists of several days of total dietary abstinence or deprivation. Glucose is the preferred energy source for cells. Once all available energy has been absorbed from the intestine, glycogen in the liver is converted to glucose through glycogenolysis or the splitting of glycogen into glucose. This process peaks within four to eight hours after glycogenolysis and gluconeogenesis in the liver begins by the formation of glucose from non-carbohydrate molecules. Both of these processes deplete stored nutrients and thus cannot meet the body's energy needs indefinitely. Proteins continue to be catabolized in gluconeogenesis to a minimal degree to provide carbon for the synthesis of glucose.

The main characteristics of **long-term starvation** are decreased dependence on gluconeogenesis and increased use of products of lipid and pyruvate metabolism for cellular energy sources. Once the supply of adipose tissue is depleted, proteolysis begins. The breakdown of muscle protein is the last process to supply energy for life. Death results from severe alteration in electrolyte balance and loss of renal, pulmonary, and cardiac function.

Adequate ingestion of appropriate nutrients is the obvious treatment for starvation. Starvation caused by chronic disease, long-term illness, or malabsorption is treated by internal or parenteral nutrition.

7. Compare ulcerative colitis and Crohn disease.

Study text pages 1340-1342; refer to Figure 36-8 and Table 36-3.

Ulcerative Colitis and Crohn Disease

	Ulcerative colitis	*Crohn disease*
Family history	Less common	More common
Location of lesions	Large intestine, no "skip" lesions, mucosal layer involved	Large or small intestine, "skip" lesions common, entire intestinal wall involved
Granulomas	Rare	Common
Anal and perianal fistulas and abscesses	Rare	Common
Narrowed lumen and possible obstruction	Rare	Common
Abdominal pain	Common, mild to severe	Common, mild to severe
Diarrhea	Common	Common
Bloody stools	Common	Less common
Abdominal mass	Rare	Common
Small intestinal malabsorption	Rare	Common
Steatorrhea	Rare	Common
Cancer risk	Increased	Not increased

8. Distinguish between diverticular disease and appendicitis.

Study text pages 1342-1343; refer to Figure 36-9.

Diverticula are herniations or saclike outpouching of mucosa through the muscle layers of the colon wall. **Diverticulosis** is asymptomatic diverticular disease. **Diverticulitis** represents symptomatic inflammation. The most frequent site of diverticula is the sigmoid colon at weak points in the colon wall where arteries penetrate the muscularis. Habitual consumption of a low-residue diet reduces fecal bulk and reduces the diameter of the colon. According to the law of Laplace, wall pressure increases as the diameter of the lumen decreases. Pressure within the narrow lumen can increase enough to rupture the diverticula and cause abscess formation or peritonitis. An increase of dietary fiber intake frequently relieves symptoms. Surgical resection may be required if there are severe complications.

Appendicitis is an inflammation of the vermiform appendix. Obstruction of the lumen with feces, tumors, or foreign bodies followed by bacterial infection is the most likely cause of appendicitis. The obstructed lumen does not allow drainage of the appendix, and as mucosal secretion continues, intraluminal pressure increases. The increased pressure decreases mucosal blood flow and the appendix becomes hypoxic. The mucosa ulcerates, which promotes bacterial inflammation and edema. Gangrene develops from thrombosis of the luminal blood vessels followed by perforation.

Epigastric or periumbilical pain is the typical

symptom of an inflamed appendix. Right lower quadrant pain that exhibits rebound tenderness is associated with extension of the inflammation to the surrounding tissues. Nausea, vomiting, and anorexia follow the onset of pain. Leukocytosis and a low-grade fever are common. Perforation, peritonitis, and abscess formation are the most serious complications of appendicitis.

Appendectomy is the treatment for simple or perforated appendicitis. This surgery is the most common surgical procedure of the abdomen.

9. Describe the complications of liver dysfunction.

Study text pages 1346-1353; refer to Figures 36-10 through 36-13 and Table 36-7.

The complications of liver disease include portal hypertension, ascites, hepatic encephalopathy, jaundice, and hepatorenal syndrome.

Liver Disease Complications

	Cause	*Manifestation*
Portal hypertension	Obstruction or impeded blood flow in portal venous system or vena cava, cirrhosis, viral hepatitis, parasitic infection, hepatic vein thrombosis, right-side heart failure	Esophageal and stomach varices with vomiting of blood, splenomegaly, ascites
Ascites	Portal hypertension and reduced serum albumin levels increase capillary hydrostatic pressure which pushes water into the peritoneal cavity, cirrhosis, heart failure, constrictive pericarditis, abdominal malignancies, nephrotic syndrome, malnutrition	Abdominal distension, displaced diaphragm and dyspnea, peritonitis
Hepatic encephalopathy	Blood that contains toxins such as ammonia are shunted from gastrointestinal tract to systemic circulation, toxins reach brain	Subtle changes in cerebral function, confusion, tremor of hands, stupor, convulsions, coma
Jaundice Hemolytic (unconjugated bilirubin)	Excessive hemolysis of red blood cells because of immune reactions, infections, toxic substances, or transfusions of incompatible blood	Dark urine, light-colored stools, anorexia, malaise, fatigue, pruritus
Obstructive (conjugated bilirubin)	Obstruction of bile flow by gall stones or tumor prevent flow into duodenum, drugs	
Hepatocellular (conjugated and un-conjugated bilirubin)	Intrahepatic disease, obstruction of bile calculi, genetic enzyme defects, infections	
Hepatorenal syndrome	Decrease in blood volume, intrarenal vasoconstriction because the liver may fail to remove excessive angiotensin, vasopressin, etc. from the blood	Oliguria, sodium and water retention, hypotension, BUN and creatinine increases

10. Compare the viral hepatitis types.
   Study text pages 1353-1356; refer to Figures
   36-14 through 36-16 and Table 36-8.

Characteristics of Viral Hepatitis

	Hepatitis A	*Hepatitis B*	*Hepatitis D*	*Hepatitis C*	*Hepatitis E*
Transmission route	Fecal-oral, parenteral, sexual	Parenteral, sexual	Parenteral, fecal-oral, sexual	Parenteral	Fecal-oral
Incubation period	30 days	60-180 days	30-180 days	35-60 days	15-60 days
Carrier state	No	Yes	Yes	Yes	No
Severity	Mild	Severe, may be prolonged	Severe	Unknown	Severe in pregnant women
Chronic hepatitis	No	Yes	Yes	Yes	No
Prophylaxis	Hygiene, immune serum globulin	Hygiene, HBV vaccine	Hygiene, HBV vaccine	Hygiene, screening blood	Hygiene, safe water

Note: Treatment is supportive, physical activity is restricted, low-fat and high-carbohydrate diet is recommended, and interferon is useful in chronic B and C types.

The clinical manifestations of the different types of hepatitis are very similar and usually consist of three phases: the prodromal, icteric, and recovery phases. The **prodromal phase** of hepatitis begins about two weeks after exposure and ends with appearance of jaundice. Fatigue, anorexia, malaise, nausea, vomiting, headache, hyperalgia, cough, and low-grade fever precede the onset of jaundice. The infection is highly transmissible during this phase. The **icteric phase** begins about one to two weeks after the prodromal phase and lasts two to six weeks. Hepatocellular destruction that prevents bilirubin conjugation and intrahepatic bile stasis causes jaundice or icterus. The icteric phase is the actual phase of illness. The liver is enlarged, smooth, and tender, and percussion over the liver causes pain. During the icteric phase, gastrointestinal and respiratory symptoms subside, but fatigue and abdominal pain may persist or become more severe. Both conjugated and unconjugated fractions increase. The posticteric or **recovery phase** begins with resolution of jaundice at about six to eight weeks after exposure. In most cases, liver function returns to normal within two to 12 weeks after the onset of jaundice.
   Fulminant hepatitis is a clinical syndrome resulting in severe impairment or necrosis of liver cells and potential liver failure. It may occur as a complication of hepatitis C or hepatitis B and is compounded by infection with the delta virus. Treatment of fulminant hepatitis is supportive. The hepatic necrosis is irreversible. Liver transplantation may be lifesaving. Survivors usually do not develop cirrhosis or chronic liver disease.

11. Describe cirrhosis and contrast various types.
   Study text pages 1356-1360; refer to Figure
   36-17 and Table 36-9.

Cirrhosis is an irreversible inflammatory disease that disrupts liver structure and function. Structural changes result from fibrosis which is a consequence of inflammation. The parenchyma of the liver becomes distorted and biliary channels may be altered or obstructed leading to jaundice. Obstruction caused by cirrhosis can cause portal hypertension. These vascular changes compromise liver function further, and the process of regeneration fails as hypoxia, necrosis, and atrophy ultimately cause liver failure.

Cirrhosis of the Liver

	Cause	*Manifestations*
Alcoholic cirrhosis	Toxic effects of chronic and excessive alcohol intake, alcohol is oxidized by the liver to acetylaldehyde which damages hepatocytes	Typical, decreased sexual function
Primary biliary cirrhosis	Unknown, possibly an auto-immune mechanism that scars ducts	Typical, circulating IgG
Secondary biliary cirrhosis	Obstruction by neoplasms, strictures, or gallstones scar the ducts proximally	Typical
Post-necrotic cirrhosis	Viral hepatitis due to HAV or hepatitis C, drugs or other toxins, autoimmune destruction	Typical, small and distorted

Note: Typical manifestations include hepatomegaly, splenomegaly, jaundice, and complications identified in Objective 9. Serologic studies reveal elevated enzymes and bilirubin, decreased albumin, and prolonged prothrombin time.

12. Compare cholelithiasis to cholecystitis.
Study text pages 1360-1361; refer to Figure 36-18.

Obstruction and inflammation are the most common disorders of the gallbladder. Obstruction is caused by gallstones, which are aggregates of substances in the bile. The gallstones may remain in the gallbladder or enter the cystic duct. If gallstones become lodged in the cystic duct, they obstruct the flow of bile into and out of the gallbladder and cause inflammation. Gallstone formation is termed **cholelithiasis,** while inflammation of the gallbladder or cystic duct is known as **cholecystitis.**

Gallstones are of two types: cholesterol and pigmented. Cholesterol stones are the most common. Cholesterol gallstones form in bile that is supersaturated with cholesterol produced by the liver. Usually within the gallbladder, supersaturation sets the stage for cholesterol crystal formation and aggregation into "macrostones." If the stones become lodged in the cystic or common duct, they cause pain and cholecystitis. The reason the hepatocytes secrete bile that is supersaturated with cholesterol may involve cholesterol synthesis or decreased secretion of bile acids which promote cholesterol solubility. Pigmented stones occur later in life and are associated with cirrhosis. Pigmented stones are created by cholesterol, calcium bilirubinate, or pigmented polymers and are associated with biliary infection and increased amounts of unconjugated bilirubin in bile. The unconjugated bilirubin precipitates in the gallbladder or bile ducts as stones. Risk factors for cholelithiasis include obesity, middle age, female gender, American Indian ancestry, and gallbladder, pancreatic, or ileal disease.

Abdominal pain and jaundice are the cardinal manifestations of cholelithiasis. Vague symptoms include heartburn, flatulence, epigastric discomfort, and fatty food intolerances. Biliary colic pain is caused by the lodging of one or more gallstones in the cystic or common duct. The pain can be intermittent or steady and located in the right upper quadrant with radiation to the mid-upper back. Jaundice indicates that the stone is located in the common bile duct.

Laparoscopic cholecystectomy is the preferred treatment for gallstones that cause obstruction or inflammation. An alternative treatment is the administration of drugs that dissolve the stones.

Cholecystitis can be acute or chronic and is almost always caused by the lodging of a gallstone in the cystic duct. Obstruction causes the gallbladder to become distended and inflamed, followed by decreased blood flow, ischemia, necrosis, and possible perforation. Fever, leukocytosis, rebound tenderness, and abdominal muscle guarding are common findings. Serum bilirubin and alkaline phosphatase levels may be elevated.

13. Describe the pathogenesis of pancreatitis.

Study text pages 1361-1362.

Pancreatitis, or inflammation of the pancreas, is a relatively rare but potentially serious disorder. It is believed that **acute pancreatitis** develops because of an injury or disruption of the pancreatic ducts or acini that permits leakage of pancreatic enzymes into pancreatic tissue. The leaked enzymes initiate autodigestion and acute pancreatitis. Bile reflux into the pancreas occurs if gallstones obstruct the common bile duct; the refluxed bile also injures pancreatic tissue. The activated trypsin, elastase, and lipases destroy tissue and cell membranes, which causes edema, vascular damage, hemorrhage, and necrosis. Toxic enzymes also are released into the bloodstream and cause injury to vessels and other organs such as the lungs and kidneys. **Chronic pancreatitis** is caused by alcohol abuse.

Mild to severe epigastric or midabdominal pain is the cardinal symptom of acute pancreatitis. The pain may radiate to the back because of the retroperitoneal location of the pancreas. The pain is caused by distended pancreatic ducts and capsule, chemical irritation and inflammation of the peritoneum, and irritation or obstruction of the biliary tract. Fever and leukocytosis accompany the inflammatory response. Nausea and vomiting are caused by hypermotility or paralytic ileus secondary to the pancreatitis or peritonitis. Hypotension and shock frequently occur because plasma volume is lost as enzymes and kinins released into the circulation increase vascular permeability and dilate vessels. The results are hypovolemia, hypotension, and myocardial insufficiency. Elevated serum amylase is a characteristic diagnostic feature. The goal of treatment for acute pancreatitis is to stop the process of autodigestion and prevent systemic complications. Parenteral fluids are given to restore blood volume and prevent hypotension and shock. Severe, unremitting pancreatitis may require peritoneal lavage to remove toxic exudates or surgical drainage of the pancreas.

To correct enzyme deficiencies and prevent malabsorption, oral enzyme replacements are taken before and during meals. Cessation of alcohol intake is essential for the management of chronic pancreatitis.

14. Characterize the various cancers of the digestive system.

Study text pages 1362-1369; refer to Figures 36-19 through 36-21 and Tables 36-10 and 36-11.

Cancers of the Digestive System

	Risks	*Manifestations*

Esophagus
  Squamous cell carcinoma
  Adenocarcinoma
	Malnutrition, alcohol, tobacco, chronic reflux	Chest pain, dysphagia

Stomach
  Adenocarcinoma
  Squamous cell carcinoma
	Dietary salty foods, nitrates, nitrosamines, gastric atrophy	Anorexia, malaise, weight loss, upper abdominal pain, vomiting, occult blood, symptoms of organ involved in metastasis from stomach

Colorectal
  Adenocarcinoma
  (left colon grows in ring: right colon grows in mass)
	Chromosomal deletions, polyps, diverticulitis, ulcerative colitis, high refined CHO, low fiber/ high fat diet	Pain, anemia, bloody stool, mass - right colon, obstruction - left colon, distention, elevated CEA

Liver	HBV, HCV, HDV, cirrhosis, intestinal parasites, aflatoxin	Pain, anorexia, bloating, weight loss, portal hypertension, ascites, +/- jaundice, elevated serum proteins and enzymes

(Continued)

Cancers of the Digestive System *(cont'd)*

	Risks	*Manifestations*

Gall bladder
    Secondary metastases
    Adenocarcinoma
    Squamous cell carcinoma
	Cholelithiasis	Steady pain, diarrhea, anorexia, vomiting, +/- jaundice

Pancreas Adenocarcinoma	Chronic pancreatitis, cigarette smoking, alcohol, diabetic women	Weight loss, weakness, nausea, vomiting, abdominal pain, depression, +/- jaundice, possible hypoglycemia if an insulin-secreting tumor

Note: Treatment for esophageal, stomach, gallbladder and pancreatic cancer is essentially surgical. Liver neoplasms are treated by surgery and chemotherapy. Colorectal cancer therapy uses surgery, radiation, and chemotherapy.

Practice Examination

1. During vomiting, there is
   a. forceful diaphragm and abdominal muscle contractions, airway closure, esophageal sphincter relaxation, and deep inspiration.
   b. deep inspiration, airway closure, forceful diaphragm and abdominal muscle contractions, and esophageal sphincter relaxation.
   c. airway closure, forceful diaphragm and abdominal muscle contractions, deep inspiration, and esophageal sphincter relaxation.
   d. esophageal sphincter relaxation, forceful diaphragm and abdominal muscle contractions, deep inspiration, and airway closure.

2. Which does not cause constipation?
   a. opiates
   b. megacolon
   c. sedentary life style
   d. hyperthyroidism
   e. emotional depression

3. Osmotic diarrhea is caused by
   a. lactase deficiency.
   b. bacterial enterotoxins.
   c. ulcerative colitis.
   d. Crohn disease.
   e. Both c and d are correct.

4. Melena is
   a. bloody vomitus.
   b. gaseous bowel distension.
   c. blood in the stool.
   d. loss of appetite.

5. A common manifestation of hiatal hernia is
   a. gastroesophageal reflux.
   b. diarrhea.
   c. belching.
   d. postprandial substernal pain.
   e. Both a and d are correct.

6. Paralytic ileus is
   a. intestinal telescoping.
   b. protrusion of intestine through a weakened abdominal wall.
   c. inflamed saccular herniations.
   d. associated with abdominal surgery.
   e. None of the above is correct.

7. Intestinal obstruction causes
   a. decreased intraluminal tension.
   b. hyperkalemia.
   c. decreased nutrient absorption.
   d. Both a and b are correct.
   e. a, b, and c are correct.

8. Peptic ulcers may be located in the
   a. stomach.
   b. esophagus.
   c. duodenum.
   d. colon.
   e. a, b, and c are correct.

9. Gastric ulcers
   a. may lead to malignancy.
   b. occur at a younger age than duodenal ulcers.
   c. always have increased acid production.
   d. exhibit nocturnal pain.
   e. Both a and c are correct.

10. Duodenal ulcers
    a. occur four times more frequently in females than in males.
    b. may be complicated by life-threatening hemorrhage.
    c. are associated with sepsis.
    d. may cause inflammation and scar tissue formation around the sphincter of Oddi.

11. In malabsorption syndrome, flatulence and abdominal distension are likely caused by
    a. protein deficiency and electrolyte imbalance.
    b. undigested lactose fermentation by bacteria.
    c. fat irritating the bowel.
    d. impaired absorption of amino acids and accompanying edema.

12. The characteristic lesion of Crohn disease is
    a. found in the ileum.
    b. precancerous.
    c. granulomatous.
    d. malignant.
    e. Both a and c are correct.

13. Low-fiber diets play a role in the pathogenesis of
    a. appendicitis.
    b. diverticulitis.
    c. ulcerative colitis.
    d. Crohn disease.
    e. cholecystitis.

14. A 14-year-old male has been admitted to the emergency room suffering with acute onset abdominal pain in the lower right quadrant. Abdominal rebound tenderness is intense and he has a fever and leukocytosis. This individual most likely is suffering
    a. acute appendicitis.
    b. diverticulitis.
    c. ulcerative colitis.
    d. cholelithiasis.
    e. cholecystitis.

15. Adult-onset obesity is
    a. both hyperplastic and hypertrophic.
    b. dispersed over the entire body.
    c. hypertrophic.
    d. unrelated to genotype.
    e. None of the above is correct.

16. Short-term starvation involves
    a. glycogenolysis.
    b. gluconeogenesis.
    c. proteolysis.
    d. Both a and b are correct.
    e. a, b, and c are correct.

17. The most common manifestation of portal hypertension is
    a. rectal bleeding.
    b. cirrhosis.
    c. intestinal bleeding.
    d. duodenal bleeding.
    e. esophageal bleeding.

18. Hepatic encephalopathy is manifested by
    a. ascites.
    b. splenomegaly.
    c. dark urine.
    d. oliguria.
    e. cerebral dysfunction.

19. Which would be consistent with a diagnosis of viral hepatitis?
    1. elevated AST serum enzymes   a. 2, 3, 5
    2. decreased serum albumin levels   b. 1, 2, 5
    3. prolonged PT and PTT coagulation times   c. 1, 2, 3
    4. increased serum bilirubin levels   d. 1, 2, 3, 4
    5. decreased ALT serum enzymes   e. 1, 2, 3, 4, 5

20. Which viral hepatitis is not associated with a chronic state or a carrier state?
    a. hepatitis A
    b. hepatitis B
    c. hepatitis C
    d. serum hepatitis
    e. hepatitis D

21. Which type of jaundice is due to increased destruction of erythrocytes?
    a. obstructive
    b. hemolytic
    c. hepatocellular
    d. Both b and c are correct.

22. Which most often causes post-necrotic cirrhosis?
    a. malnutrition
    b. alcoholism
    c. hepatitis A or C
    d. autoimmunity
    e. biliary obstruction

23. Symptoms of cholelithiasis include all except
    a. nausea and vomiting.
    b. right upper quadrant tenderness.
    c. jaundice.
    d. decreased serum bilirubin levels.
    e. abdominal distress.

24. In pancreatitis,
    a. the tissue damage likely results from release of pancreatic enzymes.
    b. high cholesterol intake is causative.
    c. diabetes is uncommon in chronic pancreatitis.
    d. bacterial infection is the etiological cause.

25. Predisposing factors in the development of colon cancer include all except
    a. familial polyposis.
    b. ulcerative colitis.
    c. low fiber/high fat diet.
    d. high fiber diet.
    e. high refined CHO diet.

Case Study

Dr. R. is a 51-year-old male professor whose department chair is an unrelenting harasser. Dr. R.'s family investments have failed and his early planned retirement is no longer possible. Persistent upper abdominal pain for the last two months has convinced him that he needs a diagnostic work-up.

At the physician's office, Dr. R. revealed a history of smoking one pack of cigarettes a day for 25 years. His eating habits are irregular. However, he indicated a pain-antacid-relief pattern. The pain was more intense right after eating. He frequently takes aspirin for headaches and to relieve rheumatoid stiffness while golfing. His family and remaining history were unremarkable except that he had lost 10 pounds during the last six weeks.

Which type of peptic ulcer do you suspect? How could your suspicion be confirmed?

CHAPTER 37

Alterations of Digestive Function in Children

Prerequisite Objective

a. Describe the structure and function of the gastrointestinal tract and accessory organs of digestion. Refer to Figure 35-1.

Remember!

• See the study guide's narrative for Prerequisite Objective **a** in Chapter 36.

Objectives

After successful study of this chapter, the learner will be able to:

1. Describe the pathophysiology and treatment associated with cleft lip and palate.

Study text pages 1377-1378; refer to Figure 37-1.

Cleft lip is caused by incomplete fusion of the nasomedial or intermaxillary process during the second month of fetal development and occurs in approximately one in 1000 births, and the incidence of cleft palate is approximately one in 1250 births; cleft lip may occur with or without cleft palate. The defect in cleft lip usually is beneath one or both nostrils and may involve the external nose, nasal cartilages, nasal septum, and alveolar processes. It also may be associated with a flattening and broadening of the facial features probably due to the absence of constraining structures which are omitted by the cleft.

Cleft palate is frequently associated with cleft lip but can occur alone. The defect may affect only the uvula and soft palate but may extend forward toward the nostrils through the hard palate. If it extends through the hard palate, open communication between the structures of the nasopharynx and the oral cavity leads to frequent sinusitis and otitis media. In most cases, cleft lip and cleft palate are caused by genetic and nongenetic factors and each contributes only a minor developmental defect. These defects may be quite disfiguring and lead to psychological problems if not repaired. Another major difficulty seen with cleft lip or palate is poor feeding. Because suckling involves both the tongue and pressure against the palate, the infant with isolated cleft lip but an intact palate may breast or bottle feed without great difficulty. On the other hand, cleft palate may significantly interfere with breast or bottle feeding. Bottle feeding may require large, soft nipples with an oversized opening. Breast feeding may be impossible for some cleft palate infants without a prosthesis for the roof of the mouth. Treatment is surgical correction that is usually accomplished in stages. Supportive therapy may include prosthodontics and orthodontics, otarlaryngological procedures, and speech and occupational therapy.

290

2. Describe the structural defects of esophageal atresia and tracheoesophageal fistula.

Study text pages 1378-1379; refer to Figure 37-2.

Congenital malformations of the esophagus occur in approximately one in 3000 to 4500 births. **Esophageal atresia** is a condition where the esophagus ends in a blind pouch and may be accompanied by a connection between the esophagus and the trachea called a **tracheoesophageal fistula** (TEF). These conditions develop from aberrant differentiation of the trachea at four to six weeks' gestation. The blind esophageal pouch in atresia fills rapidly with secretions or food and overflows, which leads to persistent drooling, poor feeding, and aspiration. TEF generally causes immediate aspiration and distress on the first feeding. Thirty percent of children with this anomaly have other associated congenital defects, particularly cardiovascular defects. If the fistula is small, diagnosis may not be made until recurrent aspiration and pneumonias become problematic. Diagnosis is confirmed by the inability to pass a catheter into the stomach as the x-ray shows the catheter coiled at the level of the defect. Treatment is surgical correction.

3. Describe the structural defect and pathophysiology associated with pyloric stenosis.

Study text pages 1379-1380.

Pyloric stenosis is an obstruction of the pylorus because of hypertrophy of the pyloric sphincter. Obstruction becomes evident between one and two weeks or three to four months of age. Boys are affected five times more frequently than girls, and whites are more frequently affected than orientals or blacks. Pyloric stenosis is seen more frequently in full-term than in premature infants. Increased gastrin secretion in the mother tends to increase the probability of pyloric stenosis and may linked to maternal stress. Hereditary factors also may be involved. Generally, stenosis is manifested in a previously healthy infant who begins to have marked projectile vomiting at three to four weeks of age that does not resolve. Weight loss and dehydration follow and may end in death if intervention is not provided. Diagnosis is usually suspected on clinical manifestations and confirmed by ultrasonography or an upper gastrointestinal series that demonstrates the lesion. A small, muscular "olive" at the site of the hypertrophic pylorus may be palpable in the left upper quadrant of the abdomen. Treatment is surgical release of the hypertrophic fibers or pyloromyotomy after stabilization of the infant's fluid and electrolyte balance.

4. Describe congenital aganglionic megacolon or Hirschprung disease.

Study text pages 1382-1383; refer to Figure 37-3.

Congenital aganglionic megacolon or **Hirschprung disease** is a condition generally associated with failure of the parasympathetic nervous system to produce intramural ganglion cells in the enteric nerve plexuses. This failed innervation causes a section of the colon to be immotile and creates a functional intestinal obstruction in the affected area. This section becomes distended with feces, thus the name "megacolon." Eighty percent of these disorders are limited to the rectal end of the sigmoid colon. Hirschprung disease accounts for one-third of all intestinal obstructions in infants and occurs in one in 5000 births with a greater incidence in boys. Clinical manifestations are mild to severe chronic constipation, although diarrhea may be the first sign because only liquid may pass the aganglionic section. Severe edema of the colon begins to obstruct blood and lymphatic flow causing **enterocolitis** and tissue destruction. Bacteria can infiltrate the bowel wall from the lumen and may case gram-negative sepsis. Severe fluid and electrolyte imbalance caused by diarrhea may become life-threatening. Diagnosis is confirmed by rectal biopsy that demonstrates the aganglionic bowel. Measurement of rectal pressures or rectal manometry is frequently helpful during diagnosis. Definitive treatment consists of resection of the aganglionic segment and constant attention to bowel hygiene thereafter.

5. Describe intussusception.

Study text page 1384; refer to Figure 37-5.

Intussusception is the telescoping or invagination of one portion of the intestine into another that causes an intestinal obstruction. The most commonly affected area is the ileum that invaginates into the cecum through the ileocecal valve. Collapse is in the direction of peristaltic flow. Eighty to 90 percent of intestinal obstructions in infants and children are caused by intussusception, and boys are more commonly affected. Intussusception generally occurs between three and 35 months of age; 75 percent occur before one year of age. The pathophysiology of intussusception is like that of megacolon because the telescoping bowel obstructs blood and lymphatic flow which causes rapid edema and tissue necrosis. Gangrene may follow. The manifestation is usually accompanied by passage of dark and gelatinous or "currant jelly" stools. Diagnosis is made on clinical manifestations and confirmed by lower gastrointestinal contrast x-rays. Reduction of the intussusception must be done immediately and is frequently performed using hydrostatic pressure of the contrast media used for x-ray or an enema to push the invaginated bowel segment from its intussusception. This is successful 60 to 70 percent of the time, although some children require surgery to correct the intussusception or related complications. This condition is fatal if untreated.

6. Describe the pathophysiology and potential complications related to gastroesophageal reflux.
Study text page 1385.

Gastroesophageal reflux (GER) is the return of gastric contents into the esophagus because of poor function of the lower esophageal sphincter. GER is more common in premature than in term newborn infants and usually resolves by six to 12 months of age without significant effect on the infant. Some children may become symptomatic with GER and develop a number of complications including poor weight gain from vomiting and apnea and reactive airways probably from aspiration. GER has been implicated as a possible factor in sudden infant death syndrome (SIDS). The cause of GER is unknown, although delayed maturation of the sphincter or impaired hormonal response mechanisms are suspected. Other factors include location of the gastroesophageal junction and the angle of the junction and mucosal gathering. Clinical manifestations include forceful vomiting with an 85 percent occurrence within the first week of life, aspiration pneumonia in one-third of those affected, and poor weight gain. **Esophagitis** may result from exposure of the esophagus to acidic gastric contents that may cause either strictures or anemia from prolonged occult blood loss. Diagnosis may be made from clinical manifestations or confirmed by barium swallow or esophageal pH probe studies that demonstrate reflux with an abrupt drop in esophageal pH during the reflux episodes. Mild GER resolves without treatment, although some children require elevated

prone positioning after feedings to help reduce reflux. Pharmacologic therapies include medication to increase lower gastrointestinal motility and decrease gastric emptying time in an effort to decrease the opportunity for reflux of gastric contents; medications that decrease gastric acidity can be used. Surgical correction or fundoplication is rarely required.

7. Describe the gastrointestinal and digestive abnormalities associated with cystic fibrosis.
Study text pages 1385-1387; refer to Table 37-1.

Cystic fibrosis (CF) is a multisystem disease that is primarily manifested in the pancreas. The classic triad of pathophysiology of cystic fibrosis includes pancreatic enzyme deficiency leading to maldigestion, overproduction of mucus in the respiratory tract leading to chronic obstructive pulmonary disease, and elevated levels of sodium and chloride in sweat. Very viscous exocrine secretions tend to obstruct glandular ducts. Although pancreatic function may range from normal to virtually absent, 85 percent of children with CF have pancreatic insufficiency. The lack of pancreatic enzymes results in maldigestion of proteins, carbohydrates, and fats leading to chronic malnutrition. Pancreatic ducts also may be blocked with viscous secretions that eventually may damage pancreatic beta cells and lead to diabetes mellitus. Maldigestion of fats causes steatorrhea or fatty stools. Other complications include anemia, biliary cirrhosis, vitamin B_{12} deficiency, vitamin K deficiency, and rectal prolapse because of the passage of large, bulky stools. Pancreatic enzyme function may be estimated by 72-hour fecal fat measurement; fecal content of trypsin and chymotrypsin also may be measured. Pancreatic enzyme replacement may be administered with meals, and a high calorie/high protein diet is usually prescribed.

Practice Examination

True/False

____ 1. Pyloric stenosis is caused by the prolapse of gastric tissue into the pylorus that results in edema and obstruction.

____ 2. Tracheoesophageal fistula is often associated with esophageal atresia.

____ 3. Poor weight gain associated with gastroesophageal reflux may be ignored because it is a self-limiting disorder.

____ 4. Intussusception involves a blind pouch in the esophagus.

___ 5. "Currant jelly" stools are a common finding in cystic fibrosis.

___ 6. Increased gastric secretion in pregnant women may contribute to pyloric stenosis in their infants.

___ 7. Diabetes mellitus may be a complication of cystic fibrosis.

___ 8. The pharmacological approach to gastroesophageal reflux includes pancreatic enzyme replacement.

___ 9. Congenital aganglionic megacolon is the result of faulty innervation of the colon.

___ 10. The pharmacological approach to cystic fibrosis includes the administration of medications that increase lower gastrointestinal motility in an effort to aid passage of large, bulky stools.

___ 11. Rectal manometry is useful in the diagnosis of aganglionic megacolon.

Fill-in-the-Blank

12. _____ has been implicated as a possible factor in sudden infant death syndrome.

13. Congenital aganglionic megacolon is diagnosed by rectal manometry and rectal _____.

14. A pH probe will demonstrate a _____ in esophageal pH during a period of reflux.

15. Cleft palate is frequently complicated by infections such as _____ and _____.

16. _____ may be a complication of cystic fibrosis secondary to passing large stools.

Match the description with the alteration.

17. involve the rectal segment of the sigmoid colon
18. acute onset of abdominal pain and distention
19. respiratory distress after first feeding
20. may initially present with diarrhea
21. copious secretions/inability to feed
22. may contribute to reactive airways
23. seen more frequently in premature infants
24. "currant jelly" stools
25. enema may be treatment

a. congenital aganglionic megacolon
b. tracheoesophageal fistula
c. intussusception
d. gastroesophageal reflux
e. esophageal atresia

Case Study

Baby B. is a full-term infant male born vaginally to a 21-year-old white woman; he is her first child. The pregnancy was complicated by moderate maternal hypertension during the last week of pregnancy. The mother was taking no medication and the family history is normal. A nurse practitioner is called to see the infant four hours after birth because he is feeding poorly; he initially took approximately 15 cc of glucose water after birth but vomited afterwards and has been "spitty" since. Baby B.'s initial physical examination is essentially normal, although he does have moderate amounts of saliva frequently exiting his mouth that occasionally require suctioning. He is not experiencing respiratory distress. His glucose levels are low.

Since Baby B. is not in respiratory distress, why is he having difficulty dealing with his secretions and what is causing his low blood sugar?

CHAPTER 38

Structure and Function of the Musculoskeletal System

Objectives

After successful study of this chapter, the learner will be able to:

1. **Identify the function and structural elements of bone.**
   Review text pages 1405-1408; refer to Table 38-1.

2. **Describe the features of compact and spongy bone; classify bones.**
   Review text pages 1408-1410; refer to Figures 38-1 through 38-3.

3. **Describe the process of bone remodeling and healing.**
   Review text pages 1410-1412; refer to Figure 38-4 and Tables 38-2 and 38-3.

4. **Structurally and functionally, classify joints; characterize articular cartilage.**
   Review text pages 1412-1418; refer to Figures 38-5 through 38-10.

5. **Describe the arrangements of muscle fiber in a skeletal muscle; explain the structure and function of a motor unit.**
   Review text pages 1419-1425; refer to Figures 38-12 through 38-15 and Tables 38-4 and 38-5.

6. **Describe skeletal muscle contraction at the molecular level.**
   Review text pages 1425-1426.

7. **Identify the energy sources for muscular contraction.**
   Review text pages 1426-1427; refer to Table 38-6.

8. **Indicate the types of skeletal muscle contractions and the interaction between groups of muscles.**
   Review text pages 1427-1428.

9. **Describe the changes in the musculoskeletal system that accompany normal aging.**
   Review text pages 1429-1430.

Practice Examination

1. The skeletal system
   1. supports tissues.
   2. binds organs together.
   3. protects CNS structures.
   4. participates in blood cell formation.
   5. lines body cavities.

   a. 1, 2, 3
   b. 2, 3, 4
   c. 2, 4, 5
   d. 1, 3, 4
   e. 1, 2, 3, 4, 5

2. Alphaglycoprotein
   a. promotes resorption.
   b. binds calcium.
   c. stabilizes the basement membrane of bones.
   d. promotes calcification.

Match the microscopic feature of bone with its description.

3. haversian canal
4. trabecular
5. lamellae

a. small canals that connect bone cells
b. concentric rings
c. cavities where bone cells are housed
d. contains blood vessels
e. irregular meshwork

6. The diaphysis is the
   a. rounded end of long bones.
   b. shaft of long bones.
   c. lattice framework of spongy bones.
   d. surface of a synovial cavity.

7. A function of the epiphyseal plate that is not a function of the articular cartilage is to
   a. enable articulation of bones.
   b. enable bone to increase in length.
   c. repair damaged bone tissue.
   d. provide sensory nerves to bone.

8. The remodeling of bone is done by basic multicellular units that consist of bone precursor cells. Precursor cells
   a. differentiate into osteoclasts and osteoblasts.
   b. are located on free surfaces of bone and along vascular channels.
   c. Neither a nor b is correct.
   d. Both a and b are correct.

9. The sequence of bone healing in fractures and surgical injuries is
   1. proccallus formation.
   2. callus formation.
   3. hematoma formation.
   4. callus replacement with lamellar or trabecular bone.
   5. periosteum and endosteum remodeling.

   a. 2, 1, 3, 4, 5
   b. 3, 1, 2, 4, 5
   c. 3, 2, 1, 4, 5
   d. 1, 2, 3, 4, 5
   e. 1, 2, 3, 5, 4

10. Joints are classified functionally and structurally. Which is a proper function and structural relationship?
    a. amphiarthrosis/fibrous
    b. diarthrosis/synovial
    c. synarthrosis/synchondrosis
    d. diarthrosis/fibrous
    e. synarthrosis/cartilaginous

11. In older individuals, the bone remodeling cycle
    a. is faster because osteoclastic activity is enhanced.
    b. is enhanced because mineralization increases.
    c. has more precursor cells.
    d. has fewer precursor cells because the bone marrow becomes infiltrated with fat.
    e. Both a and b are correct.

12. When an individual spreads his or her fingers, the movement is
    a. hypertension.
    b. adduction.
    c. flexion.
    d. abduction.
    e. extension.

13. The perimysium is to a fasciculus as the
    a. periosteum is to a bone.
    b. muscle is to epimysium.
    c. myofibril is to a muscle fiber.
    d. epimysium is to the endomysium.
    e. muscle cell is to the endomysium.

Match the microscopic feature of muscle fibers with its description.

14. sarcomere
15. sarcolemma
16. sarcoplasmic reticulum

    a. membrane covering the muscle fiber
    b. flattened, tube-like network
    c. stacks of myofilaments, unit of contraction
    d. calcium transport system
    e. tube-like structure that runs perpendicular to muscle fibers.

17. Which is not a characteristic of type I muscle fibers?
    a. sparse capillary supply
    b. slow contraction speed
    c. high resistance to fatigue
    d. profuse capillary supply
    e. oxidative metabolism

18. Which protein is found in the thick myofilaments?
    a. actin
    b. myosin
    c. troponin
    d. tropomyosin
    e. a, c, and d are correct.

19. An important function of the T-tubule is to
    a. provide organic nutrients to muscle fibers.
    b. initiate fiber contraction.
    c. enable regeneration of muscle fibers.
    d. carry the electrical action potential deeper into the muscle fiber.

20. The cation necessary for cross-bridging is
    a. sodium.
    b. calcium.
    c. potassium.
    d. magnesium.
    e. phosphate.

296

21. Aerobic respiration
    a. permits the body brief periods during which it does not require oxygen.
    b. causes an increase in the amount of lactic acid.
    c. yields more molecules of ATP than anaerobic respiration.
    d. uses more glycogen to produce ATP than anaerobic respiration.
    e. leads to oxygen debt.

22. Repayment of oxygen debt
    a. converts lactic acid to glycogen.
    b. replenishes ATP stores.
    c. replenishes phosphocreatine stores.
    d. Both b and c are correct.
    e. a, b, and c are correct.

23. The strength of muscle contraction depends on the
    a. extent of the load.
    b. initial length of muscle fibers.
    c. recruitment of additional motor units.
    d. nerve innervation ratios.
    e. All of the above are correct.

24. Attempting to push an object too heavy to move is an example of a/an _____ contraction.
    a. isotonic
    b. concentric
    c. flaccid
    d. tetanic
    e. isometric

25. Which does not happen with muscle as individuals grow older?
    a. A reduction of the size of motor units occurs.
    b. Up to 30 percent of skeletal muscles may be lost by age 80.
    c. The synthesis of acetylcholine increases to compensate for muscle bulk loss.
    d. a, b, and c all occur with advancing age.

Alterations of Musculoskeletal Function

Prerequisite Objectives

a. Describe the processes that maintain bone integrity.
   Review text pages 1410-1412.

Remember!

- The internal structure of bone is maintained by a remodeling process in which existing bone is resorbed and new bone is laid down to replace it. Remodeling is accomplished by clusters of bone cells termed basic multicellular units. These units are made up of bone precursor cells located on the free surfaces of bones and along the vascular channels and marrow cavities. The precursor cells differentiate into osteoclasts and osteoblasts.

- In the first phase of the remodeling cycle, a stimulus such as hormone, drug, vitamin, or physical stressor activates the osteoclasts. In phase two, the osteoclasts resorb bone and leave in its place an elongated cavity termed a resorption cavity. The resorption cavity in compact bone follows the longitudinal axis of the haversian system; whereas in spongy bone the resorption cavity parallels the surface of the trabeculae. In phase three, new bone or secondary bone is laid down by osteoblasts lining the walls of the resorption cavity. In compact bone, successive layers are laid down until the resorption cavity is reduced to a narrow haversian canal around a blood vessel. This process destroys old haversian systems and forms new haversian systems. New trabeculae are formed in spongy bone.

- The remodeling process is capable of repairing microscopic bone injuries, but gross injuries such as fractures and surgical wounds heal by a different process. In bone wound healing, the stages are as follows:

  1. Hematoma formation occurs when damaged vessels hemorrhage. Fibrin and platelets within the hematoma form a meshwork. Hematopoietic growth factors such as platelet-derived growth factor and transforming growth factor are involved in this stage.

  2. Procallus formation occurs as fibroblasts, capillary buds, and osteoblasts move into the wound and produce granulation tissue; this is the procallus. Enzymes and growth factors aid in this stage of healing.

(Continued)

Remember! *(cont'd)*

3. Callus formation occurs as osteoblasts in the procallus form membranous or woven bone. Enzymes increase the phosphate content and it joins with calcium as a deposit of mineral which hardens the callus.

4. Osteoblasts continue to replace the callus with either lamellar bone or trabecular bone.

5. Synthesis of type I bone collagen predominates at this stage. This final remodeling stage is vital to ensure good mechanical properties for weight bearing and mobility.

---

b. Describe the types of joints.
   Review text pages 1412-1418; refer to Figures 38-5 through 38-10.

Remember!

- Joints are classified by the degree of movement they permit or by the connecting tissues that hold them together. Based on movement, a joint is classified as a (1) synarthrosis or an immovable joint, (2) an amphiarthrosis or a slightly movable joint, or (3) a diarthrosis or a freely movable joint. On the basis of connective structures, joints are classified as fibrous, cartilaginous, or synovial.

- A joint united directly to bone by fibrous connective tissues is called a fibrous joint. Generally, fibrous joints are synarthroses, or immovable, but many fibrous joints allow some movement. The degree of movement depends on the distance between the bones and the flexibility of the fibrous connective tissue.

- There are two types of cartilaginous joints or amphiarthroses. A symphysis is a cartilaginous joint in which bones are united by a pad or disk of fibrocartilage. The articulating surfaces are usually covered by a thin layer of hyaline cartilage and a thick pad of fibrocartilage which acts as a shock absorber and stabilizer. Examples of symphyses are the symphysis pubis and the intervertebral discs. A synchondrosis is a joint in which hyaline cartilage connects the two bones. The joints between the ribs and the sternum are synchondroses. Slight movement at the synchondroses between the ribs and the sternum allows the chest to move outward and upward during breathing.

- Synovial joints or diarthroses are the most movable and complex joints in the body. A synovial joint consists of a fibrous joint capsule or articular capsule, a synovial membrane, a joint cavity or synovial cavity, synovial fluid, and an articular cartilage. The joint capsule consists of parallel, interlacing bundles of dense, white fibrous tissue. It has a rich supply of nerves, blood vessels, and lymphatic vessels. The nerves are sensitive to the rate and direction of motion, compression, tension, vibration, and pain.

- The synovial membrane is the smooth, delicate inner lining of the joint capsule. It lines the nonarticular portion of the synovial joint and any ligaments or tendons that traverse the joint cavity. The synovial membrane is capable of rapid repair and regeneration.

- The joint cavity or synovial cavity is an enclosed, fluid-filled space between the articulating surfaces of the two bones that enables the two bones to move "against" one another. Synovial fluid within the cavity lubricates the joint surfaces, nourishes the pad of the articular cartilage, and contains free-floating synovial cells and various leukocytes that phagocytose joint debris and microorganisms.

- Articular cartilage is a layer of hyaline cartilage that covers the end of each bone. The function of articular cartilage is to reduce friction and to distribute the weight-bearing forces. Articular cartilage has no blood vessels, lymph vessels, or nerves. Therefore, it is insensitive to pain and regenerates slowly and minimally after injury. Regeneration occurs primarily at sites where the articular cartilage meets the synovial membrane.

---

c. Define terms associated with muscle fibers.
Review text pages 1420-1425; refer to Figures 38-12 through 38-15.

Remember!

- Each anterior horn cell, its axon, and the innervated muscle fibers is called a **motor unit**. The motor unit behaves as a single entity and contracts as a whole when it receives an adequate electrical impulse. A **muscle fiber** is a single muscle cell. This long cell is cylindrical in structure surrounded by a membrane capable of excitation and impulse propagation. The muscle fiber contains bundles of **myofibrils** in a parallel arrangement along the longitudinal axis of the muscle. The myofibrils contain **sarcomeres** that are the actual contracting units. The sarcomeres consist of **actin** and **myosin** which are the contractile proteins.

- Besides the myofibrils, the major components of the muscle fiber include the muscle membrane, sarcotubular system, sarcoplasm, and mitochondria. The muscle membrane is a two-part membrane. It includes the **sarcolemma** which contains the plasma membrane of the muscle cell and the cell's **basement membrane**. At the motor nerve endplate, where the nerve impulse is transmitted, the sarcolemma forms the highly convoluted **synaptic cleft**. The protein systems of the sarcolemma transport nutrients and synthesize proteins. They also provide the sodium-potassium pump and include the cell's cholinergic receptor. The basement membrane serves as the cell's microskeleton and maintains the shape of the muscle cell.

- The **sarcoplasm** is the cytoplasm of the muscle cell and contains numerous enzymes and proteins that are responsible for the cell's energy production, protein synthesis, and oxygen storage. Unique to the muscle is the **sarcotubular system** which includes the **transverse tubules** and the **sarcoplasmic reticulum**. The sarcoplasmic reticulum is involved in calcium transport that initiates muscle contraction at the sarcomere. The sarcoplasmic reticulum is composed of tubules that run parallel to the myofibrils and are termed sarcotubules. The transverse tubules are closely associated with the sarcotubules and run across the sarcoplasm and communicate with the extracellular space. Both tubules allow for intracellular calcium uptake, regulation, release during muscle contraction, and storage of calcium during muscle relaxation.

---

d. Identify the major events of muscle contraction and relaxation.
Review text pages 1425-1427; refer to Figures 26-17 and 38-15.

Remember!

Major Events of Muscle Contraction and Relaxation

Excitation and Contraction

A nerve impulse reaches the end of a motor neuron and releases acetylcholine
↓

Acetylcholine diffuses across the neuromuscular junction and binds to acetylcholine receptors on the muscle fiber
↓

Stimulation of acetylcholine receptors initiates an impulse that travels along the sarcolemma, through the T-tubules, and to the sarcoplasmic reticulum
↓

Calcium is released from the sarcoplasmic reticulum into the sarcoplasm; calcium binds to troponin molecules in the thin myofilaments
↓

Tropomyosin molecules shift to expose actin's active engagement sites

(Continued)

Remember! *(cont'd)*

↓

Energized myosin cross-bridges of the thick myofilaments bind to actin and use their ATP energy to pull the thin myofilaments toward the center of each sarcomere

↓

As the thin filaments slide past the thick myofilaments, the entire muscle fiber shortens

Relaxation

After the impulse passes, the sarcoplasmic reticulum begins actively pumping calcium back into the sarcoplasm

↓

As calcium leaves the troponin molecules of the thin myofilaments, tropomyosin returns to its position and blocks actin's active engagement sites

↓

Myosin cross-bridges cannot bind to actin and can no longer sustain the contraction

↓

The thick and thin myofilaments are no longer connected, so the muscle fiber returns to its longer, resting length

---

Objectives

After successful study of this chapter, the learner will be able to:

1. Compare the types of fractures; describe the manifestations and treatment of fractures.

Study text pages 1435-1439; refer to Figures 39-1 through 39-5 and Table 39-1.

Fractures are classified as complete or incom-
plete and open or closed. In a **complete** fracture, the bone is broken all the way through; whereas, in an **incomplete** fracture, the bone is damaged but remains one piece. Complete or incomplete fractures also are considered **open** if the skin is broken or as **closed** if it is not. Fractures also are classified according to the direction of the fracture line. A fracture wherein the bone breaks into two or more fragments is termed a **comminuted** fracture.

Types of Fractures

	Characteristic	*Cause*
Common Fractures		
Open Fracture	Communicating wound between bone and skin	Moderate to severe energy that exceeds tissue tolerance
Oblique Fracture	Fracture line at 45° angle to long axis of bone	Angulation and compressive energy
Spiral Fracture	Fracture line encircling bone	Twisting energy with distal part unable to move
		(Continued)

Types of Fractures (cont'd)

	Characteristic	*Cause*
Transverse Fracture	Fracture line perpendicular to long axis of bone	Energy directly toward bone
Impacted	Fracture fragments are pushed into each other	Compressive energy directly to distal fragment
Pathologic	Fracture occurs at any point in the bone	Minor energy to already weakened bone
Common Incomplete Fractures		
Greenstick Fracture	Break on one cortex of bone with spongy bone splintering	Minor direct or indirect energy in children or elderly
Stress Fracture	Microfracture	Bone is subjected to repeated stress beyond its strength, muscles are stronger than bone

The signs and symptoms of a fracture include unnatural alignment, swelling, muscle spasm, tenderness, pain, and impaired sensation. The immediate pain of a fracture is severe and usually due to the traumatic injury. Subsequent pain often is produced by muscle spasm. Numbness is caused by the pinching of a nerve by the trauma or by bone fragments. Pathologic fractures are not usually associated with trauma or trauma-related pain. Stress fractures are painful because of accelerated remodeling and are usually relieved by rest. Range of motion in the joint is limited and movement may evoke audible clicking sounds or crepitus.

Fracture treatment involves realigning the bone fragments to their normal or anatomic position and holding the fragments in place so that bone union can occur. Several methods are available to reduce or align a fracture, including closed manipulation, traction, and open surgical reduction. Splints and plaster casts are used to immobilize and hold a reduction in place. Improper reduction or immobilization of a fractured bone may result in nonunion, delayed union, or malunion.

2. Define terms associated with skeletal system stress.

Study text pages 1440-1445; refer to Figures 39-6 and 39-7 and Table 39-2.

Dislocation is the temporary displacement of two bones in which the articular cartilage loses contact entirely. If the contact between the surfaces is only partially lost, the injury is called **subluxation.** Dislocations and subluxations are often accompanied by fracture. As the bone separates from the joint, it may bruise or tear adjacent nerves, blood vessels, ligaments, supporting structures, and soft tissue.

A tear in a tendon is a **strain.** Major trauma or excessive stress can tear a tendon at any site in the body. The tendons of the hands, feet, knee, upper arm, thigh, ankle, and heel are frequently injured sites. Ligament tears are known as **sprains.** Ligaments tears and ruptures can occur at any joint but are most common in the wrist, ankle, elbow, and knee joints. A complete separation of a tendon or ligament from its attachment is an **avulsion.** An avulsion is the result of abnormal stress on the ligament or tendon and is commonly seen in young athletes, especially sprinters, hurdlers, and runners.

Trauma can also cause painful inflammation of tendons or **tendinitis** and bursae or **bursitis.** Besides trauma, causes of tendinitis include crystal deposits, postural misalignment, and hypermobility in a joint. **Epicondylitis** is inflammation of a tendon where it attaches to a bone. Examples of epicondylitis include tennis elbow, which is an inflammation of the lateral epicondyle of the humerus, and medial epicondylitis, which is referred to as golfer's elbow. Acute **bursitis** occurs primarily in the middle years and is caused by repeated trauma. Septic bursitis is caused by wound infection or bacterial infection of the skin overlying the bursae. The shoulder is the most common site of bursitis.

Muscle strain is often the result of sudden, forced motion causing the muscle to become stretched beyond its normal capacity. Muscles are injured more often than tendons in young people; the opposite is true in older populations. Regardless of the cause of trauma, muscle cells are usually able to regenerate, although regeneration may take up to six weeks.

Myositis ossificans is thought to be caused by scar tissue calcification and subsequent ossification. An example is seen in football players after injury to thigh muscles.

Myoglobinuria can be a life-threatening complication of severe muscle trauma manifested by excess myoglobin, an intracellular muscle protein, in the urine. Muscle damage releases the myoglobin. The most severe form is often called crush syndrome. Less severe and more localized forms are called compartment syndromes, which can lead to Volkmann ischemic contracture in the forearm or leg. Crush syndrome first gained notoriety in injuries seen following the London air raids in World War II. More recently, it has been reported in individuals found unresponsive because of drug overdoses and those who are immobile for long periods of time. Myoglobinuria can also be seen following viral infections, administration of certain anesthetic agents, strychnine poisoning, tetanus, excessive muscular activity, heat stroke, electrolyte disturbances, fractures, status epilepticus, electroconvulsive therapy, and high-voltage electrical shock.

3. Differentiate between osteoporosis, osteomalacia, Paget disease, and osteomyelitis.
Study text pages 1445-1452; refer to Figures 39-8 through 39-10.

Common Disorders of Bone

	Cause	Pathophysiology	Manifestations
Osteoporosis	Decreased levels of estrogen and testosterone, reduced physical activity lessens muscle stress on bone, insufficient calcium, corticosteroid use	Reduced bone mass or density, imbalance in bone resorption and formation	Pain and bone deformity, fracture, increased radiolucency
Osteomalacia (adult) Rickets (children)	Deficiency of vitamin D lowers absorption of calcium from intestines	Inadequate and delayed mineralization, osteoid tissue is not mineralized	Pain, bone fractures, vertebral collapse, radiolucent bands perpendicular to bone surface, pseudofracture
Paget disease	Unknown	Excessive resorption of spongy bone followed by accelerated formation of softened bone	Thickening of bones, radiographic findings of irregular bone trabeculae with thickened and disorganized patterns
Osteomyelitis	Most often a staphylococcal infection, contaminated open wound	Acute inflammation of marrow and bone, necrosis	Acute and chronic inflammation, fever, pain, lymphadenopathy, necrotic bone by radionuclide bone scanning

4. **Classify bone tumors by tissue of origin, whether benign or malignant, and their pattern of bone destruction.**

Study text pages 1452-1458; refer to Figures 39-11 through 39-15 and Table 39-3.

Bone tumors may originate from bone cells, cartilage, fibrous tissue, marrow, or vascular tissue. On the basis of mesodermal tissue of origin, bone tumors are classified as osteogenic, chondrogenic, collagenic, or myelogenic. The mesoderm contributes to primitive fibroblasts and reticulum cells. The fibroblast is the progenitor of the osteoblast, the chondroblast, and the fibrous connective tissue cell.

Benign bone tumors destroy small areas of bone, tend to be limited to the anatomic confines of the host bone, and have a well-demarcated border. Benign bone tumors push against neighboring tissue, have a symmetrical, controlled growth pattern, and tend to compress and displace neighboring normal bone tissue which weakens the bone's structure until it leads to pathologic fracture.

The geographic pattern, the moth-eaten pattern, and the permeative pattern are patterns of bone destruction in bone tumors. Tumors exhibiting the geographic pattern have well-defined margins that can be easily separated from the surrounding normal bone. There is a uniform and well-defined lytic area in the bone of these benign lesions.

In the moth-eaten pattern, the tumorous lesion has a less-defined or demarcated margin that cannot be easily separated from normal bone. Areas of partially destroyed bone adjacent to completely lytic areas are found. This pattern of bone destruction is characteristic of rapidly growing, malignant bone tumors. An aggressive, malignant tumor causes the permeative pattern of bone destruction. The margins of the tumor are poorly demarcated and abnormal bone merges with surrounding normal bone tissue. Malignant bone tumors tend to be large and aggressive in their bone destruction, to invade surrounding tissue, and to metastasize.

Origin of Benign and Malignant Bone Tumors

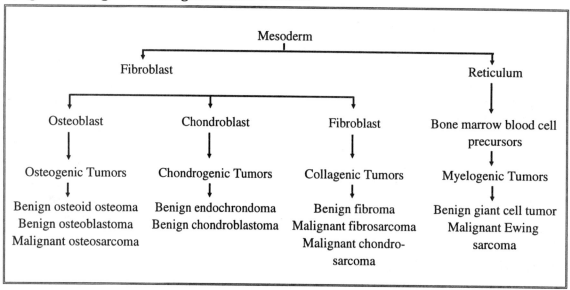

Note: Diagnosis depends on serum metabolite and enzyme levels, radiologic studies, CT scans, MRI, blood counts, and biopsy.

5. **Characterize the common types of bone tumors.**

Study text pages 1454-1458.

Osteosarcomas or osteogenic tumors account for 38 percent of bone tumors and occur more frequently in males than in females. Adolescents and young adults are the predominant victims. In the 50 to 60 age group, individuals with a history of Paget disease and radiation therapy also develop osteosarcomas.

Osteosarcoma is a malignant bone-forming tumor that is large and destructive and most often found in bone marrow; it has a moth-eaten pattern of bone destruction. Osteosarcomas always contain osteoid and callus and also may contain chondroid and fibrinoid tissue. The osteoid is deposited between the trabeculae of the callus. The "streamers" of osteoid infiltrate the normal compact bone, destroy it, and replace it with dense callus and masses of osteoid. The bone tissue never matures to compact bone. Ninety percent of osteosarcomas are located in the metaphyses of long bones. Fifty percent of osteosarcomas occur around the knee area. The tumor breaks through the cortex, lifts the periosteum, and forms a soft tissue mass that is not covered by new bone.

Common initial symptoms are pain and swelling;

pain is usually worse at night. Systemic symptoms are uncommon. Surgery is a major treatment of choice. The location of the tumor, its size, malignancy grade, and evidence of metastasis dictate the type and extent of surgery. Preoperative chemotherapy has increased the number of individuals whose limbs can be saved. Chemotherapy can be given both preoperatively and postoperatively.

Chondrosarcoma, a chondrogenic tumor, is a tumor of middle-aged and older adults. A chondrosarcoma is a large, ill-defined malignant tumor that infiltrates trabeculae in spongy bone. It occurs most often in the metaphysis or diaphysis of long bones. The tumor contains large lobules of hyaline cartilage that are separated by bands of fibrous tissue and anaplastic cells. It expands and enlarges the contour of the bone, causes extensive erosion of the cortex, and expands into the soft tissues.

Symptoms associated with the chondrosarcoma have an insidious onset. Local swelling and pain are usual symptoms. At first, the pain is intermittent; then, it gradually intensifies and becomes constant. Surgical excision is generally regarded as the treatment of choice; however, individuals demonstrate recurrences and so amputation is considered.

Fibrosarcoma, a malignant collagenic tumor, is seen in middle-aged adults. It is a solitary tumor that most frequently affects the metaphyseal region of the femur or tibia. The tumor is composed of a firm, fibrous mass of tissue containing collagen, malignant fibroblasts, and occasional osteoclast-like giant cells. Pain and swelling are the usual symptoms and indicate that the tumor has broken through the cortex. Local tenderness, a palpable mass, limitation of motion, or a pathologic fracture are other symptoms and signs. Radical surgery and amputation are the treatments of choice for fibrosarcoma.

Giant cell tumors have a wide age distribution with the majority found in persons between 20 and 40 years of age. Unlike most other bone tumors, giant cell tumors affect females more frequently than males.

The giant cell tumor is a solitary, circumscribed tumor that causes extensive bone resorption because of its osteoclastic origin. The tumor is rich in osteoclast-like giant cells and anaplastic stromal cells and is found in the center of the epiphysis in the femur, tibia, radius, or humerus. The tumor has a slow, relentless growth rate and is usually contained within the original contour of the affected bone. It may extend into the articular cartilage. It has recurrence rate as high as 80 percent.

The most common symptoms associated with the giant cell tumor are pain, local swelling, and limitation of movement. Cryosurgery and resection of the tumor decrease recurrence and are more successful treatments than curettage and radiation; amputation may be necessary.

Myeloma is a malignant neoplastic proliferation of plasma cells; incomplete antibodies are formed. The tumor may be solitary or multifocal. If multifocal, it is known as a multiple myeloma. The myeloma is common in persons over 40 years of age and affects males twice as frequently as females; blacks have a higher incidence rate than whites.

Myelomas cause cortical and medullary bone lysis and infiltrate the bone marrow. The most common symptom of myeloma is pain that is initially aching, intermittent, and aggravated by weight bearing. As the disease progresses, the pain becomes severe and prolonged. Myeloma has a poor prognosis and the treatment is generally palliative. Radiotherapy and chemotherapy have very limited success.

6. Compare osteoarthritis to rheumatoid arthritis; characterize other inflammatory joint diseases.

Study text pages 1458-1471; refer to Figures 39-16 through 39-21.

Noninflammatory and Inflammatory Joint Disease

	Osteoarthritis	*Rheumatoid arthritis*
Pathologic Feature	Noninflammatory, loss of proteoglycans from articular cartilage in synovial joints, bone sclerosis, bone spurs	Inflammatory, damage or destruction of synovial membrane, extends to articular cartilage joint capsule and surrounding ligaments and tendons, pannus *(Continued)*

	Osteoarthritis	*Rheumatoid arthritis*
Onset Age	> 40, increases with age, equal sex distinction	Middle age, prevalence in females
Risk Factors	Primary: autosomal recessive Secondary: joint stress, congenital abnormalities, joint instability	Genetics, environmental
Joints Affected	Peripheral and central, weight bearing	Phalangeal, wrists, knee
Joint Fluid	Proteoglycans/fragments, normal mucin, few cells	Inflammatory exudate, poor mucin
Cause	Cytokines, collagenases	Microbial invasion, autoimmunity
Manifestations	Pain, stiffness, enlargement, tenderness, limited motion, muscle wasting, dislocation, deformity	Same as OA with systemic involvement, synovial, and subcutaneous modules, deviation of joints, rheumatoid factor and circulating immune complexes

Ankylosing spondylitis is a chronic, inflammatory joint disease characterized by stiffening and fusion or ankylosis of the spine and sacroiliac joints. Like rheumatoid arthritis, ankylosing spondylitis is a systemic, immune inflammatory disease. The disease is strongly associated with the presence of histocompatibility antigen HLA-B27 on the chromosomes of affected individuals; this suggests a genetic predisposition to the disease. In ankylosing spondylitis, the primary pathologic site is at the point where ligaments, tendons, and the joint capsule are inserted into bone rather than in the synovial membrane as in rheumatoid arthritis. The end result of ankylosing spondylitis is fibrosis, ossification, and fusion of the joint.

Ankylosing spondylitis begins with inflammation of fibrocartilage in cartilaginous joints, particularly in the vertebrae. As inflammatory cells infiltrate and erode fibrocartilage in joint structures, repair begins to occur. Repair begins with the proliferation of fibroblasts. The collagen synthesized by fibroblasts becomes organized into fibrous scar tissue. Eventually, the scar tissue calcifies and ossifies. With time, all the cartilaginous structures of the joint are replaced by ossified scar tissue and the joints fuse or lose flexibility.

The most common symptoms of early ankylosing spondylitis are low back pain and stiffness. The pain, initially is insidious but progressively becomes persistent. Forward flexion, rotation, and lateral flexion of the spine are restricted and painful. As the disease progresses, the individual becomes increasingly stooped. The thoracic spine becomes rounded, the head and neck are held forward on the shoulders, and the hips are flexed. Along with low back pain, many individuals may have peripheral joint involvement, uveitis or inflammation of eye structures, fibrotic changes in the lungs, cardiomegaly, aortic incompetence, amyloidosis, and Achilles tendinitis.

Treatment of individuals with ankylosing spondylitis consists of physical therapy to maintain skeletal mobility and prevent the natural progression of contractures. Anti-inflammatory and analgesic medications are prescribed to suppress some of the pain and stiffness and to facilitate exercise. Surgical procedures and radiotherapy are sometimes used to provide relief for individuals with end-stage disease or intolerable deformity.

Gout is a metabolic disorder that disrupts the body's control of uric acid production or excretion. High levels of uric acid accumulate in the blood and in other body fluids including synovial fluid. When the uric acid reaches a certain concentration in fluids, it crystallizes. The crystals are deposited in connective tissues throughout the body.

When crystallization occurs in synovial fluid, painful inflammation of the joint develops. This condition is known as gouty arthritis. With time, crystal deposition in subcutaneous tissues causes the formation of small, white nodules or **tophi** and their inflammatory sequelae. Crystal aggregates deposited in the kidneys can form urate renal stones and lead to renal failure. In classic **gouty arthritis**, inflammation of the joint is caused by the formation of monosodium urate crystals. In **pseudogout**, the crystals are of calcium pyrophosphate-dihydrate. Either crystal causes the onset of acute inflammatory response.

Approximately 95 percent of affected individuals, almost always men, have **primary gout** wherein the hyperuricemia is due to an overproduction of uric acid. The defect in primary gout in unknown but is likely an inherited enzyme defect. In **secondary gout**, the hyperuricemia is the result of an acquired chronic disease or a drug that interferes with balance between production and excretion of uric acid. Hyperuricemia from overproduction of uric acid can be due to increased metabolic processes such as leukemia, increased cellular breakdown like hemolytic anemia, neoplastic processes, and genetic metabolic disorders in which hyperuricemia is just one of many clinical manifestations. Diuretics are thought to cause secondary gout as they decrease the renal tubular excretion of urate. Chronic renal disease, hypertension, and starvation also decrease uric acid excretion.

The pathophysiology of gout is closely linked to purine metabolism, cellular metabolism of purines, and kidney function. Uric acid is a break down product of purine nucleotides. Some individuals with gout have an accelerated rate of purine synthesis and other individuals break down purine nucleotides at a accelerated rate. Both conditions result in an overproduction of uric acid. Kidney function is involved in the pathophysiology of gout because most uric acid is eliminated from the body through the kidneys. Urate undergoes both reabsorption and excretion within the renal tubules. Sluggish urate excretion by the kidney may be caused by decreased glomerular filtration of urate or an acceleration in urate reabsorption.

The presence of urate crystals anywhere triggers the acute inflammatory response as the neutrophils are attracted to phagocytose the crystals. Tissue damage occurs when the phagocytizing neutrophils release the contents of their digestive lysosomes. Lysosomal contents are released from neutrophils as they die following their lifespan of about two days, by leakage after injury by biochemical reactions with ingested urate crystals or through rupture of neutrophils during attempts to ingest exceptionally large urate crystals.

Attacks of gouty arthritis occur abruptly, usually in a peripheral joint. The primary symptom is severe pain. Approximately 50 percent of the initial attacks occur in the metatarsophalangeal joint of the great toe. Other involved joints are the heel, ankle, instep of the foot, knee, wrist, or elbow.

Tophaceous gout, the chronic stage of disease, can begin as early as three years or as late as 40 years after the initial attack of gouty arthritis. Progressive inability to excrete uric acid expands the urate pool until tophi appear in cartilage, synovial membranes, tendons, and soft tissue. The helix of the ear is the most common site of tophi, which are the diagnostic lesions of chronic gout. Each tophus consists of a deposit of urate crystals surrounded by a granuloma made of mononuclear phagocytes that have developed into epithelial giant cells. Tophaceous deposits appear in other areas and produce irregular swellings of the fingers, hands, knees, and feet. Though the tophi themselves are painless, they often cause progressive stiffness and persistent aching of the affected joint.

Acute gouty arthritis is treated with anti-inflammatory drugs. The individual should have a low purine diet and high fluid intake to increase urinary output. Antihyperuricemic drugs can be given to reduce serum urate concentrations.

7. Describe examples of secondary muscular dysfunction.
Study text pages 1471-1473.

Muscular symptoms arise from causes unrelated to the muscle itself. These secondary muscular phenomena include contracture, stress-related muscle tension, and immobility.

Several conditions cause the muscle fibers to shorten without contracting; this is called a **contracture**. A physiologic muscle contracture occurs without muscle action potential in the sarcolemma and is explained as failure of the calcium pump even in the presence of plentiful adenosine triphosphate (ATP). A physiologic contracture is seen in McArdle disease, which is an enzyme deficiency, and malignant hyperthermia. The contracture is usually temporary if the underlying pathology can be corrected.

A pathologic contracture is considered a permanent muscle shortening due to muscle spasm or weakness. It is associated with plentiful ATP and will occur in spite of a normal action potential. The most common form of contracture is seen in muscular dystrophy and central nervous system (CNS) injury. Contractures may also develop secondary to scar tissue contraction in the flexor tissues of a joint.

Stress-induced muscle tension has been associated with chronic anxiety as well as a variety of stress-related muscular symptoms including neck stiffness, back pain, and headache. The underlying pathophysiology presumably is caused by increased activity of the reticular-activating system and increased firing of the efferent loop of the gamma fibers which produce further muscle contraction and increased muscle tension.

Progressive relaxation training and biofeedback are possible ways to treat muscle tension. The hope is to enhance the individual's ability to relax specific muscle groups in order to relieve tension. This could reduce CNS and ANS arousal.

The term **disuse atrophy** describes the pathologic reduction in normal size of muscle fibers following inactivity due to bed rest, trauma, casting, or local nerve damage. It is possible that a marked reduction in mitochondrial oxidative metabolism leaves less energy available for muscle protein synthesis and explains the reduction in volume and number of myofibrils. Atrophy may be prevented by frequent forceful isometric muscle contractions and passive lengthening exercises.

8. Distinguish between muscle membrane abnormalities.
Study text page 1473.

The hyperexcitable membrane seen in myotonic disorders and the intermittently unresponsive membrane seen in the periodic paralyses are defects in the plasma membrane of the muscle fiber. **Myotonia** is a delayed relaxation after voluntary muscle contraction such as gripe, eye closure, or muscle percussion. It is due to the prolonged depolarization of the muscle membrane. Myotonia is seen mostly in inherited disorders. Its symptoms are mild except in myotonic muscular dystrophy where there is progressive atrophy of skeletal muscles. Myotonia is treated by drugs that reduce muscle fiber excitability.

In **periodic paralysis**, the muscle membrane is unresponsive to neural stimuli. Periodic paralysis is triggered by exercise and any process or medication that alters serum potassium. The disorder is often inherited in an autosomal dominant pattern. The flaccid paralysis does not affect the respiratory muscles. Because of changes in serum potassium, cardiac dysrhythmias are possible during attacks. Oral and intravenous potassium can relieve acute attacks. Drugs and a low-salt diets are useful for long-term therapy.

9. Compare the metabolic, inflammatory, and acquired metabolic and toxic myopathies.
Study text pages 1473-1477.

Myopathies

	Cause	Manifestations
Metabolic Myopathy		
	Altered thyroid hormone levels change muscle protein synthesis and electrolyte balance	
	Thyrotoxicosis	Proximal weakness, paresis of extraocular muscles
	Hypothyroidism	Flabby and weak muscles, sluggish movements
	Hyperparathyroidism	Proximal weakness, wasting and fatigue, brisk reflexes
McArdle disease	Absence of muscle phosphorylase, unable to catabolize glycogen or produce lactic acid	Exercise intolerance, fatigue, painful muscle cramps, muscle weakness and wasting
Acid maltase deficiency	Autosomal recessive, absence of acid maltase, accumulation of glycogen in lysosomes of muscle and other cells	
		(Continued)

Myopathies *(cont'd)*

	Cause	*Manifestations*
Pompe disease (Infantile)		Hypotonia, areflexia, enlarged heart and tongue and liver, early death Adult: similar to muscular dystrophy or polymyositis, severe respiratory muscle weakness
Myoadenylate deaminase deficiency	Absence of myoadenylate deaminase, cannot form phosphocreatine and ATP during exercise	Exercise intolerance
Carnitine palmitoyl transferase (CPT) and carnitine deficiency	Absence of CPT and carnitine, fatty acid byproducts and energy are not transported to the myofibrils	CPT: mild muscular symptoms, bouts of renal failure because of myoglobinuria Carnitine: progressive muscle weakness
Inflammatory myopathy		
Infectious		
Tuberculosis and sarcoidosis	Granulomas in muscle and other tissues
Trichinosis	Larvae from infected pork migrate to host lymphatics: pain, rash, and muscle stiffness
Viral infections	Muscle pain and tenderness similar to symptoms of influenza
Polymyositis (generalized muscle inflammation) Dermatomyositis (polymyositis with skin lesions)	Cell-mediated and humoral immune systems abnormalities	Necrosis of muscle fibers, malaise, fever, muscle swelling pain and tenderness, lethargy, symmetric proximal muscle weakness; both diseases show dysphagia, vasculitis, Raynaud phenomenon, cardiomyopathy, fibrosis, coexisting pulmonary collagen disorders; dermatomyositis exhibits skin rash, calcinosis, and eyelid edema

(Continued)

	Cause	Manifestations
	Toxic Myopathy	
	Alcohol abuse, direct toxic effect and nutritional deficiency causes necrosis of muscle fibers	Benign cramps and pain, severe weakness, myoglobinuria and renal failure
	Antimalarial and amebicidal agents impair lysomal processes	Generalized muscle weakness
	Sedatives and narcotics	Myoglobinuria
	Repeated therapeutic drug injection	Local muscle fiber necrosis, fibrotic bands

10. Identify the incidence, manifestations, treatment, and prognosis of rhabdomyosarcoma.
Study text page 1477.

The malignant tumor of striated muscle is a **rhabdomyosarcoma.** The incidence of rhabdomyosarcoma ranges from 10 to 20 percent of all soft tissue cancers and is highly malignant because of its rapid metastasis. Two age peaks occur, at two to six years and the early to late teens, although rhabdomyosarcoma also can occur in adults and the elderly population. These tumors are located in the muscle tissue of the head, neck, and genitourinary tract 75 percent of the time. The remainder are in the trunk and extremities.

The diagnosis of rhabdomyosarcoma is made by incisional biopsy and histological examination of the specimen. Pleomorphic, embryonal, and alveolar types can be differentiated. The pleomorphic type is a highly malignant tumor of the extremities of adults.

Treatment consists of a combination of surgical excision, radiation therapy, and systemic chemotherapy. Patients with regionally involved tumors of the orbit and genitourinary tract have been reported to have a five-year survival rate of 75 percent if vigorously treated. Childhood rhabdomyosarcoma of any type with only regional involvement can be controlled 60 percent of the time. Tumors of the trunk and extremities have less favorable prognosis, and cure in those with distant metastasis is unlikely.

Practice Examination

1. In a complete fracture,
   a. the fracture crosses or involves the entire width or thickness of the bone.
   b. more than two bone fragments are present.
   c. separation of ligaments exists.
   d. post-traumatic infection is always present.
   e. the surface opposite the break is intact.

2. In an oblique fracture, the energy or force is
   a. twisting with the distal part unable to move.
   b. compressive and at an angle.
   c. directly at an already weakened bone.
   d. directly to the distal fragment.

3. Which is a definite sign of a fracture?
   a. abrasion
   b. shock
   c. muscle spasm
   d. unnatural alignment
   e. All of the above are correct.

Match the term with its characteristic.

4. subluxation
5. sprain

   a. articular cartilages lose contact entirely
   b. articular cartilages are partially separated
   c. complete separation of a tendon or a ligament
   d. a ligament tear
   e. painful inflammation of bursitis

6. Compartment syndromes
   a. involve large compartments of hemorrhage.
   b. bleed into joints.
   c. lead to ischemic contracture in muscles.
   d. may result from myoglobinuria.
   e. Both c and b are correct.

7. The most common cause of osteomyelitis is
   a. hematogenous spread of infection.
   b. rheumatoid disease.
   c. by direct contamination of an open wound.
   d. deficiency of calcium.
   e. deficiency of vitamin D.

8. Osteoporosis is
   a. inadequate mineralization.
   b. impaired synthesis of bone organic matrix.
   c. reduced bone mass or density.
   d. formation of sclerotic bone.
   e. None of the above is correct.

9. Osteomalacia causes
   a. loss of bone matrix.
   b. inadequate mineralization.
   c. radiolucency.
   d. All of the above are correct.
   e. Both b and c are correct.

10. Bone tumors may originate from all except
    a. epithelial tissue.
    b. cartilage.
    c. fibrous tissue.
    d. vascular tissue.
    e. mesoderm.

11. In benign bone tumors, there is
    a. a uniform and well-defined lytic area.
    b. a moth-eaten pattern of bone destruction.
    c. abnormal bone merging with surrounding normal bone tissue.
    d. an area of partially destroyed bone adjacent to completely lytic areas.

12. An osteosarcoma is a/an
    a. collagenic, malignant bone tumor.
    b. myelogenic, benign tumor.
    c. myelogenic, malignant tumor.
    d. osteogenic, benign bone tumor.
    e. osteogenic, malignant tumor.

13. The major symptom of bone cancer is a
    a. flattering gait.
    b. persistent pain that worsens at night.
    c. lack of sensation.
    d. general swelling over a bone.
    e. coolness over a bone.

14. Giant cell tumors
    a. affect males more frequently than females.
    b. are located in the diaphysis of a long bone.
    c. have extensive osteoblastic activity.
    d. have high recurrence rates.
    e. are multifocal.

15. Myeloma
    a. is a malignant proliferation of plasma cells.
    b. may be solitary or multifocal.
    c. infiltrates the bone marrow.
    d. Both a and c are correct.
    e. a, b, and c are correct.

16. Rheumatoid arthritis begins with
    a. destruction of the synovial membrane and subsynovial tissue.
    b. inflammation of ligaments.
    c. destruction of articular cartilage.
    d. softening of the articular cartilage.
    e. destruction of the joint capsule.

17. The causes of osteoarthritis include
    1. collagenases.   a. 1, 3, 4
    2. cytokines.   b. 1
    3. rheumatoid factor.   c. 2, 3
    4. circulating immune complexes. d. 1, 2
    5. infections.   e. 3, 4, 5

18. Ankylosing spondylitis
    1. is a systemic immune inflammatory disease.   a. 1, 2
    2. is characterized by stiffening or fusion of the spine. b. 1, 2, 5
    3. causes instability of synovial joints.   c. 2, 5
    4. begins with inflammation of fibrocartilage.   d. 1, 2, 4, 5
    5. in manifested early by low back pain and stiffness. e. 3

19. In gout,
    a. the pathogenesis is formation of monosodium urate crystals in joints and tissues.
    b. metatarsophalangeal joints are usually involved.
    c. approximately 95 percent of affected individuals likely have an inherited enzyme defect.
    d. the hyperuricemia can be the result of acquired chronic disease or a drug.
    e. All of the above are correct.

20. A muscle contracture is
    a. likely caused by increased activity in the reticular activating system and the gamma loop in the muscle fiber.
    b. permanent muscle shortening due to spasticity that might be seen in CNS injury.
    c. often helped by relaxation training and biofeedback.
    d. a consequence of reduced muscle protein synthesis.
    e. All of the above are correct.

21. Myotonia is all except
    a. delayed relaxation after voluntary muscle contractions.
    b. prolonged depolarization of the muscle membrane.
    c. mostly inherited.
    d. unresponsiveness to neural stimulation.
    e. progressive atrophy of skeletal muscle.

Match the myopathy with its cause.

22. McArdle disease
23. acid maltase deficiency
24. polymyositis

a. hypothyroidism
b. hyperparathyroidism
c. accumulation of glycogen in lysosomes
d. unable to catabolize glycogen
e. immune system abnormality

25. Rhabdomyosarcomas have all except
    a. a poor prognosis.
    b. aggressive invasion.
    c. early, widespread dissemination.
    d. two age peaks, at six years and the teens.
    e. All of the above are characteristics of this sarcoma.

Case Study

Mrs. B.B. is a 52-year-old homemaker who has complained of bilateral knee and hand pain for seven years. The pain has progressively worsened and persists during rest and limits her walking, climbing stairs, and weight bearing. Her physical examination showed slight ulnar deviation of the digits and swelling of the metacarpal, phalangeal, and proximal interphalangeal joints with limited range of motion and some instability of both knees.

Laboratory studies revealed:

CBC = normal, except for mild anemia
Rheumatoid factor = high titer
Synovial fluid analysis = turbid appearance
Radiographic examination of knees = joint narrowing on both knees, thinning of the articular cartilage, cystic areas, and bony spurs

Which arthritis is Mrs. B.B. experiencing? Explain your answer.

Alterations of Musculoskeletal Function in Children

Prerequisite Objective

a. Describe the processes of bone and muscle growth from birth to maturity.
   Review text pages 1482-1485; refer to Figure 40-1.

Remember!

- Until adult stature is reached, growth in the length of bone occurs at the epiphyseal plate through endochondral ossification. Cartilage cells in the proximal layer of the epiphyseal plate multiply and enlarge and then are destroyed and replaced by bone at the metaphyseal side of the plate. In the shaft of new bone, the slow growing bone is produced by accretion and is compact and dense. The longitudinal growth rate of the extremities is greater at birth than at any other time. Growth in the diameter of bone occurs by deposition of new bone on an existing bone surface. Bone matrix is laid down by osteoblasts on the periosteal surface and subsequently becomes calcified. While bone resorption occurs on the endosteal surface, endosteal resorption increases the diameter of the medullary cavity and its spongy bone. When the skeleton is mature, the epiphyseal plate is replaced by bone. This epiphyseal closure that unites the diaphysis and epiphysis occurs earlier in females than males because of the accelerating influence of estrogens on cartilage growth and matrix formation. Throughout life, bone is constantly being destroyed and reformed. The process is at its maximum in children about two and one-half years of age. By young adulthood, bone turnover or remodeling occurs at a relatively low rate.

- The axial skeleton changes shape with growth. In a newborn, the entire spine is concave anteriorly; the child's natural posture is "curled up." In the first three months of life as the ability to control the head develops, the upper or cervical spine begins to "arch" or become convex anteriorly. The normal arch in the spine begins to develop with sitting. The appendicular skeleton, or the extremities, grows faster during childhood than does the axial skeleton. The neonate has a relatively large head and long spine with disproportionately shorter limbs than an adult. By age one, 50 percent of the total growth of the spine has occurred.

(Continued)

Remember! *(cont'd)*

- After birth, the muscle fibers enlarge by accumulating cytoplasm. Between birth and maturity, the number of muscle nuclei in the body increases 14 times in boys and 10 times in girls. Muscle fibers reach their maximal size in girls about the age of 10 and in boys by the age of 14. The length of a muscle fiber is the direct consequence of the range of movement it is called on to perform. In the infant, muscle accounts for approximately 25 percent of total body weight compared with 40 percent in the adult. The respiratory and facial muscles are well developed at birth so that the infant can perform the vital functions of breathing and sucking. Other muscle groups such as the pelvic muscle take several years to develop fully. Throughout life, the weight of the skeletal muscles can be increased by exercise. Visceral muscle fibers increase both in number and size; fiber enlargement alone can increase the bulk of visceral muscle by as many as eight times. Cardiac muscle also grows mainly by enlargement of existing fibers.

Objectives

After successful study of this chapter, the learner will be able to:

1. Describe the most common congenital musculoskeletal defects in children.
Study text pages 1485-1488; refer to Figures 40-2 through 40-4 and Table 40-1.

Syndactyly, or webbed fingers, is the most common congenital defect of the upper extremity and may involve simple, soft tissue webbing of the fingers or true syndactyly, which is actual fusion of the bone. Simple webbing is best surgically corrected at three to four years of age; whereas true syndactyly requires correction beginning at six to 12 months and completion of treatment before starting school. Syndactyly may accompany other congenital defects and should prompt a thorough examination to rule out others.

Developmental dysplasia of the hip (DDH) is also known as congenital hip dislocation and is an anomaly of the development of the proximal femur, acetabulum, or both. The hip may be subluxed, dislocatable, or dislocated. The subluxed femur maintains contact with the acetabulum but is not well seated within it. The dislocatable hip may be located properly but may be dislocated with manipulation. The dislocated hip has no contact between the femur or acetabulum. Incidence is approximately one in 1000 live births, with girls being affected 6:1 over boys. The exact cause of this disorder is unknown and is probably multifactorial. Risk factors include breech presentation, family history, first pregnancy, and oligohydramnios. Presence of other lower extremity deformities may increase the risk of DDH. Clinical findings include leg length discrepancy, limitation of hip abduction, asymmetry of gluteal folds, positive Ortolani and Barlow signs, positive Trendelenburg

sign, abnormal gait, and pain. Early diagnosis by physical examination and x-ray imaging is extremely important because permanent joint deterioration results from treatment delay. Treatment generally consists of bracing the joint in flexion and abduction. Surgery is occasionally required.

Metatarsus adductus (MTA) is the most common congenital defect of the lower extremity and is believed to be due to intrauterine positioning of the feet. In this deformity, the bones of the forefoot are inwardly rotated and may be easily flexed back into position or may be fairly fixed. Most cases are self-correcting, but the more fixed forms require physical therapy or serial casting.

Talipes equinovarus or **clubfoot** occurs in approximately one to two per 1000 live births in the United States and is bilateral in approximately 50 percent of cases; boys are more frequently affected than girls. The foot normally goes through a period of flexion and eversion early in development and arrest of development at this stage is generally thought to be the cause of this defect. The forefoot is abducted and the hindfoot is adducted and inverted. The entire foot points downward. The foot is in rigid fixation. Treatment consists of early serial casting and frequently requires surgery for full correction.

Congenital myopathies are rare and mild defects in muscular development which are usually present in hypotonic infants or infants who are developmentally delayed in attaining motor development. The defects include congenital absence of muscles, hypo- or hyperplasia of muscles, faulty intrinsic development leading to disfigurement of fibers, and presenile degeneration. Diagnosis is confirmed by muscle biopsy and histologic appearance. Treatment is nonspecific and usually requires aggressive physical therapy programs to maximize potential.

2. Describe the pathophysiology and common clinical features related to osteogenesis imperfecta.

Study text pages 1488-1490; refer to Figure 40-5.

Osteogenesis imperfecta is primarily a defect in collagen production resulting in easily fractured, "brittle" bones. Incidence is approximately one in 40,000 live births, and it is usually inherited by the autosomal dominant route but may be autosomal recessive. In the most severe form, fractures may occur in utero but usually do not become a problem until ambulation is attained. Other clinical features include osteoporosis and bowed or deformed limbs. Short stature, curvature of the spine, or a bluish discoloration of the sclera also may be a feature. Diagnosis is based on clinical findings and serologic tests. Alkaline phosphatase is elevated in all forms of the disease. Prenatal diagnosis is available through ultrasound and chorionic villus sampling. No clear benefits have been demonstrated for most therapies, although supplemental calcium, fluoride, vitamin C, magnesium oxide, and calcitonin have all been tried.

3. Describe two major forms of scoliosis and describe their pathophysiology.

Study text pages 1490-1492; refer to Figure 40-6.

Scoliosis or lateral curvature of the spine may be classified as (1) nonstructural occurring from causes extrinsic to the spine, such as posture, pain, or leg length discrepancy; (2) structural that is associated with vertebral rotation; or (3) idiopathic. Idiopathic scoliosis may be further classified as infantile, juvenile, or adolescent according to age of onset. Adolescent idiopathic scoliosis is the most common. Girls most frequently have severe curvature and require treatment. Pathophysiologic change includes shortening of ligaments on the concave side of the curve; this eventually results in vertebral deformity. The deformity is due to unequal stress on the epiphyseal centers of the vertebral bodies. Eventually, progressive deformity of the vertebral column and ribs develop. The curvature progresses most rapidly during times of rapid skeletal growth. In curvature greater than 50 degrees, the spine is mechanically unstable and the curvature will probably progress throughout life. Curvature greater than 60 degrees results in pulmonary dysfunction. Clinical manifestations include asymmetry of hip and shoulder height, shoulder and scapular prominence, rib prominence, and posterior humping of ribs or hips. These findings are noted when the child bends forward from the waist. Diagnosis is confirmed by x-ray. Treatment includes bracing of curvatures between 25 and 35 degrees in

the skeletally immature but is not effective in curvatures greater than 40 degrees or in the skeletally mature. These individuals require surgery and instrumentation of the vertebrae. An alternative treatment in appropriate cases is transcutaneous muscle stimulation.

4. Describe the pathophysiology and common pathogens related to osteomyelitis in children.

Study text pages 1492-1494; refer to Figure 40-7.

Osteomyelitis is an inflammation of the bone marrow which occurs most frequently between three and 12 years of age with a predilection for boys. In this process, bacteria enter the bone through the bloodstream and lodge in the medullary cavity. This is frequently where the process is halted by the immune system because of a rich supply of phagocytes in this area. In other cases, however, bacteria invade the epiphyseal plate where phagocytes are absent, and resultant infection develops. Osteomyelitis may be preceded by trauma which may then predispose to infection. The infection usually begins as a bloody abscess in the metaphysis of the bone that ruptures under the periosteum and spreads along the shaft or into the medullary cavity. The microorganism usually gains access to the subperiosteal space through the metaphysis, which is the path of lease resistance because of the porous nature of the bone in that area. If infection occurs near a joint, the accumulated pressure of inflammatory products may cause pus and bacteria to rupture through the bone and into the joint space causing a **secondary suppurative arthritis**. The spread of infection into joint spaces is also aided because the epiphyseal plates in infants less than one month of age are penetrated by capillaries that communicate directly into joints. Severe infection in infants and young children rapidly leads to permanent damage of the joints and disruption of the blood supply to the bone with subsequent growth arrest. In the child 12 years of age or older, the epiphyseal plate helps prevent the spread of infection.

The most common etiologic agents in osteomyelitis are *Staphylococcus aureus*, Group B strep, and *E. coli* in the newborn. *Staph aureus* and *H. influenzae* are the common agents in older children. Clinical presentation of the illness tends to be somewhat variable. Osteomyelitis is frequently abrupt in onset in young children and infants as the child displays signs of toxicity, fever, and refusal to move the affected limb. This process may be more subacute in older children and adults and may involve the vertebrae; whereas in young children and infants it usually involves the long bones. Diagnosis is usually confirmed by an elevated white blood cell count and erythrocyte sedimentation rate; radiologic imaging, although findings on plain x-ray may take two weeks to become apparent; and culture aspirations of the blood and affected tissues. Treatment includes long-term, appropriate antibiotic therapy and surgical intervention where warranted.

tion, casting, or surgical intervention if necessary. Outcome depends on the age of the child, the extent of necrosis, and disease staging at the beginning of therapy. Approximately 70 to 80 percent of treated children have satisfactory hip function at the completion of therapy.

5. Describe the pathophysiology, evaluation, and treatment of Legg-Calve-Perthes disease.
Study text pages 1496-1497; refer to Figure 40-8.

Legg-Calve-Perthes disease (LCP) is a process of interrupted blood supply to the femoral head. It commonly occurs between three and 10 years of age with a peak incidence at six years of age. It is most frequently seen in boys and is self-limiting in nature, running its course in two to five years. The deformation that results is permanent. In this process, interruption of blood flow to the femoral head results in necrosis of the femoral head. Inflammation and new bone formation follow over time with a resultant flattening of the femoral head and distortion of the hip joint. The first necrotic stage lasts only a few weeks; however, the healing phase lasts from two to four years. The etiology of LCP is unknown, although familial occurrence is known as is a history of antecedent trauma. It is probable that an antecedent synovitis causes increased hydrostatic pressure within the joint and interferes with blood flow. Birth weight tends to be low in children with LCP disease and skeletal maturation is delayed as well. Presentation of LCP disease may be fairly incipient with the child complaining of lower extremity pain for weeks to months. A limp then follows known as the antalgic abductor lurch. The child frequently demonstrates pain when the hip is externally rotated while in extension. Diagnosis is confirmed by radiologic imaging, and treatment is accomplished by bracing the legs in abduc-

6. Describe the pathophysiology, evaluation, and treatment of Duchenne muscular dystrophy.
Study text pages 1499-1500; refer to Figure 40-9 and Table 40-3.

Duchenne muscular dystrophy is an x-linked inherited disorder that is caused by a deletion of a segment of DNA. This deletion results in an absence of dystrophin that is found in normal muscle cells. The lack of dystrophin apparently causes loss of muscle bulk and fibers. In the late stages, interstitial connective tissue and fat may replace muscle fibers. The disease is frequently diagnosed at approximately three years of age when parents notice slow motor development, problems with coordination and walking, and generalized weakness. Weakness always begins in the pelvic girdle and hypertrophy is present in the calf muscles of approximately 80 percent of affected children. Gower sign, a peculiar manner of standing from sitting by climbing up the legs, is often evident. Within three to five years, the shoulder girdle muscle becomes involved with constant progression of the illness until cardiac involvement is seen. Pulmonary and cardiac failure may follow and, eventually, death results by age 20. Diagnosis is confirmed by serum enzyme studies and electromyelography. Creatine phosphokinase (CPK) may be 10 times normal and histologic examination of biopsied muscle fibers will be abnormal as well. Treatment is chiefly supportive with the goal being to preserve function of remaining muscle groups for as long as possible.

Practice Examination

True/False

_____ 1. A fused finger in syndactyly is best treated by being "clipped" at birth.

_____ 2. Developmental dysplasia of the hip is often noted shortly after birth due to a positive Gower sign.

_____ 3. Osteogenesis imperfecta is a disease related to overcalcification of the bone that causes it to be brittle and break easily.

_____ 4. Metatarsus abductus is a positional deformity of the foot that may be self-correcting.

_____ 5. Legg-Calve-Perthes disease may be suspected when a positive Ortolani or Barlow maneuver is noted.

___ 6. Osteomyelitis is an infection of bone that can be spread to the site through the blood.

___ 7. Breech presentation is not a risk factor for developmental hip dysplasia because traction on the feet during the birth process negates undue pressure on the hip joint.

___ 8. Club foot is not self-limiting and requires casting with or without surgery for successful treatment.

___ 9. Congenital myopathy may include congenital absence of muscles.

___ 10. Treatment of club foot is usually delayed as the bones of the infant are generally not well ossified at birth and may be easily corrected later.

Fill-in-the-Blank

11. The disease process of Legg-Calve-Perthes disease is self-limited but the destruction that it causes is

_____.

12. Gluteal folds in developmental dysplasia of the hip may be _____.

13. Duchenne muscular dystrophy results from a lack of _____ in muscle cells.

14. DDH is treated by bracing the hips in _____ and _____.

15. Talipes equinovarus is also known as _____.

Match the outcome with the alteration.

16. fractures present at birth
17. death by 20 years of age
18. positive Barlow or Ortolani maneuver or both
19. Gower sign
20. antalgic abductor lurch
21. subluxed, dislocated, dislocatable
22. pain in external rotation with affected limb
23. frequently caused by *S. aureus*
24. defect in collagen synthesis
25. lateral curvature of the spine

a. scoliosis
b. osteogenesis imperfecta
c. osteomyelitis
d. Legg-Calve-Perthes disease
e. developmental hip dysplasia
f. Duchenne muscular dystrophy

Case Study

Ashley G. is a 5-year-old caucasian girl visiting the nurse practitioner's office today because of her mother's latent curiosity about the shape of her child's chest. As best as can be determined, Ashley has had fairly unremarkable past medical, prenatal, and family histories. She has seen health care providers only sporadically for minor illness and has not had a complete physical examination since birth. Although fully immunized, she never had any well-child visits. On physical examination, Ashley is found to have a "sunken" appearance to her left chest with an unusually shaped and low placed nipple. Her examination is otherwise noncontributory.

What syndrome is suspected?

Structure, Function, and Disorders of the Integument

Prerequisite Objectives

a. Describe the skin and its layers.
   Review text pages 1513-1515; refer to Figure 41-1 and Table 41-1.

Remember!

- The skin is the largest organ of the body; it covers the entire body and accounts for approximately 20 percent of the body's weight. Outer skin serves as a barrier against microorganisms, ultraviolet radiation, and loss of body temperature; it is involved in the production of vitamin D; and its touch and pressure receptors provide important protective functions and pleasurable sensations. The skin has two major layers: a superficial **epidermis** and a deeper layer, the **dermis**. The subcutaneous tissue or **hypodermis** is an underlying layer of connective tissue which contains macrophages, fibroblasts, and fat cells.

- The epidermis grows continually by shedding its superficial layer of stratum corneum which consists of keratinocytes and melanocytes. **Keratinocytes** produce keratin, which is a scleroprotein. Keratin is the main constituent of skin, hair, and nail cells. Keratinocytes are formed in the basal layer or stratum basale and move upward and differentiate to form the spinous layer or stratum spinosum. Together, these two layers form the germinative layer or stratum germinativum. The cells enlarge and then become flattened, stacked, and cornified as they move to the skin surface to become the stratum corneum. Cornification or keratinization of this layer prevents dehydration of deeper skin layers.

- The **melanocytes** are usually located near the base of the epidermis and synthesize and secrete the pigment melanin when exposed to sunlight in response to melanocyte-stimulating hormone of the pituitary gland. Melanin provides a protective shield against ultraviolet radiation and determines skin color. Other cells contribute to the function of the epidermis. **Langerhans cells** migrate to the dermis from the bone marrow to provide protection against environmental antigens. **Merkel cells** are associated with touch receptors and function when stimulated by deformation of the epidermis.

- The dermis is composed of connective tissue containing collagenous and elastic fibers. Their arrangement permits the skin to be mobile, stretch, and contract with body movement. Hair follicles, sebaceous glands, sweat glands, blood vessels, lymphatic vessels, and nerves are contained in the dermis. Projections of the papillary dermis interface with the epidermis and are known as **rete pegs**. The cells of the dermis include fibroblasts, mast cells, and macrophages.

(Continued)

Remember! *(cont'd)*

Fibroblasts secrete the connective tissue matrix. Mast cells release histamine and play a role in hypersensitivity reactions in the skin. Macrophages are phagocytic and participate in immune responses.

- The dermal appendages include the nails, hair, sebaceous glands, and the eccrine and apocrine sweat glands. The **nails** are protective keratinized plates that appear at the ends of fingers and toes. **Hair follicles** arise from the matrix located deep in the dermis. Hair growth begins in the bulb with cellular differentiation occurring as the hair progresses up the follicle. Hair is fully cornified by the time it emerges at the skin surface. The **sebaceous glands** open onto the surface of the skin through a canal and secrete sebum composed primarily of lipids, which oils the skin and hair and prevents drying.

- The **eccrine sweat glands** are distributed over the body and are important in cooling of the body through evaporation. The **apocrine sweat glands** are fewer in number and are located in the axillae, scalp, face, abdomen, and genital area.

- The blood supply to the skin is by the papillary capillaries or plexus of the dermis. Arteriovenous anastomoses in the dermis facilitate the regulation of body temperature. Heat loss can be regulated by varying blood flow through the skin by opening or closing the arteriovenous anastomoses to modify evaporative heat loss through sweat. The sympathetic nervous system regulates both vasoconstriction and vasodilation as there are only adrenergic receptors in the skin. The lymphatic vessels of the skin arise in the dermis and drain into larger subcutaneous trunks; these vessels remove cells, proteins, and immunologic mediators.

b. Identify the changes that occur in skin during aging.
    Review text pages 1515-1516.

Remember!

- Structurally, the skin becomes thinner, dryer, and wrinkled and changes in pigmentation during aging. Fewer melanocytes decrease the protection against ultraviolet radiation. Fewer Langerhans cells decrease the skin's immune response during aging. The thickness of the dermis decreases and the skin becomes translucent and assumes a paper-thin quality. Loss of the rete pegs gives the skin a smooth, shiny appearance. The decreased vasculature probably contributes to the atrophy of eccrine, apocrine, and sebaceous glands so the skin becomes drier with age. Loss of elastin fibers is associated with wrinkling. The collagen fibers become less flexible and decrease the ability of the skin to stretch and regain shape. Decreased cell generation, blood supply, and depressed immune responses delay wound healing in aging skin. Greying of hair color is due to loss of melanocytes from hair bulbs and thinning hair occurs from a gradual decline in the number of hair follicles. As the barrier function of the stratum corneum is reduced, there is increased permeability and decreased clearance of substances from the dermis. The accumulation of such substances can cause skin irritation. Temperature regulation is less effective in the elderly and there is increased risk for both heat stroke and hypothermia. The pressure and touch receptors and free nerve endings all decrease in number and reduce sensory perception.

c. Summarize diagnostic skin procedures.
     Refer to Table 41-2.

Remember!

Diagnostic Skin Procedures

Test	*Purpose*
Skin biopsy	Differential diagnosis of benign or malignant lesions, chronic infections, blistering diseases, or vasculitis
Microscopic immunofluorescence	Identification of antibodies, immunoglobulins, and complement components for diseases
Gram stain	Differentiation of gram-positive from gram-negative bacteria
Culture	Identification of chronic bacterial and fungal infections
Wood's lamp examination	Examination of skin or hair to identify fungus that fluoresces under ultraviolet light
Patch and scratch tests	Application of suspected allergens to skin patch or scratch for evaluation of immune system response to known allergens
Skin scrapings	Application of potassium hydroxide and low heat to identify fungi
Side lighting	Indirect lighting to the side of the lesions to evaluate patterns of depression and elevation of skin lesions
Diascopy	Pressure on the skin to differentiate dilated capillaries by blanching from extravasation of blood that does not blanch

Objectives

After successful study of this chapter, the learner will be able to:

1. Distinguish between skin lesions.
    Study text pages 1516 and 1522-1524; refer
    to Table 41-3.

Basic Lesions of the Skin

Type	Characteristics	Example
Flat Lesions		
Macule	A flat, circumscribed discolored lesion of any size less than 5 mm in diameter	Hyperpigmentation, erythema, telangiectasias, purpura
Patch	A flat, irregular lesion larger than a macula	Vitiligo
Petechiae	A circumscribed area of blood less than 0.5 cm in diameter	Thrombocytopenia, bacteremia, vasculitis (inflamed vessel)
Purpura	A circumscribed area of blood greater than 5.0 cm in diameter	Same as petechiae
Telangiectasia	Dilated, superficial blood vessels	Rheumatoid arthritis, hepatitis
Elevated Lesions		
Papule	Lesions 1 cm or less in diameter because of infiltration or hyperplasia or the dermis	Verruca (warts), lichen planus, nevus
Plaque	Lesions with a large surface area, larger laterally than in height	Psoriasis, eczema
Nodule	Palpable circumscribed lesion 1-2 cm in diameter located in the epidermis, dermis, or hypodermis; smooth to ulcerated	Benign or malignant tumors, foreign body inflammation, calcium deposits
Wheal	A transient lesion with well defined and often changing borders caused by edema of the dermis	Hives, angioedema
Vesicle & bulla	A fluid-filled, thin-walled lesion; a bulla is a vesicle greater than 0.5 cm in diameter	Herpes zoster, impetigo, pemphigus, second-degree burns

(Continued)

Basic Lesions of the Skin *(cont'd)*

Type	Characteristics	Example
Pustule	Lesion containing an exudate of white blood cells	Acne, pustular psoriasis
Comedone	Plugged hair follicle	Blackhead, whitehead
Scale	Accumulation of loose stratum corneum from cellular retention or cellular over-production	Psoriasis
Crust	Accumulation of dried blood or serum, size varies	Eczema, impetigo
Lichenification	Thickening, toughening of the skin with accentuation of skin lines caused by scratching	Chronic dermatitis
Cyst	An encapsulated mass of dermis or subcutaneous layers, solid or fluid filled	Sebaceous cyst
Tumor	A well-demarcated solid lesion greater than 2 cm in diameter	Fibroma, lipoma melanoma, hemangioma
Scar	Thin or thick fibrous tissue	Healed laceration, burn, surgical incision
Depressed Lesions		
Atrophy	Thinning of the epidermis or dermis caused by decreased connective tissue	Thin facial skin of elderly, striae of pregnancy
Ulcer	Loss of epidermis and dermis	Pressure sores, basal cell carcinoma
Excoriation	Loss of epidermis with exposed dermis	Scratches
Fissure	Linear crack or break exposing dermis	Athlete's foot, cheilosis
Erosion	Moist, red break in epidermis, follows rupture of vesicle or bulla, larger than fissure	Chickenpox, diaper dermatitis

2. Identify the cause and lesion of inflammatory disorders of the skin.

Study text pages 1524-1531; refer to Figures 41-4 through 41-12.

Inflammatory Skin Disorders

	Cause	*Lesion*
Allergic contact dermatitis	Allergen binds to carrier protein to form a sensitizing antigen, T-cell hypersensitivity	Pruritic (itching) vesicles
Irritant contact dermatitis	Nonimmunologic inflammation due to chemicals	As above
Atopic dermatitis	Mast cell and IgE, T-lymphocytes, and monocytes interact	Red, weeping crusts, lichenification
Stasis dermatitis	Venous stasis and edema	Initial erythema and pruritus; then, scaling, petechiae, and hyperpigmentation
Seborrheic dermatitis	Unknown	Scaly plaques with mild pruritus
Psoriasis	Unknown, genetic or immunologic	Thick, silvery, scaly, erythematous, plaque surrounded by normal skin; rapid shedding of epidermis
Pityriasis rosea	Unknown, virus?	Pruritus, demarcated salmon-pink scale within a plaque
Lichen planus	Unknown, exposure to drugs?	Nonscaling, violet-colored pruritic papules
Acne vulgaris	Increased activity of sebacceous glands or sebum inability to escape through the narrow opening	Comedones
Acne rosacea	Unknown, associated with chronic flushing and sensitivity to sun	Erythema, papules, pustules and telangiectasia
Discoid lupus erythematosus	Immune response to unknown antigen	Cutaneous manifestations of elevated red plaque with brown scale, hair loss, urticaria (hives), telangiectasis
Systemic lupus erythematosus	Unknown, genetics or autoimmunity	Systemic manifestations of connective tissue degeneration; stiffness and pain in hands, feet, or large joints; patchy atrophy of skin with diffuse facial erythematous rash in a butterfly pattern over the nose and face

3. Contrast pemphigus and erythema multiforme.

Study text pages 1531-1532; refer to Figure 41-13.

Pemphigus is a rare, chronic blister-forming disease of the skin and oral mucous membranes with several different types that include pemphigus vulgaris, pemphigus foliaceus, and pemphigus erythematosus. The blisters form in the epidermis and occur deeply in pemphigus vulgaris and superficially in pemphigus foliaceus and pemphigus erythematosus.

Pemphigus is an autoimmune disease caused by circulating IgG autoantibodies. Serum autoantibodies are formed that react with the intracellular cement of substance that holds the epidermal cells together. The antibody reaction likely causes the intraepidermal blister formation and acantholysis or loss of cohesion between epidermal cells.

Pemphigus vulgaris is the most common form of the disease and begins with the formation of a blister in the mouth or on the scalp. Within six months to one year, flaccid bullous lesions appear that rupture easily and leave crusty, denuded skin. Pressure on the blister may cause it to spread to adjacent skin; this is the Nikolsky sign. In **pemphigus foliaceus** and **pemphigus erythematosus**, oral lesions are usually absent and erythema with localized crusting, scaling, and occasional bullae develop.

In the diagnosis of pemphigus, immunofluorescence demonstrates the presence of antibodies at the site of blister formation. The primary treatment for pemphigus is systemic corticosteroids usually in high doses to suppress the immune response during acute episodes or when there is widespread involvement.

Erythema multiforme is an acute, recurring, inflammatory disorder of the skin and mucous membranes. It is associated with allergic or toxic reactions to drugs or microorganisms such as *Mycoplasma pneumoniae* and herpes simplex. Immune complex formation and deposition of C3, IgM, and fibrinogen around the superficial dermal blood vessels, basement membrane, and keratinocytes can be observed in most individuals with erythema multiforme. The characteristic "bull's eye" lesion occurs on the skin surface with a central erythematous region surrounded by concentric rings or alternating edema and inflammation. A vesiculobullous form is characterized by mucous membrane lesions and erythematous plaques on the extensor surfaces of the extremities.

The most common form expressed in children and young adults is **Stevens-Johnson syndrome** wherein there are numerous erythematous, bullous lesions on both the skin and mucous membranes. The bullous lesions form erosions and crusts when they rupture. The mouth, air passages, esophagus, urethra, and conjunctiva may be involved. Mild forms of the disease require no treatment as they are self-transmitting; underlying infections should be treated.

4. Identify the causes and lesions of cutaneous infection.

Study text pages 1532-1537; refer to Figures 41-14 through 14-17 and Tables 41-5 and 41-6.

Cutaneous Infections

	Cause	*Lesion*
Folliculitis	Bacterial infection of hair follicles usually by *Staphylococcus aureus*	Pustules with surrounding erythema
Furuncle	Infection from folliculitis spreading into dermis	Deep, red, firm, painful nodule changes to fluctuant and tender cystic nodule
Carbuncle	Collection of infected hair follicles	Erythematous, painful mass that drains through many openings
Cellulitis	Infection of dermis and subcutaneous tissue; extension from skin wound, ulcer, furuncle, or carbuncle	Erythematous, swollen, and painful area

(Continued)

Cutaneous Infections *(cont'd)*

	Cause	*Lesion*
Erysipelas	Group A streptococci	Systemic manifestations, red spots progress to pruritic vesicles
Impetigo	Coagulase positive staphylococci; beta-hemolytic streptococci	Serous and purulent vesicles that rupture and crust
Herpes simplex virus-1 (HSV-1)	Primary and secondary infections (sensory nerve ganglion latency) on nongenital sites such as cornea, mouth, and labia	Clusters of vesicles on an erythematous base that become purulent and crusty
HSV-2	Primary and secondary infection (sensory nerve ganglion latency) genital herpes	Vesicles that progress to painful ulceration, pruritus, and weeping
Varicella (chickenpox) primary Herpes Zoster (shingles) secondary	Varicella-Zoster virus	Varicella: pink papules with reddened halo that is dry and crusty Zoster: erythema followed by grouped vesicles along a unilateral dermatome that later crust
Warts (verrucae)	Human papillomavirus	Round, elevated with a rough, grayish surface
Tinea capitis (scalp) Tinea pedis (athlete's foot) Tinea corporis (ringworm) Tinea cruris ("jock itch")	Dermatophytes (fungi) that invade and thrive on keratin	Scaling and erythema, vesicles and fissures
Candidiasis	Candida albicans (yeastlike fungus) changes from a skin and mucous membrane commensal to a pathogen	Thin walled pustule with inflammatory pruritic base

5. Contrast vasculitis and urticaria.

Study text page 1537.

Vasculitis, or angiitis, is an inflammation of the blood vessels. Cutaneous vasculitis develops from the deposit of immune complexes in small blood vessels as a response to drugs, allergens, or streptococcal or viral infection. The deposit of immune complex likely activates complement which is chemotactic for polymorphonuclear leukocytes. The lesions appear as palpable purpura and progress to hemorrhagic bullae with necrosis and ulceration because of occlusion of the vessel. Identifying and removing the antigen is the first step in treatment. Prednisone may be used if symptoms are severe.

Urticarial lesions are most commonly associated with type one hypersensitivity reactions to drugs, certain foods, intestinal parasites, or physical agents. The lesions are mediated by histamine release which causes the endothelial cells of skin blood vessels to contract and increase their permeability. The fluid from the vessel appears as wheals, welts, or hives. Antihistamines usually reduce the hives and provide relief of itching. Corticosteroids may be required for treatment of severe attacks.

6. Compare the benign tumors of the skin.

Study text pages 1539-1540; refer to Figures 41-19 and 41-20 and Table 41-7.

Seborrheic keratosis is a benign proliferation of basal cells that produces elevated smooth or warty lesions. Multiple lesions are seen on the chest, back, and face in older people. The color varies; it may be tan to waxy yellow, flesh-colored, or dark brown-black, and the lesions are often oval and greasy appearing with a hyperkeratotic scale. Lesion size varies from a few millimeters to several centimeters. Cryotherapy with liquid nitrogen is an effective treatment and the lesions usually slough in two to three weeks after treatment.

A **keratoacanthoma** is a benign, self-limiting tumor that arises from hair follicles. It usually occurs on sun-exposed surfaces and develops in individuals between 60 and 65 years of age. The lesion develops in stages. The proliferative stage produces a rapid growing domeshaped nodule with a central crust. In the mature stage, the lesion is filled with whitish colored keratin. The mature lesion requires differentiation from squamous cell carcinoma. The involution stage usually occurs over a three to four month period as the lesion regresses.

Although the lesion will resolve spontaneously, it can be removed surgically.

Actinic keratosis is a premalignant lesion found on skin surfaces exposed to ultraviolet radiation of the sun. The lesions can progress to squamous cell carcinoma. The prevalence is highest in individuals with unprotected, light-colored skin. The lesions appear as pigmented patches of rough, adherent scale and surrounding areas may have telangiectasias. Freezing with liquid nitrogen provides quick, effective treatment. Excisions provide tissue for biopsy.

Nevi or moles are pigmented or nonpigmented lesions that form from melanocytes beginning at ages three to five years. During early development, the melanocytes accumulate at the junction of the dermis and epidermis and become macular lesions. Over time, the cells move into the dermis and become nodular and palpable. Nevi may appear anywhere on the skin singly or in groups and they vary in size. Nevi may undergo transition to malignant melanoma; if irritated, they can be excised.

7. Describe malignant skin lesions.

Study text pages 1540-1544; refer to Figures 41-21 through 41-26.

Cancerous Skin Lesions

	Cause	Growth Rate/ Metastasis	Appearance
Basal cell carcinoma	Sunlight exposed skin, cellular shedding by keratinization is prevented	Slow growth; almost never metastasize, invasive destruction	Smooth surface with pearly border, ulcerated center, telangiectasis
Squamous cell carcinoma	Sunlight exposed skin, immunosuppression, arise from premaligant lesions	Moderate growth; some metastasize	Rough, hyperkeratotic nodule with an indurated base, ulcer
Malignant melanoma	Genetic predisposition, solar radiation and steroid hormones, precursor nevi	Fast growth, highly invasive; rapid metastasis	Nevi that change color, size, or margins; pruritus, bleeding, nodule formation or ulceration
Kaposi sarcoma	Immunodeficient states, genetics—black, Jewish, or Italian males	Slow spread through skin, some aggressive change	Multifocal purplish, brown vascular macules that develop into plaques and nodules which may be painful and pruritic; may affect gastrointestinal and respiratory tracts

Note: Treatment consists of surgery, electrodesiccation, radiation, or cryosurgery. For malignant melanomas, wide and deep excisions and removal of lymph nodes is required. For basal cell and squamous cell skin cancers, cure is virtually assured with early detection and treatment. The survival is poor for malignant melanoma because it metastasizes quickly. The general response to treatment of Kaposi sarcoma is poor.

8. Classify burns according to the extent of injury.

Study text pages 1544-1549; refer to Figures 41-27 through 41-32 and Tables 41-8 and 41-9.

Burn Injury

	First degree	Second degree		Third degree
		Superficial partial-thickness	Deep partial-thickness	Full-thickness
Morphology	Destruction of epidermis only	Destruction of epidermis and some dermis	Destruction of epidermis and dermis	Destruction of epidermis, dermis, and subcutaneous tissue
Skin function	Yes	No	No	No
Tactile and pain sensors	Yes	Yes	Diminished	No
Blisters	Present after 24 hours	Present within minutes	May or may not appear, a flat dehydrated layer that lifts off in sheets	Blisters are rare: a flat dehydrated layer that lifts off easily
Appearance of wound after initial debridement	Skin peels after 24 to 48 hours, normal or slightly red	Red to pale ivory, moist surface	Mottled with areas of waxy white, dry surface	White, cherry red, or black: may contain visible thrombosed veins; dry, hard leathery surface
Healing time	3 to 5 days	21 to 28 days	30 days to many months, excision and grafting	Will not heal, may close from edges as secondary healing if wound is small, excision and grafting
Scarring	None	May be present, influenced by genetic predisposition	Highest incidence, influenced by genetic predisposition	Scarring minimized by early excision and grafting, influenced by genetic predisposition

9. Characterize the cardiovascular and cellular response to burn injury.

Study text pages 1549-1554; refer to Figures 41-33 through 41-35 and Table 41-10.

Hypovolemic shock develops quickly following major burn injury. The severity of burn shock is directly proportional to the extent of the total body surface area (TBSA) that is burned. Burns involving 25 to 40 percent TBSA in adults or 15 to 25 percent TBSA in children require cardiovascular support with intravenous fluid. Within minutes of a major burn injury, the capillary bed opens not only in the burn area but also in the entire capillary system. This increased capillary permeability is the mechanism for fluid, electrolyte, and protein loss into the interstitium; this leads to the ensuing hypovolemic shock and massive edema. If the profound hypovolemic shock is not treated, irreversible shock and death may occur within a few hours.

Burn shock resuscitation involves infusion of intravenous fluid at a rate faster than the loss of circulating volume fluid for 24 hours after burn injury. The massive edema associated with burn shock is an iatrogenic complication, but failure to administer resuscitation fluid results in irreversible hypovolemic shock and death. The most reliable criterion to determine adequate resuscitation of burn shock is the urine output. If the individual does not have adequate urine output, sufficient fluid is not being administered. As burn shock ends, fluid administered remains in the circulating volume and is reflected as increased urine output.

Major burn injury affects the entire physiologic system; however, survival depends on its ultimate impact at the **cellular level.** The cellular response to burn injury has a metabolic response and an immunologic response. The cellular dysfunction of burn injury involves disruption of transmembrane potential and sodium-potassium pump impairment and includes loss of intracellular magnesium and phosphate and elevated serum lactic dehydrogenase (LDH) levels. The decrease in the efficiency of the pump can be reversed by adequate fluid resuscitation of burn shock. Metabolic reactions to the stress of a major burn injury involve systemic alterations of the sympathetic nervous system and other homeostatic regulators. Catecholamines are found in elevated amounts in both the serum and urine of burned individuals. Burn injury induces an almost immediate hypermetabolic state that persists until wound closure; there is persistent elevation of core body temperatures. Evaporative water loss and surface cooling are not the primary stimulus for the hypermetabolic state; rather, the hypermetabolism is related to an increase and resetting of the hypothalamic thermal regulatory set point. A reflex arc mobilizes neural and/or hormonal afferent stimuli to the hypothalamus that produces a catecholamine response which is manifested as hypermetabolism, hyperthermia, and hyperglycemia; gluconeogenesis is promoted. Vasodilation, increased capillary permeability, and edema facilitate healing of the local area by transporting both heat and glucose preferentially to the wound. The extensive **evaporative water loss** that occurs in burn tissue is a heat-consuming process and the energy need is met in part by increased visceral heat production. Hypothalamic function alterations cause the elevation of human growth hormone (HGH) serum levels and hyperglycemia. A hepatic response to burn injury is characterized by alterations in the clotting factors. A **hypercoagulable state** develops, which is manifested by elevated plasma fibrinogen concentration in the presence of shortened prothrombin time (PT) and activated partial thromboplastin time (PTT).

In summary, these systemic alterations occur because of the cutaneous inflammatory process and are believed to facilitate wound repair. The neural component of this alteration is in response to sympathetic reaction that releases catecholamines in large amounts. In individuals surviving burn shock, **immunosuppression** and increased susceptibility to potentially fatal systemic burn wound sepsis develop. Translocation of microbes and endotoxins across the intestinal wall may be a mechanism of infection leading to septic shock following burn injury and other major trauma. Natural resistance to infection in burn wounds depends on the nonspecific immune system and relies on the ability of phagocytic cells to leave the bloodstream, migrate to the site of infection, and ingest and kill microorganisms. The burned individual's serum contains an inhibitor of complement conversion that leads to decreased opsonization of bacteria and less polymorphonuclear neutrophil chemotaxis. Individuals with altered immunocompetence who are burned are at additional risk for complications.

10. Characterize frostbite.

Study text pages 1554-1555.

Frostbite is an injury to the skin caused by exposure to extreme cold. The mechanism of injury appears to be direct cold injury to cells, indirect injury from ice crystal formation, or impaired circulation from anoxia to the exposed area. Frozen skin becomes white or yellowish, is waxy, and has no sensation of pain. With mild frostbite during rewarming, there is redness and discomfort followed by a return to normal in a few hours. Cyanosis and mottling develop followed by redness, swelling, and burning pain on rewarming in more severe cases. The most severe cases result in gangrene and loss of the affected part. Frostbite may be classified by depth of injury. Superficial frostbite includes partial skin freezing and is known as first degree;

full-thickness skin freezing is second degree; full-thickness skin and subcutaneous freezing is third degree. Immersion in a warm water bath until frozen tissue is thawed is the best treatment. Pain during the thawing period is severe and should be treated with potent analgesics. Gentle cleansing and avoidance of pressure on the skin should be maintained during healing. Amputation of necrotic tissue is delayed until a clear line of demarcation appears.

11. Define terms used in disorders of the hair and nails.

Study text pages 1555-1556.

Male-pattern alopecia is an inherited form of irreversible baldness where hair is lost in the central scalp and recession of the temporofrontal hairline occurs. **Female-pattern alopecia** is a thinning of the central hair of the scalp that begins in women at 20 to 30 years of age. **Alopecia areata** is patchy loss of hair usually associated with stress or metabolic diseases; it is usually reversible. **Hirsutism** is a male pattern of hair growth in women; it may be normal or the result of excessive secretion of androgenic hormones. **Paronychia** is an inflammation of the cuticle that can be acute or chronic and is usually caused by staphylococci or streptococci or occasionally by *Candida*. **Onychomycosis** is a fungal infection of the nail plate; the plate turns yellow or white and accumulates hyperkeratotic debris.

Practice Examination

1. The major differentiating cell of the epidermis is the
   a. mast cell.
   b. histocyte.
   c. keratinocyte.
   d. melanocyte.
   e. fibroblast.

2. The dermis is composed of all except
   a. melanocytes.
   b. collagen.
   c. elastin.
   d. mast cells.
   e. fibroblasts.

3. Which does not occur as the skin ages?
   a. more melanocytes
   b. decreased Langerhans cells
   c. loss of rete pegs
   d. loss of elastin fibers
   e. depressed immune response

4. The application of KOH and low heat to skin scrapings on a glass slide identifies
   a. chronic bacterial infections.
   b. vasculitis.
   c. antibodies.
   d. fungi.
   e. None of the above is correct.

Match the lesion with its descriptor.

5. macule
6. nodule
7. scale
8. wheal

a. hardened, adherent serum
b. changed color, not raised nor depressed
c. accentuated skin lines caused by scratching
d. palpable, elevated solid lesion
e. flaky, accumulated stratum corneum
f. ridge-like, reddened elevation caused by edema and congestion

9. The cause of atopic dermatitis is
   a. unknown.
   b. venous stasis.
   c. increased activity of sebaceous glands.
   d. mast cell, T-cells, and monocyte interaction.
   e. non-immunologic inflammation to chemicals.

10. The skin lesion of psoriasis is a
    a. nonscaling, violet-colored pruritic papule.
    b. comedone.
    c. pruritic vesicle.
    d. erythematous, butterfly shaped rash.
    e. thick, scaly, erythematous plaque.

11. A circular, demarcated salmon-pink scale within a plaque is characteristic of
    a. psoriasis.
    b. seborrheic dermatitis.
    c. acne rosacea.
    d. pityriasis rosea.
    e. lichen planus.

12. The Nikolsky sign is seen in
    a. herpes simplex.
    b. pemphigus.
    c. erythema multiforme.
    d. Stevens-Johnson syndrome.
    e. Both c and d are correct.

13. The cause of impetigo is
    a. *Staphylococcus aureus.*
    b. group A streptococci.
    c. coagulase-positive staphylococci.
    d. beta-hemolytic streptococci.
    e. Both c and d are correct.

14. The usual transmission mode of type II herpes simplex is by
    a. fomites.
    b. kissing and touching.
    c. sexual encounters.
    d. contaminated food or water.
    e. b, c, and d are correct.

15. Of the benign tumors of the skin, keratoacanthomas are characterized by
    a. proliferation of basal cells.
    b. hyperkeratotic scales.
    c. origination from hair follicles.
    d. a proliferative stage that produces a nodule with a central crust.
    e. Both c and d are correct.

16. Which are most likely to undergo malignant transition?
    a. seborrheic keratosis and keratoacanthoma
    b. seborrheic keratosis and actinic keratosis
    c. nevi and keratoacanthoma
    d. nevi and actinic keratosis
    e. None of the above is correct.

17. The cause of Kaposi sarcoma is likely
    a. solar radiation.
    b. steroidal hormones.
    c. precursor nevi.
    d. immunodeficiency.
    e. keratinization.

18. Squamous cell carcinoma of the skin is manifested as
    a. irregular pigmentation.
    b. ulcerated, hyperkeratotic nodules with dermal invasion.
    c. a smooth, pearly lesion with multiple telangiectasia.
    d. multifocal purplish, brown macules.

19. An untreated basal cell carcinoma
    a. metastasizes frequently.
    b. often involves regional lymphatics.
    c. ulcerates and involves local tissue.
    d. grows rapidly.
    e. will eventually require removal of nearby lymph nodes.

20. Which malignant skin lesion metastasizes the earliest?
    a. basal cell carcinoma
    b. squamous cell carcinoma
    c. malignant melanoma
    d. Kaposi sarcoma

21. In which burn does skin function continue?
    a. first degree
    b. superficial partial-thickness
    c. deep partial-thickness
    d. full-thickness

22. A burn that destroys the epidermis and dermis is a
    a. first degree burn.
    b. superficial partial-thickness burn.
    c. deep partial-thickness burn.
    d. full-thickness burn.

23. Hypovolemic shock in severely burned individuals is the result of
    a. dilation of capillaries.
    b. increased capillary permeability.
    c. increased peripheral resistance.
    d. Both a and b are correct.
    e. a, b, and c are correct.

24. In individuals surviving burn shock, increased wound sepsis is due to
    a. altered complement conversion.
    b. translocation of microbes and endotoxins across the intestinal wall.
    c. inability of phagocytes to migrate to the site of infection.
    d. All of the above are correct.
    e. Both b and c are correct.

25. Onychomycosis is
    a. a fungal infection of the nail plate.
    b. caused by staphylococci or streptococci.
    c. an inflammation of the cuticle.
    d. None of the above is correct.

Case Study

Mr. E. is 26-year-old caucasian male who sustained severe burns while welding an automobile gasoline tank that had been removed from a truck. Mr. E.'s friend, for whom the welding was being done, took him immediately to a regional burn center located 20 miles away. On admission to the burn unit, it was determined that Mr. E. neither smokes cigarettes nor drinks alcohol and has never been seriously ill or had any surgical operations. His family history was noncontributory.

Initial assessment revealed that Mr. E. had received full-thickness burns on his face, to both arms and hands bilaterally and circumferentially, and to the anterior trunk; the burned total body surface area (TBSA) was 35 percent.

What are the major and immediate concerns of the burn unit?

Alterations of the Integument in Children

Prerequisite Objectives

a. Identify the structures of the integumentary system and describe their function.
   Refer to Figure 41-1 and Table 41-1.

Remember!

- See the study guide's narrative for Prerequisite Objective **a** in Chapter 41.

---

b. Identify diagnostic skin procedures.
   Refer to Table 41-2.

Remember!

- See the study guide's narrative for Prerequisite Objective **c** in Chapter 41.

Objectives

After successful study of this chapter, the learner will be able to:

1. Differentiate between atopic and diaper dermatitis in infants and children.
   Study text pages 1562-1564; refer to Figures 42-2 and 42-3.

   Diaper dermatitis is an inflammation of the skin in the diaper area that is caused by many factors including lengthy exposure to wet and soiled diapers. It is mostly localized in the perineal area but may extend from the abdomen to the thighs and usually affects infants and young children. Diaper dermatitis is characterized by an erythematous rash of varying degrees of severity and often is complicated by a secondary fungal infection caused by the microorganism *Candida albicans*. The characteristic rash of *C. albicans* is very erythematous and papular and is associated with **papulovesicular satellite lesions**. This condition can become very painful. The best treatment is preventive by keeping the perineal area clean and dry with frequent diaper changes and routine hygiene. Topical barriers may become necessary once the rash develops. If *C. albicans* is present, a topical antifungal agent should be included in the treatment.

Atopic dermatitis or eczema is an inflammation of the skin of unknown etiology. There is, however, an increased incidence of 75 to 80 percent in individuals who have allergies and reactive airways. Onset is usually in infancy with 85 percent of cases occurring by five years of age. Positive allergy tests, increased serum IgE levels, and eosinophilia are common findings but are not diagnostic. The distribution and occurrence of the skin lesions vary with the age of the child. The face, scalp, trunk, and extensor surfaces of the extremities are commonly affected in younger children; the neck, hands, feet, and flexor surfaces are commonly affected in older children. In the infant, the characteristic rash is erythematous with weeping and crusting lesions. In older children, the rash is frequently erythematous with scaling and thick, leather-like lesions. Atopic dermatitis is chronic in nature with acute exacerbations of variable frequency and intensity. Pruritus or itching leads to rubbing and scratching and more damage to the skin. Scratching causes microscopic cracking in the skin that allows water loss and exposes the lower layers to irritants which, in turn, lead to increased pruritus and scratching. Treatment includes avoiding known irritants, hydration of the skin, antihistamines to relieve pruritus, and topical steroids to decrease inflammation. Antibiotics or antifungal agents may be necessary for secondary skin infections.

2. Describe the etiology and pathophysiology of staphylococcal scalded-skin syndrome.
     Study text pages 1565-1566; refer to Figure 42-5.

Staphylococcal scalded-skin syndrome is an interesting illness because the severe skin lesions it causes are a manifestation of a staphylococcal infection, usually group II staphylococci, at a body site other than the skin. The primary site of infection is the throat or chest with the onset of lesions usually preceded by an upper respiratory infection that is characterized by fever, rhinorrhea, and malaise. This severe infection is an illness of children under 10 years of age and is frequently seen in newborns because their immune systems are immature. Manifestations are caused by an epidermolytic toxin produced by the staphylococcal microorganisms at the primary site of infection; the toxin circulates to the skin where it produces the classic effects. The toxin splits the epidermis away from the underlying layers. The first sign of skin involvement is the acute onset of generalized erythema and tenderness over the entire body except the palms, soles of the feet, and the mucous membranes. Blisters and bullae form over the next several days which rupture and denude the skin leaving the child at risk for dehydration and secondary infection. In severe cases, generalized skin sloughing may occur. Diagnosis is confirmed by culture and histologic studies. Lesions are treated like severe burns and the primary infection is treated with oral or parenteral antibiotics. Healing in uncomplicated cases usually requires 10 to 14 days.

3. Categorize and characterize the infectious processes of impetigo, tinea capitis, tinea corporis, molluscum contagiosum, and chickenpox.
     Study text pages 1564-1570; refer to Figures 42-4, 42-6, 42-7, and 42-9 and Table 42-1.

Impetigo is a common bacterial skin infection in children and is either bullous or vesicular.

Impetigo

	Bullous	*Vesicular*
Etiologic agent	*Staphylococcus aureus*	Streptococcus pyogenes or combined with staphylococcus
Source	Other infected individuals or contaminated objects	Other infected individuals, contaminated objects, insect bites
Regional lymphadenitis	Uncommon	Common
Treatment	Systemic antibiotics	Systemic antibiotics
Potential complications	Uncommon	Acute glomerulonephritis

Tinea capitis and **tinea corporis** are caused by dermatophytes or fungal infections of the skin. Dermatophytes invade the stratum corneum and release toxins that cause skin inflammation.

Fungal Infections

	Tinea capitis	*Tinea corporis*
Etiologic Agent	*Microsporum canis, Trichophyton tonsurans*	Microsporum canis, Trichophyton *mentagrophytes*
Source	*M. canis* from cats, dogs, or rodents *T. tonsurans* from humans	*M. canis* and *T. mentagrophytes* from kittens or puppies
Lesion	Circular, slight erythema, scaling raised border	Oval or round with scale, central clearing, mild erythema or ringworm
Diagnostic test	KOH examination	KOH examination
Treatment	Oral antifungals (topicals do not penetrate hair bulb)	Topical antifungals

Molluscum contagiosum is a contagious, viral disease characterized by a 1 cm to 5 cm diameter pearlescent, dome-shaped lesion that may appear anywhere on the body but most frequently affects the face, trunk, and extremities. The lesions are asymptomatic and are not inflamed. No specific treatment is recommended because it is self-limiting, although recurrence is common.

Chickenpox is caused by the varicella zoster virus, a member of the complex family of herpes DNA viruses. It is a highly contagious disease of early childhood and is primarily spread by droplet transmission from an infected person to others. Household infection rates approach 90 percent in susceptible individuals. The incubation period is approximately 14 days with infected persons contagious for approximately 24 hours prior to the onset of the rash and for five to six days after the rash appears. Chickenpox is usually an illness of late winter or early spring. The first signs of illness are pruritus or itching or the appearance of vesicles. There may be no prodromal symptoms.

Characteristically, the rash undergoes a process of maturation with lesions starting as macules that progress to superficial papules and vesicles which then rupture and heal. The rash lasts for four to five days and may consist of up to 300 lesions distributed over the body. Complications from chickenpox are fairly rare but may include pneumonia due to the varicella virus. Treatment is asymptomatic with treatment consisting of cool baths, wet dressings, and oral antihistamines.

4. Compare and contrast the infestations of scabies and lice.

Review text pages 1570-1572; refer to Figure 42-10.

Insect Infestations

	Scabies (mite)	*Pediculosis (lice)*
Etiologic agent	*Sarcoptes scabiei*	*Pediculus capitis* (head), *Pediculus corporis* (body), *Phthirius pubis* (pubic)
		(Continued)

Insect Manifestations *(cont'd)*

	Scabies (mite)	*Pediculosis (lice)*
How spread	Contact with infested person	Contact with infested person or object (hat, clothing)
Symptoms	Severe pruritis and burrows in the intertriginous areas	Pruritus, ova (nits) may be seen on hair shafts, mature lice may be seen
Cause of symptoms	Sensitization to larva buried in the skin	Irritation from toxic saliva from louse bites
Treatment	Permethrin/lindane, treatment of exposed persons and infested objects	Permethrin/lindane, treatment of exposed persons and infested objects

5. Compare and contrast the congenital vascular disorders.

Study text pages 1572-1574; refer to Figures 42-12 and 42-13.

Vascular Disorders

	Strawberry hemangioma	*Cavernous hemangioma*	*Salmon patches*	*Portwine stain*
Description	Raised vesicular	Raised vesicular with larger mature vessels	Macular, most common	Flat, becomes papular and cavernous
Manifestations	At birth or emerges in three to five weeks	At birth	At birth	At birth or in a few days
Color	Bright red (capillary projections)	Bluish, less distinct borders	Pink, distended dermal capillaries	Pink to dark reddish purple
Location	One lesion on head, neck or trunk	Head, neck	Nap of neck, forehead, upper eyelid	Face and other body surfaces
Growth	Initially rapid then at child's rate of growth	Rapid first six months, matures at one year	Fades in one year	Does not fade

(Continued)

Vascular Disorders *(cont'd)*

	Strawberry hemangioma	*Cavernous hemangioma*	*Salmon patches*	*Portwine stain*
Involution	Begins by 12 to 16 months, complete by five to six years	Begins by six to 12 months, complete by nine years	N/A	N/A
Treatment	None	May require surgery, laser surgery, or liquid nitrogen depending on location of lesion	None	Cryosurgery, laser surgery

Practice Examination

True/False

____ 1. Diaper dermatitis is caused by *Candida albicans*.

____ 2. Impetigo is contracted only by human-to-human contact.

____ 3. Molluscum contagiosum is a very painful viral infection.

____ 4. Atopic dermatitis is also called eczema.

____ 5. Staphylococcus scalded-skin syndrome is a contagious disease of the skin.

____ 6. Tinea capitis must be treated with systemic antifungal agents.

____ 7. Salmon patches are commonly called stork bites and fade over time.

____ 8. Portwine stains will involute by adulthood.

____ 9. Acute glomerulonephritis is a complication of bullous impetigo.

____ 10. The microorganism that causes bullous impetigo is *Streptococcus pyogenes*.

Match the description with the alteration.

11. viral skin infection contracted during the first decade
12. positive allergy tests, increased IgE, and eosinophilia
13. erythematous lesions in the perineal area with secondary papulovesicular satellites
14. raised, erythemic, scaling lesions on the scalp
15. dome-shaped lesions ranging from 1 cm to 5 cm on the extremities without pruritus
16. macules, fever, itching, papules, and rupturing and healing vesicles
17. crusted lesion
18. mite burrowing in the stratum corneum
19. present at birth or shortly after birth
20. entire skin sloughing
21. nits on hair shaft
22. chronic condition with acute exacerbations, pruritus, thick leathery skin
23. oval or circular lesions, peripheral spreading, central clearing (ringworm)
24. action of a epidermolytic toxin
25. parasitic in nature, epidemic in elementary schools

a. staphylococcus scalded-skin syndrome
b. tinea capitis
c. atopic dermatitis
d. pediculosis
e. diaper dermatitis with *Candida albicans*
f. chickenpox
g. vascular disorders
h. impetigo
i. molluscum contagiosum
j. scabies
k. tinea corporis

Case Study

Lance D. is a five-year-old caucasian boy who visits the nurse practitioner's office with a "runny" nose that started about one week ago but has not resolved. He has been blowing his nose quite frequently and "sores" have developed on his face. His mother states that the sores started as "big blisters" that rupture; sometimes, a scab forms with a crust that looks like "dried maple syrup" but continues to weep and drain. She is becoming worried because the lesions are also now on his forearm. Lance's past medical and family histories are normal. He has been febrile but is otherwise asymptomatic. The physical examination is unremarkable except for moderate, purulent rhinorrhea and 0.5 cm to 1 cm diameter weeping lesions around the nose and mouth and on the radial surface of the right forearm. There is no regional lymphadenopathy.

Is the crust and character of these lesions significant? Is the lack of lymphadenopathy significant? Why have these lesions spread to his arm?

Answers

Chapter 1

1.	c	6.	a	11.	g	16.	b	21.	e
2.	e	7.	c	12.	e	17.	b	22.	e
3.	a	8.	d	13.	f	18.	b	23.	b
4.	e	9.	h	14.	j	19.	e	24.	c
5.	d	10.	d	15.	i	20.	c	25.	d

Chapter 2

1.	d	6.	a	11.	d	16.	c	21.	c
2.	b	7.	a	12.	b	17.	b	22.	a
3.	d	8.	b	13.	a	18.	d	23.	d
4.	e	9.	a	14.	d	19.	a	24.	b
5.	e	10.	d	15.	d	20.	e	25.	e

Chapter 3

1.	e	6.	e	11.	d	16.	c	21.	e
2.	c	7.	b	12.	d	17.	e	22.	b
3.	e	8.	b	13.	c	18.	b	23.	a
4.	c	9.	a	14.	b	19.	d	24.	c
5.	d	10.	c	15.	e	20.	a	25.	b

Chapter 4

1.	a	6.	d	11.	d	16.	f	21.	h
2.	b	7.	b	12.	d	17.	h	22.	d
3.	d	8.	c	13.	b	18.	g	23.	f
4.	d	9.	c	14.	c	19.	i	24.	g
5.	d	10.	a	15.	a	20.	b	25.	c

Chapter 5

1.	True	6.	False	11.	False	16.	True	21.	False
2.	True	7.	True	12.	False	17.	True	22.	e
3.	True	8.	True	13.	False	18.	False	23.	g
4.	True	9.	True	14.	True	19.	True	24.	a
5.	False	10.	False	15.	False	20.	True	25.	h

Chapter 6

1.	c	6.	e	11.	d	16.	d	21.	c
2.	a	7.	b	12.	e	17.	a	22.	a
3.	d	8.	d	13.	d	18.	b	23.	a
4.	e	9.	d	14.	e	19.	c	24.	b
5.	f	10.	a	15.	d	20.	f	25.	a

Chapter 7

1.	e	6.	a	11.	d	16.	d	21.	b
2.	b	7.	a	12.	a	17.	c	22.	d
3.	d	8.	b	13.	b	18.	e	23.	e
4.	b	9.	e	14.	b	19.	e	24.	g
5.	d	10.	d	15.	c	20.	e	25.	f

Chapter 8

1.	b	6.	b	11.	c	16.	a	21.	e
2.	c	7.	d	12.	d	17.	d	22.	e
3.	a	8.	c	13.	c	18.	a	23.	d
4.	c	9.	d	14.	d	19.	c	24.	a
5.	d	10.	d	15.	a	20.	b	25.	d

Chapter 9

1.	c	6.	a	11.	c	16.	a	21.	c
2.	f	7.	b	12.	a	17.	c	22.	e
3.	d	8.	c	13.	d	18.	a	23.	g
4.	e	9.	b	14.	a	19.	c	24.	h
5.	g	10.	d	15.	d	20.	a	25.	i

Chapter 10

1.	c	6.	a	11.	c	16.	b	21.	e
2.	e	7.	d	12.	d	17.	e	22.	c
3.	f	8.	e	13.	e	18.	e	23.	d
4.	c	9.	b	14.	c	19.	a	24.	a
5.	c	10.	f	15.	e	20.	d	25.	f

Chapter 11

1.	e	6.	e	11.	c	16.	d	21.	g
2.	c	7.	b	12.	d	17.	d	22.	c
3.	d	8.	e	13.	a	18.	a	23.	e
4.	e	9.	d	14.	e	19.	d	24.	f
5.	e	10.	c	15.	c	20.	b	25.	a

Chapter 12

1.	c	6.	a	11.	c	16.	c	21.	a
2.	d	7.	c	12.	a	17.	a	22.	b
3.	c	8.	a	13.	a	18.	d	23.	a
4.	b	9.	b	14.	c	19.	c	24.	d
5.	e	10.	d	15.	a	20.	a	25.	c

Chapter 13

1.	b	6.	b	11.	e	16.	b	21.	c
2.	a	7.	e	12.	b	17.	a	22.	j
3.	e	8.	e	13.	d	18.	e	23.	i
4.	b	9.	c	14.	c	19.	e	24.	h
5.	c	10.	b	15.	b	20.	e	25.	g

Case Study Discussion

Her history and response to medication were typical of *depression*. Depression causes sleep disturbances characterized by insomnia, early morning awakenings, or multiple awakenings during the night. The improvement in the quality of sleep following antidepressants often occurs before other appropriate behavioral changes are seen. It seems likely that her insomnia may return, and an appropriate course of action might include seeking assistance from a sleep disorder center and/or a social worker, psychiatrist, or psychologist.

Chapter 14

1.	c	6.	c	11.	c	16.	c	21.	l
2.	e	7.	e	12.	b	17.	a	22.	b
3.	b	8.	d	13.	a	18.	e	23.	e
4.	a	9.	e	14.	b	19.	j	24.	f
5.	b	10.	d	15.	c	20.	k	25.	g

Case Study Discussion

Normal laboratory values and the normal CSF likely exclude the possibility of an infection such as meningitis and other causes known to precipitate seizures. The skull X-ray ruled out the possibility of a skull fracture. The absence of slow-wave activity on the EEG likely excludes intracranial pressure from brain masses. Since EEG may be normal between seizures, the episodal pattern suggests a *generalized grand mal seizure*. A judicious administration of anticonvulsant medications is likely indicated.

Chapter 15

1.	d	6.	d	11.	a	16.	d	21.	b
2.	b	7.	e	12.	b	17.	b	22.	d
3.	e	8.	a	13.	c	18.	c	23.	g
4.	c	9.	b	14.	e	19.	b	24.	c
5.	b	10.	e	15.	c	20.	b	25.	f

Case Study Discussion

Mrs. B. exhibits risk factors for a CVA. She smokes cigarettes, is overweight, has used estrogen for 20 years, and is hypertensive. Her mother and siblings each had a history of diabetes, CVA, and hypertension; all of these indicate a family history that increases the risk for CVA.

Her symptoms and signs suggest a *thrombotic stroke* with ischemia rather than a hemorrhagic or embolic stroke. Mrs. B.'s elevated blood pressure is likely caused by atherosclerosis which can lead to a thrombus formation. The absence of blood in CSF rules out a hemorrhagic stroke. Since there was no fibrillation on the electrocardiogram, the heart was an unlikely source for emboli, thus ruling out an embolic stroke.

Chapter 16

1.	False	6.	True	11.	False	16.	craniosynostosis	21.	e
2.	False	7.	True	12.	Reye, hepatic	17.	i	22.	d
3.	False	8.	True	13.	posterior	18.	h	23.	c
4.	True	9.	False	14.	anterior	19.	g	24.	b
5.	False	10.	False	15.	meningitis	20.	f	25.	a

Case Study Discussion

X-rays reveal an absence of spinal processes on the vertebrae from L3 to L5! MRI is then ordered revealing a **meningomyelocele** at the same level with tethering of the cord. A neurosurgical consultation is ordered and surgery is planned. However, one week before surgery, some loss of bladder control is noted. This is a rather unusual presentation for a meningomyelocele but illustrates that these problems may be fairly obscure and only become apparent later in childhood.

Chapter 17

1.	a	6.	b	11.	b	16.	d	21.	a
2.	e	7.	a	12.	d	17.	e	22.	c
3.	c	8.	c	13.	e	18.	b	23.	e
4.	b	9.	d	14.	c	19.	d	24.	d
5.	d	10.	d	15.	d	20.	e	25.	f

Chapter 18

1.	c	6.	a	11.	a	16.	c	21.	a
2.	a	7.	a	12.	b	17.	a	22.	c
3.	a	8.	a	13.	b	18.	e	23.	e
4.	d	9.	b	14.	b	19.	c	24.	d
5.	b	10.	d	15.	c	20.	e	25.	b

Case Study Discussion

Scott's symptoms, signs, and laboratory values are classic for *diabetes hetoacidosis*. The serum values indicated metabolic acidosis with some accompanying respiratory compensation. His elevated glycosylated hemoglobin showed that he likely had been hyperglycemic for several months. This diabetes is Type I (IDDM) and will require insulin administration and personal instructions regarding recognition of future signs and symptoms of hyperglycemia and hypoglycemia, self-blood glucose monitoring, insulin therapy, diet, and exercise.

Chapter 19

1.	e	6.	d	11.	a	16.	c	21.	a
2.	a	7.	a	12.	e	17.	e	22.	c
3.	e	8.	b	13.	b	18.	c	23.	c
4.	d	9.	e	14.	c	19.	e	24.	e
5.	c	10.	b	15.	a	20.	a	25.	a

Chapter 20

1.	a	6.	e	11.	c	16.	d	21.	d
2.	d	7.	d	12.	d	17.	d	22.	b
3.	c	8.	e	13.	a	18.	d	23.	a
4.	e	9.	d	14.	e	19.	a	24.	b
5.	d	10.	b	15.	b	20.	d	25.	b

Case Study Discussion

Mrs. B.'s history and examination are indicative of *breast cancer* in her left breast. A positive familial history of breast cancer has a strong, confirmed causal link to breast cancer. A chromosome 17 defect has been implicated as a genetic causal factor in breast cancer as well. Other associated risk factors for breast cancer that Mrs. B. exhibits include late age at first delivery, early menarche, birth control pills, and benign breast tumors. Other possible risk factors such as high dietary fat and alcohol intake and hypothyroidism are not present for Mrs. B.

The cardinal manifestation of breast cancer was a hard, fixed mass palpable in Mrs. B.'s left breast. The freely moveable, soft masses of the right breast are likely benign as they display different, fluctuating patterns of tissue proliferation than the left breast. The palpation of the axillary lymph node indicated that cancer cells have metastasized through the lymphatic channels surrounding the breast.

The mammographic confirmation of the mass dictates the need for modified radical mastectomy in order to remove, stage, and classify the tumor and do an estrogen receptor assay. The results of these procedures and tests will enable the selection of further treatment modalities.

Chapter 21

1.	c	6.	False	11.	False	16.	False	21.	True
2.	e	7.	False	12.	False	17.	True	22.	False
3.	f	8.	True	13.	False	18.	True	23.	False
4.	h	9.	True	14.	True	19.	False	24.	True
5.	i	10.	True	15.	False	20.	True	25.	True

Case Study Discussion

Cervicitis is common in the STDs of gonorrhea, chlamydia, and herpes. No blisters are observed, suggesting herpes is unlikely. The vaginal discharge indicates gonorrhea or chlamydial infection. The absence of diplococci inside neutrophils rules out gonorrhea and leads to a presumptive diagnosis of *Chlamydia trachomatis* as the cause of this STD. A test on a sample of cervical discharge could be used to establish a definitive diagnosis of chlamydial infection. Such a test would use fluorescein - labeled monoclonal antibody against *Chlamydia trachomatis*. The test would be read microscopically.

Chapter 22

1.	e	6.	c	11.	d	16.	b	21.	e
2.	b	7.	c	12.	e	17.	c	22.	e
3.	e	8.	c	13.	e	18.	a	23.	b
4.	d	9.	d	14.	d	19.	a	24.	d
5.	a	10.	e	15.	d	20.	b	25.	d

Chapter 23

1.	e	6.	a	11.	b	16.	b	21.	e
2.	d	7.	c	12.	b	17.	b	22.	b
3.	c	8.	c	13.	c	18.	a	23.	a
4.	a	9.	c	14.	a	19.	e	24.	e
5.	b	10.	c	15.	a	20.	b	25.	c

Case Study Discussion

Three anemias have erythrocytes that are microcytic and hypochromic: iron deficiency, sideroblastic anemia, and thalassemia. Ann's ancestral history suggests she may have thalassemia; however, blood loss is the major cause of *iron deficiency anemia*. Her history has some factors that could contribute to anemia from blood loss. The menorrhagia causes more iron loss than is normal with each menstrual period and excessive aspirin intake irritates the gastrointestinal mucosa and can precipitate chronic mucosal microhemorrhage.

Ann's homeostatic mechanisms are trying to compensate in several ways, including shunting blood to more critical organs, increasing erythropoiesis, increasing the heart rate to handle increased venous return, and increased breathing to make oxygen available to the remaining erythrocytes. The last two signs are relevant compensation efforts in Ann's circumstance.

The impression of an iron deficiency anemia can be verified by providing oral iron replacement and checking her hemoglobin values in one month. If the hemoglobin deficit is being corrected, it is likely that the correct diagnosis was made. The source of bleeding should be corrected, if possible, a substitute for aspirin should be used, and iron supplementation should be used for at least one year.

Chapter 24

1.	b	6.	d	11.	c	16.	a	21.	e
2.	c	7.	d	12.	b	17.	b	22.	d
3.	d	8.	e	13.	b	18.	b	23.	e
4.	f	9.	d	14.	a	19.	c	24.	e
5.	g	10.	d	15.	a	20.	a	25.	e

Case Study Discussion

The physician would likely conclude that L.L. has *acute lymphocytic leukemia* since the onset is usually insidious in children and is initially manifested by general malaise. The pale skin with petechiae and ecchymoses is abnormal, as is the gingival bleeding from minor trauma. These are highly suggestive of blood disorders. Also, past viral infection may cause leukemia. Although the abnormal values for RCBs, hemoglobin, total leukocyte count, and platelet count have many possible causes, the presence of blasts in peripheral blood indicates a bone marrow dysfunction. At this time, the physician will likely refer L.L. to a pediatric oncologist for extensive diagnostic tests and treatment.

Chapter 25

1.	False	6.	False	11.	d	16.	b	21.	e
2.	True	7.	False	12.	c	17.	e	22.	c
3.	True	8.	a	13.	e	18.	e	23.	d
4.	False	9.	b	14.	d	19.	a	24.	c
5.	True	10.	d	15.	d	20.	b	25.	d

Case Study Discussion

Steven has the typical manifestations of *idiopathic thrombocytopenia purpura* (ITP), although it has come to medical attention in a very round-about manner. He likely will be started on oral steroid therapy to suppress the immune attack on platelets and followed closely for the next few weeks until his signs clear. About 90% of affected children regain normal platelet counts.

Chapter 26

1.	b	6.	b	11.	a	16.	b	21.	a
2.	b	7.	e	12.	a	17.	c	22.	d
3.	b	8.	a	13.	c	18.	b	23.	b
4.	c	9.	c	14.	d	19.	d	24.	b
5.	b	10.	e	15.	a	20.	a	25.	b

Chapter 27

1.	d	6.	b	11.	e	16.	f	21.	e
2.	e	7.	d	12.	a	17.	b	22.	d
3.	c	8.	e	13.	b	18.	c	23.	b
4.	b	9.	c	14.	c	19.	b	24.	c
5.	a	10.	b	15.	e	20.	c	25.	b

Case Study Discussion

Alterable myocardial infarction risk factors for W.S. are essential hypertension and cigarette smoking. If hypertension is medically controlled and smoking is discontinued, the atherosclerotic process is slowed. Unalterable risk factors for W.S. include advancing age, male sex, and family history of early cardiac death. Atherosclerosis in the anterior descending branch of the left coronary artery was the beginning process leading to this infarction. The location of infarction was verified by electrocardiogram.

The precipitating event in this myocardial infarction was complete occlusion of the coronary artery. Ischemia from dysrhythmia and valvular changes occur but seldom decrease myocardial perfusion enough to cause infarction. Dysrhythmias are common complications of myocardial infarctions rather than being the cause. The history of hypertension also supports occlusion of the coronary artery as the cause for this myocardial infarction.

Pulmonary thromboembolism is a common cause of death from myocardial infarction as emboli disseminate from debris or clots from the infarcted endocardium. Deep venous thrombi of the legs are common sources for systemic emboli. Prophylactic heparin therapy decreases the risk of pulmonary embolism and deep vein thrombosis by interfering with the conversion of prothrombin to thrombin so thrombi are less likely to form.

Chapter 28

1. False
2. True
3. False
4. True
5. False
6. Shunt
7. left, right
8. right, left
9. oxygenated, unoxygenated
10. equal
11. constricting
12. 10-21 days
13. pulmonary stenosis
14. afterload, congestive heart failure
15. coarctation of the aorta
16. e
17. a
18. a
19. b
20. c
21. c
22. c
23. d
24. d
25. a

Case Study Discussion

After consultation, the echocardiogram demonstrates a moderate *coarctation of the aorta* in the aortic arch. This discrepancy in the quality of upper and lower extremity pulses is because of well-developed collateral circulation to the descending aorta; the femoral pulses will be decreased as blood fills the collateral vessels. Although this boy is presently asymptomatic, the degree of coarctation will cause symptoms later in life such as headache, hypertension, and epistaxis.

Chapter 29

1. d	6. e	11. c	16. d	21. a
2. d	7. d	12. a	17. a	22. e
3. c	8. c	13. c	18. b	23. a
4. d	9. a	14. d	19. b	24. b
5. d	10. b	15. b	20. e	25. a

Chapter 30

1. g	6. d	11. c	16. d	21. b
2. c	7. e	12. e	17. e	22. d
3. h	8. f	13. d	18. d	23. e
4. l	9. j	14. e	19. b	24. b
5. i	10. m	15. a	20. b	25. a

Case Study Discussion

Mr. S. presents the classic symptoms and signs of *emphysema*. His long-term, extensive smoking is consistent with most cases of emphysema, as is his dyspnea on exertion progressing to dyspnea even at rest. Leaning forward with arm bracing on knees when sitting often is seen in individuals with emphysema. Hyperinflation of lungs causes the anteroposterior chest diameter to increase. The chest radiograph is consistent with findings in emphysema. Prolonged forced expiratory volume, decreased tidal volume, and increased total lung capacity are also present in emphysema. These tests indicate the walls of alveoli have been destroyed, the lungs have become more distended or less compliant, and have less elastic recoil. Therefore, air is trapped and expiration flow is diminished.

Chapter 31

1. False	6. True	11. c	16. d	21. e
2. False	7. e	12. d	17. a and b	22. c
3. False	8. e	13. c	18. a and b	23. d
4. True	9. d	14. e	19. f	24. c
5. False	10. e	15. d	20. f	25. a

Case Study Discussion

Tyler has classic manifestations of *bronchiolitis*. The most likely etiologic agent in Tyler's illness is respiratory syncytial virus to which his parents likely exposed him during their "colds." He is displaying the classic signs of respiratory distress in an infant and is unable to feed due to this respiratory distress. He is becoming dehydrated, and his lethargy is probably due to the dehydration, mild hypoxia and hypercapnia, and general fatigue from prolonged ventilatory effort. He may suffer respiratory failure if left untreated. Hospitalization for oxygen therapy, rehydration, and respiratory therapy should support him through the worst of his illness, and he should improve within a few days.

Chapter 32

1.	c	6.	b	11.	e	16.	d	21.	b
2.	a	7.	b	12.	b	17.	a	22.	c
3.	d	8.	c	13.	b	18.	e	23.	c
4.	a	9.	d	14.	d	19.	d	24.	d
5.	d	10.	c	15.	b	20.	a	25.	d

Chapter 33

1.	d	6.	d	11.	d	16.	b	21.	c
2.	b	7.	b	12.	e	17.	d	22.	b
3.	a	8.	b	13.	d	18.	c	23.	d
4.	a	9.	b	14.	d	19.	a	24.	a
5.	e	10.	d	15.	e	20.	d	25.	e

Case Study Discussion

Eddie's history of sore throat, back pain, and his laboratory values suggest *post-streptococcal glomerulonephritis.* Proteinuria is a sensitive indicator of glomerular dysfunction. In glomerulonephritis, the glomerulus is injured and its permeability increased enough to permit protein to enter into the filtrate and urine. Blood and RBC casts also are seen in glomerulonephritis. BUN and creatinine are excreted entirely by the kidneys and therefore are directly related to renal excretion. The creatinine level should remain constant because it is associated with muscle mass which fluctuates little. Whenever the BUN and creatinine ratio remain constant, renal disease is the cause rather than hydration alterations, gastrointestinal bleeding, malnutrition, or liver abnormalities. Measurements of the ASO liter is used in the differential diagnosis of poststreptococcal diseases such as glomerulonephritis, rheumatic fever, bacterial endocarditis, and scarlet fever. It indicates that a streptococcal infection is or recently has been present. Eddie's pediatrician will most likely place him on penicillin and may prescribe an antihypertensive medication and monitor his blood pressure, electrolyte balance, and BUN and creatinine levels.

Chapter 34

1.	False	6.	False	11.	e	16.	d	21.	b
2.	True	7.	c	12.	e	17.	e	22.	d
3.	False	8.	a	13.	d	18.	e	23.	c
4.	False	9.	e	14.	d	19.	d	24.	a
5.	True	10.	c	15.	d	20.	f	25.	g

Case Study Discussion

The laboratory values reveal an anemia and thrombocytopenia; the child is losing red blood cells and platelets. Her protein and albumin are low, which alters the osmotic pressure for fluid balance; thus, the generalized edema. Since she has not voided any urine, acute renal failure is very likely. These results suggest the diagnosis of *hemolytic uremic syndrome*. She will require hospitalization for blood transfusions and dialysis. Other supportive care would be close monitoring of laboratory values, intake and output of fluids, vital signs, and good skin care.

Chapter 35

1.	d	6.	d	11.	d	16.	d	21.	b
2.	d	7.	d	12.	b	17.	a	22.	c
3.	b	8.	a	13.	a	18.	b	23.	e
4.	e	9.	d	14.	c	19.	a	24.	c
5.	e	10.	b	15.	c	20.	c	25.	a

Chapter 36

1.	b	6.	d	11.	b	16.	d	21.	b
2.	d	7.	c	12.	e	17.	e	22.	c.
3.	a	8.	e	13.	b	18.	e	23.	d
4.	e	9.	a	14.	a	19.	d	24.	a
5.	e	10.	b	15.	c	20.	a	25.	d

Case Study Discussion

A *gastric ulcer* is likely. Factors associated with these ulcers include smoking, stress, and use of aspirin or other ulcerogenic drugs. Although, the clinical manifestations of gastric ulcers are similar to those of duodenal ulcers, the pain of gastric ulcers is more likely to occur immediately after eating. Also, gastric ulcers tend to be chronic rather than alternate between periods of remission and exacerbation. An upper gastrointestinal study using barium sulfate as a contrasting medium and endoscopy can detect the location of the ulcer and confirm that Dr. R. has a gastric ulcer.

Chapter 37

1.	False	10.	False	18.	c
2.	True	11.	True	19.	b
3.	False	12.	gastroesophageal reflux	20.	a
4.	False	13.	biopsy	21.	e
5.	False	14.	decrease	22.	d
6.	True	15.	otitis media, sinusitis	23.	d
7.	True	16.	rectal prolapse	24.	c
8.	False	17.	a	25.	c
9.	True				

Case Study Discussion

Baby B.'s problem was somewhat diagnosed when an attempt to pass a catheter from the infant's mouth into the stomach failed. X-ray shows a "kink" in the esophagus. Both observations are fairly characteristic manifestations of *esophageal atresia*. He was hypoglycemic because of his inability to feed. The defect probably did not have any relationship to the mother's hypertension. Baby B. is transferred to a pediatric surgeon for surgical correction.

Chapter 38

1.	d	6.	b	11.	d	16.	d	21.	c
2.	d	7.	b	12.	d	17.	a	22.	e
3.	d	8.	d	13.	a	18.	b	23.	e
4.	e	9.	b	14.	c	19.	d	24.	e
5.	b	10.	b	15.	a	20.	b	25.	c

Chapter 39

1.	a	6.	e	11.	a	16.	a	21.	d
2.	b	7.	c	12.	e	17.	d	22.	d
3.	d	8.	c	13.	b	18.	d	23.	c
4.	b.	9.	e	14.	d	19.	e	24.	e
5.	d	10.	a	15.	e	20.	b	25.	e

Case Study Discussion

The presenting symptoms of Mrs. B.B. might be compatible with either osteoarthritis or rheumatoid arthritis. The laboratory studies support a diagnosis of *rheumatoid arthritis.* The presence of rheumatoid factor is helpful in the diagnosis of rheumatoid arthritis. It is positive in about 80 percent of individuals who have rheumatoid arthritis. Although other diseases may show a positive test, osteoarthritis will not. Synovial fluid analysis showing poor mucin precipitates and inflammatory exudates satisfies the diagnostic criteria for rheumatoid arthritis. In osteoarthritis, few cells and normal mucin would be expected. The radiograph is more representative of rheumatoid arthritis than osteoarthritis. In osteoarthritis, deformity of articular cartilage, bone sclerosis, cystic areas, and bony spurs would be likely observations.

Chapter 40

1.	False	6.	True	11.	permanent	16.	d	21.	e
2.	False	7.	False	12.	asymmetric	17.	f	22.	d
3.	False	8.	True	13.	dystrophin	18.	e	23.	c
4.	True	9.	True	14.	abduction, flexion	19.	f	24.	b
5.	True	10.	False	15.	club foot	20.	d	25.	a

Case Study Discussion

This child has the most common of the *congenital myopathies*, congenital absence of the pectoral muscle. This is more common in Duchenne muscular dystrophy than in the general population and is known as Poland syndrome when combined with syndactyly in the affected side. This is not the case with Ashley. Although the defect is permanent, referrals are made to plastic surgeons who may be helpful in the future.

Chapter 41

1.	c	6.	d	11.	d	16.	d	21.	a
2.	a	7.	e	12.	b	17.	d	22.	c
3.	a	8.	f	13.	e	18.	b	23.	d
4.	d	9.	d	14.	c	19.	c	24.	d
5.	b	10.	e	15.	e	20.	c	25.	a

Case Study Discussion

Adults with burns involving 25 to 40 percent TBSA require cardiovascular support through intravenous fluid since *hypovolemic shock* develops quickly following major burn injury. Within minutes of a major burn injury, the capillary bed not only at the site of the burn but throughout the entire body becomes more permeable to water, sodium, and proteins. This leads to fluid loss from the intravascular spaces into the interstitial spaces and massive edema; the blood volume and cardiac output diminish. Nasotracheal intubation is required to avoid edematous obstruction of the upper airway. The infusion of intravenous fluid or burn shock resuscitation for the first 24 hours must be faster than the rate of loss of circulatory volume. To determine adequate levels of infusion, urine output must be measured so Mr. E. will require a catheter into his bladder.

Although hypovolemic shock is the immediate concern for major burn patients, other alterations are very important; monitoring and maintenance of electrolytes is required. Circulation to burned extremities may be impaired as the circumferential nature of the burns and the edema may act as a tourniquet. Therefore, a surgical cut through the circumferential area may be required to restore adequate blood supply to the limbs. Cleansing and hydrotherapy of burned areas should not draw vital electrolytes from cells because of altered toxicity. The hypermetabolic rate of burned individuals requires adequate nutrition to provide a positive nitrogen balance. Finally, excision and grafting procedures require meticulous care.

Chapter 42

1.	False	6.	True	11.	f	16.	f	21.	d
2.	False	7.	True	12.	c	17.	h	22.	c
3.	False	8.	False	13.	e	18.	j	23.	k
4.	True	9.	False	14.	b	19.	g	24.	a
5.	False	10.	False	15.	i	20.	a	25.	d

Case Study Discussion

This is a fairly classic case of *bullous impetigo* caused by a *Staphylococcus aureus* infection in Lance's nasopharynx. Abrasion from blowing his nose frequently has opened the skin and allowed the bacteria to enter the skin and cause the lesions. The infection spread to his arm because he has been wiping his nose on his arm. Lance is treated with oral antibiotics and the infection resolves.